D0624681

Diabetes Mellitus
and Hypertension

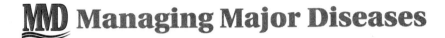 **Managing Major Diseases**

Diabetes Mellitus and Hypertension

CONTRA COSTA COLLEGE DISCARD LIBRARY SAN PABLO, CALIFORNIA

CONTRA COSTA COLLEGE LIBRARY

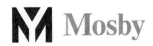 Mosby

St. Louis Baltimore Boston Carlsbad Chicago Minneapolis New York Philadelphia Portland
London Milan Sydney Tokyo Toronto

JUN 3 0 2010

RC
660
D517
1999

M Mosby

Dedicated to Publishing Excellence

A Times Mirror
Company

Publisher Stanley Loeb
Editorial Director William J. Kelly
Clinical Director Cindy Tryniszewski, RN, MSN
Associate Editor Kevin Dodds
Editors Laura Ninger, Nancy Priff, Marcia Ringel
Clinical Editors Marcy Caplin, RN, MSN, CS; Marlene Ciranowicz, RN, MSN, CDE; Kathy Donnelly, RN; Maryann Foley, RN, BSN; Karen E. Michael, RN, MSN; Helene Nawrocki, RN, MSN, CNA; Joyce Okawa, RN, MA; Colleen Seeber-Combs, RN, MSN, CCRN
Copy Editor Stacey Ann Follin
Production Coordinator Marie C. Fusco
Manufacturing Manager William A. Winneberger, Jr.
Art and Design Manager Guy Jacobs
Designers Lynn Foulk, Jennifer Marmarinos
Illustrators Neverne Covington, Rolin Graphics, Inc.
Composition Specialist Camillo M. Gonsalves

Copyright © 1999 by Mosby, Inc.

All rights reserved. No part of this publication may be reproduced, stored in a retrieval system, or transmitted, in any form or by any means, electronic, mechanical, photocopying, recording, or otherwise, without written permission of the publisher.

Permission to photocopy or reproduce solely for internal or personal use is permitted for libraries or other users registered with the Copyright Clearance Center, provided that the base fee of $4.00 per chapter plus $.10 per page is paid directly to the Copyright Clearance Center, 222 Rosewood Drive, Danvers, MA, 01923. This consent does not extend to other kinds of copying, such as copying for general distribution, for advertising or promotional purposes, for creating new collected works, or for resale.

Printing and binding by R.R. Donnelley & Sons, Inc./CTP
Printed in the United States of America

Mosby, Inc.
11830 Westline Industrial Drive
St. Louis, Missouri 63146

Library of Congress Cataloging-in-Publication Data
Diabetes mellitus and hypertension.
  p. cm. — (Managing major diseases)
 Includes bibliographical references and index.
 ISBN 0-8151-2040-0
 1. Diabetes. 2. Hypertension. I. Series.
 [DNLM: 1. Diabetes Mellitus. 2. Hypertension. WK 810D53817
1999]
 RC660.D517 1999
 616.4'62—dc21
 DNLM/DLC
 for Library of Congress   98-27919
              CIP

99 00 01 02 03 04 / 9 8 7 6 5 4 3 2 1

Gift 6/30/2010

Contents

Advisory Board

Kathleen Gainor Andreoli, RN, DSN, FAAN
Vice-President, Nursing Affairs
Rush-Presbyterian-St. Luke's Medical Center
Dean, Rush University College of Nursing
Rush University
Chicago, Ill.

Maria Connolly, RN, CCRN, DNSc,
Past Associate, National Board of AACN
Directors
Regional Director, Academy of Medical-Surgical
Nurses
Associate Professor
Department of Medical-Surgical Nursing
Loyola University
Maywood, Ill.

Sheila S. Griffin, RN, MSN, CS, CETN
Regional Director, Academy of Medical-Surgical
Nurses
Clinical Nurse Specialist, Enterostomal Therapy
Harris Methodist Hospital
Fort Worth, Tex.

Sarah B. Keating, RN, EdD, C,PNP, FAAN
Chair, California Strategic Planning Committee
for Nursing
Dean of Nursing, Professor
Samuel Merritt–Saint Mary's Intercollegiate
Program in Nursing
Oakland, Calif.

Janet C. Ross-Kerr, RN, PhD
Professor, Nursing
University of Alberta
Edmonton, Alberta, Canada

Annette Levitt, RN, MS, CNA
Past President, Academy of Medical-Surgical
Nurses
Nurse Manager
Massachusetts General Hospital
Boston, Mass.

Kathryn L. McCance, RN, PhD
Member of Huntsman Cancer Institute
Professor, College of Nursing
University of Utah
Salt Lake City, Utah

Sally Russell, RN,C, MN
Education Director
St. Elizabeth School of Nursing
Lafayette, Ind.

Marilyn Sawyer Sommers, RN, PhD, CCRN
Past President, Greater Cincinnati AACN
Associate Professor, College of Nursing
University of Cincinnati Medical Center
Cincinnati, Ohio

Carol Will, RN,C, MA, CMC
Nurse Gerontologist and Consultant
Will's Consulting
Keokuk, Iowa

Contributors

Jean Betschart, RN, MS, MN, CRNP, CDE
Pediatric Nurse Practitioner, Endocrinology
Children's Hospital of Pittsburgh
Pittsburgh, Pa.

Sandra J. Bixler, RN, MSN, CCRN
Clinical Nurse Specialist
Berks Cardiologists
Reading, Pa.

Dee Deakins, RN, MS, CDE
Diabetes Educator, Patient Care Services
Department of Veterans Affairs Medical Center
Lexington, Ky.

James A. Fain, RN, PhD, FAAN
Associate Professor
Director, Collaborative PhD Program in Nursing
Graduate School of Nursing
University of Massachusetts Medical Center
Worcester, Mass.

Martha Mitchell Funnell, RN, MS, CDE
Associate Director for Administration
Diabetes Research and Training Center
University of Michigan
Ann Arbor, Mich.

Mary Jo Gerlach, RN, MSNEd
Assistant Professor in Adult Nursing
Medical College of Georgia School of Nursing
Athens, Ga.

Dawna Martich, RN, MSN
Clinical Manager
University of Pittsburgh Medical Center-USO
Moon Township, Pa.

Denise Max, RN,CS, MSN, CNS,C
Advance Practice Nurse, Cardiology
Robert Wood Johnson University Hospital
New Brunswick, N.J.

Leanna Miller, RN, MN, CCRN, CEN, CPNP
Nurse Practitioner, Clinical Nurse Specialist
LRM Consulting
Juliette, Ga.

Charlotte L. Nath, RN, MSN, EdD, CDE
Professor, Department of Family Medicine
West Virginia University
Morgantown, W.Va.

Judy Singley, RD, MA, CDE
Clinical Specialist and Registered Dietitian
Rushland, Pa.

Geralyn Spollett, RN, MSN, C,ANP, CDE
Assistant Professor
Yale School of Nursing
New Haven, Conn.

Dee Trottier, RN, BSN, CCRC
Case Manager
Pharmacia & Upjohn, Inc.
Kalamazoo, Mich.

Consultants

Debbie Bordwell, RN, BSN, CDE
Diabetes Educator
Hoag Memorial Hospital Presbyterian
Newport Beach, Calif.

Theresa Coons, RN, MSN, CCRN
Clinical Nurse Specialist
Critical Care Services
Thomas Jefferson University Hospital
Philadelphia, Pa.

Marilyn R. Graff, RN, BSN, CDE
Program Coordinator, Diabetes Care Team
Longmont Clinic
Longmont, Colo.

Stephanie Schwartz, RN, MPH, CDE
Diabetes Nurse Specialist
The Children's Mercy Hospital
Kansas City, Mo.

Ann Smith-Gregoire, RN, MSN, CRNP, CCRN
Tertiary Care Nurse Practitioner
The Milton S. Hershey Medical Center
Hershey, Pa.

Robin Hillmer-Thomas, RN, MN
Medical-Surgical Clinical Nurse Specialist
Providence Medical Center
Seattle, Wash.

DIABETES MELLITUS

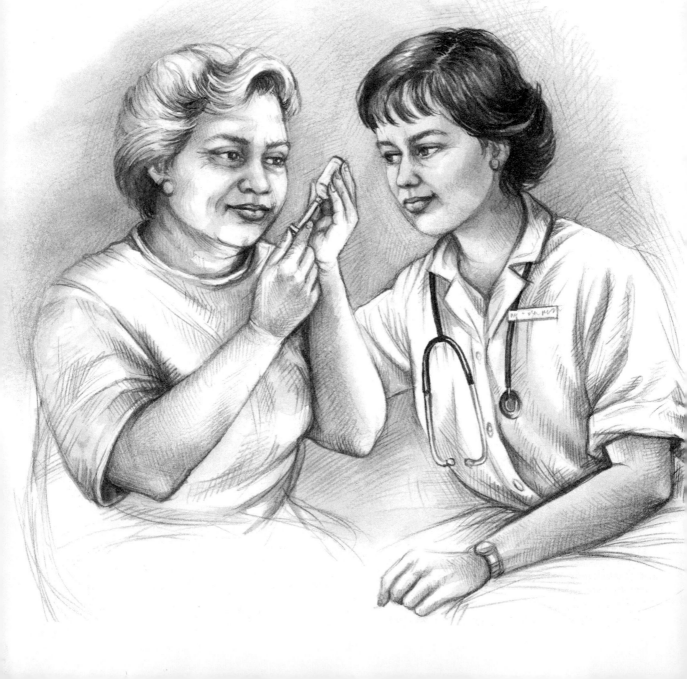

DIABETES MELLITUS

Overview

Diabetes looks different in different patients. The signs and symptoms, the severity, and even the type of diabetes can vary. But one thing is always the same: hyperglycemia.

Any patient with diabetes has one or both of these problems: She either produces little or no insulin, or her body can't use insulin effectively. As a result, she has difficulty metabolizing carbohydrates, fats, and proteins, so hyperglycemia develops.

To diagnose diabetes, a physician needs to determine if a patient has hyperglycemia. Depending on the patient's history and her signs and symptoms, one of three tests may be performed. For a patient with the typical signs and symptoms of diabetes, such as polydipsia, polyuria, polyphagia, blurry vision, and unexplained weight loss, a physician can base the diagnosis on a single random blood glucose level of 200 mg/dl or more. If a patient doesn't have the typical signs and symptoms of diabetes, the physician needs a fasting blood glucose level of 126 mg/dl or more to make the diagnosis. For a patient who is at risk for developing diabetes (for example, someone who has a family history of diabetes or who is obese) and who has a normal fasting blood glucose level, a physician will use the 2-hour oral glucose tolerance test. He'll make a diagnosis of diabetes if an initial test and one follow-up test reveal blood glucose levels of 200 mg/dl or more.

Treating diabetes consists of keeping blood glucose levels as close to normal as possible, using a combination of medication, diet, exercise, and stress control. By closely monitoring blood glucose levels and keeping them as close to normal as possible, a patient can reduce the risks of

acute and long-term complications. The acute life-threatening complications of diabetes include hypoglycemia, diabetic ketoacidosis (DKA), and hyperglycemic hyperosmolar nonketotic (HHNK) syndrome. Long-term complications, which develop because chronic hyperglycemia causes damage to organs and tissues, include nephropathy, cardiovascular disease, peripheral vascular disease, cerebral vascular disease, neuropathy, and retinopathy.

Types of diabetes mellitus

After a patient has been diagnosed with diabetes mellitus, a physician determines the type so that treatment can begin. In some cases, a physician can determine the type only after evaluating the patient's initial response to treatment.

The four types are Type 1, or insulin-dependent diabetes mellitus; Type 2, or non–insulin-dependent diabetes mellitus; gestational diabetes mellitus; and diabetes secondary to other medical conditions. Borderline and chemical diabetes are now called impaired glucose tolerance and aren't classified as diabetes at all (see *Comparing Type 1 and Type 2 diabetes,* page 2).

Type 1 diabetes mellitus

Patients with Type 1 diabetes produce no insulin, and their blood glucose levels can be controlled only with daily insulin injections. These patients account for about 10% of all those with diabetes. Previously called juvenile-onset diabetes, Type 1

Comparing Type 1 and Type 2 diabetes

Characteristics	Type 1	Type 2
Onset	• Usually rapid	• Insidious
Age at onset	• Before age 30, usually in early adolescence • Appears earlier in females than in males	• Usually after age 35
Body weight	• Normal or below normal	• Typically overweight but may be normal
Symptoms	• Polydipsia, polyphagia, polyuria	• Usually mild or not noticeable
Diabetic ketoacidosis	• Typical	• Atypical
Islet beta cell function	• Severely reduced	• Moderately reduced
Dietary management and exercise program	• Essential • Used with insulin therapy	• Essential • May control glucose levels without medication
Insulin	• Required	• Required in about 33% of patients
Oral antidiabetic drugs	• Ineffective	• Effective or partially effective

generally appears before age 30, but it appears most commonly during early adolescence. The disease may appear slightly earlier in females than in males.

The signs and symptoms of Type 1 diabetes seem to begin abruptly. Patients with Type 1 diabetes are prone to DKA and are at risk for developing vascular complications.

No one fully understands what causes Type 1 diabetes. Some theories suggest a genetic susceptibility linked to an environmental trigger. Genetic studies have shown that a family history of Type 1 diabetes may put a person at risk for developing the disease. Yet, about 80% of children with Type 1 diabetes have no family history of the disease. Human leukocyte antigens, which appear on genes that control immune response, may cause the genetic susceptibility. However, many people have these antigens and never develop diabetes.

Various environmental causes may trigger diabetes in a person who's genetically susceptible to the disease. For example, children who drink cow's milk at a young age may be at increased risk for developing Type 1 diabetes because of an autoimmune response to milk proteins. Viruses also seem to play a role in triggering diabetes. The disease appears more commonly in the fall and winter during viral outbreaks, but the time between exposure to the virus and the first signs and symptoms of diabetes makes it difficult to identify the triggering virus.

Islet cell antibodies also have been linked to Type 1 diabetes. Some patients with Type 1 diabetes have islet cell antibodies years before their symptoms begin. These antibodies cause active autoimmunity against beta cells—the cells that produce insulin.

Despite the many theories about the cause of Type 1 diabetes, there's no way to predict who will develop the disease.

Type 2 diabetes mellitus

Patients with Type 2 diabetes mellitus have insulin resistance and impaired insulin secretion;

many of them don't require insulin injections. These patients account for about 90% of all patients with diabetes. In the United States, Type 2 diabetes affects more women than men, more African-Americans than whites, and more people with low incomes and limited education. Previously called adult-onset diabetes, Type 2 diabetes usually appears in people over age 35.

Patients with Type 2 diabetes aren't prone to DKA, but like those with Type 1 diabetes, they're at risk for developing vascular complications. Because the signs and symptoms of Type 2 diabetes develop over time, the disease may go unnoticed for many years.

The cause of Type 2 diabetes isn't known. As with Type 1 diabetes, genetic susceptibility and environmental triggers, such as viruses, seem to play a role. However, there's no evidence that autoimmunity or islet cell antibodies play any role.

Severe obesity significantly increases a patient's risk of developing Type 2 diabetes. Other risk factors include age, a sedentary lifestyle, a high-fat diet, stress, and a family history of diabetes. Type 2 diabetes occurs more commonly in women who have been pregnant more than once and who have a history of gestational diabetes. Also, it commonly appears in the children of women who develop gestational diabetes.

Gestational diabetes

Gestational diabetes, a complication in about 4% of all pregnancies in the United States, develops as glucose intolerance during pregnancy. If a woman had diabetes before she became pregnant, the disorder isn't considered gestational diabetes.

During pregnancy, a woman's insulin requirements increase, and between the 24th and 28th weeks of pregnancy, her insulin requirements rise sharply. In some women, insulin production is limited, and the demand for insulin exceeds the supply, resulting in hyperglycemia. After delivery, insulin supply and demand return to normal.

Between the 24th and 28th weeks of pregnancy, all women should have an oral glucose tolerance test to detect gestational diabetes. Detecting this condition and controlling blood glucose levels reduce the woman's risk of complications, including pregnancy-induced hypertension, hydramnios, premature delivery, and cesarean delivery. Risks to the fetus include hypoglycemia, respiratory distress syndrome, hypocalcemia, polycythemia, hyperbilirubinemia, and intrauterine death.

The chances that a woman will develop gestational diabetes increase with these risk factors: advanced age, obesity, previous gestational diabetes, a family history of diabetes, and a previous stillborn delivery, spontaneous abortion, or delivery of an abnormally large baby. Women who develop gestational diabetes have an increased risk of developing Type 2 diabetes within 15 years. A small percentage of women develop Type 1 diabetes.

Secondary diabetes

Diabetes also can result from pancreatic disease and surgery; endocrine disorders, such as acromegaly, pheochromocytoma, and Cushing's syndrome; and therapy with drugs, such as glucocorticoids, streptozocin, pentamidine, and estrogen. Secondary diabetes usually resolves after the primary condition is treated successfully.

How the pancreas works

The pancreas helps regulate and maintain homeostasis by performing both exocrine and endocrine functions. As part of the exocrine system, the pancreas aids in the digestion of proteins, fats, and carbohydrates. As part of the endocrine system, the pancreas plays an important role in metabolizing glucose and regulating blood glucose levels. In people with diabetes, a dysfunction in glucose metabolism leads to hyperglycemia.

Location and structure

The pancreas lies in the upper abdominal cavity behind the stomach and in front of the first and second lumbar vertebrae. It also lies over the inferior vena cava and the two large renal arteries. Measuring 12 to 15 cm in length and weighing about 60 grams, the pancreas is divided into a head, body, and tail. The head of the pancreas lies in and is attached to the C-shaped duodenal loop. The body of the pancreas extends horizontally across the upper abdomen, and the tail touches the spleen (see *Two views of the pancreas,* page 4).

Two views of the pancreas

The main illustration shows the pancreas and the C-shaped duodenal loop. The inset gives you a microscopic view of the exocrine and endocrine tissue.

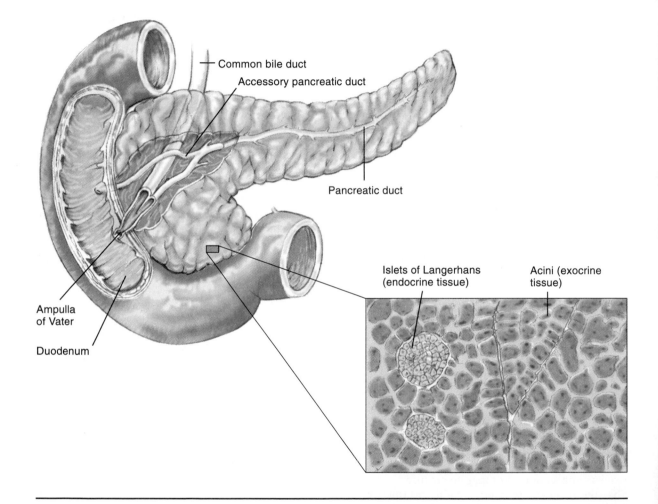

Common bile duct

Accessory pancreatic duct

Pancreatic duct

Islets of Langerhans (endocrine tissue)

Acini (exocrine tissue)

Ampulla of Vater

Duodenum

Exocrine function

Most of the pancreas is made up of exocrine tissue, which is arranged in small saclike structures called acini. The cells of these acini release secretions into tiny ducts that eventually unite with the pancreatic duct, which extends from the tail to the head of the pancreas. The pancreatic duct gets larger as it passes through the pancreas. This duct joins the common bile duct and then empties into the duodenum at the ampulla of Vater. The accessory pancreatic duct, also known as the duct of Santorini, extends from the head of the pancreas into the duodenum.

When food enters the stomach, the intestinal mucosa releases the hormone secretin into the bloodstream. Secretin in turn stimulates the acinar cells and ducts to secrete pancreatic juice. An alkaline solution, the pancreatic juice consists of water, bicarbonate, electrolytes, and enzymes for food digestion. These pancreatic enzymes fall into three categories: proteolytic enzymes (trypsin and chymotrypsin), which break down proteins; pancreatic lipase, which helps digest fat; and pancreatic amylase, which helps digest carbohydrates. The digestive enzymes and the other components of the pancreatic juice pass from the microscopic ducts into the pancreatic duct and then enter the duodenum. In the duodenum, the pancreatic juice neutralizes the acidic chyme from the stomach.

The pancreas protects itself from these digestive enzymes by secreting them in inactive forms. They don't become active until they reach the digestive tract, where activating enzymes convert them. For example, trypsin is released from the pancreas as the zymogen trypsinogen, which is then converted to active trypsin by enterokinase in the intestine.

Endocrine function

Clusters of about one million endocrine cells lie embedded between the acini. These endocrine cells, also known as pancreatic islets or islets of Langerhans, make up about 2% of the total mass of the pancreas. The endocrine cells function as glucose regulators by secreting various hormones that work together to maintain balance among food molecules—glucose, fatty acids, and amino acids.

The islets of Langerhans contain three main types of hormone-secreting cells:
- glucagon-secreting alpha cells
- insulin-secreting beta cells
- somatostatin-secreting delta cells.

These islets also contain F cells that secrete pancreatic polypeptide, an exocrine hormone. Unlike exocrine cells, the endocrine cells release their secretions into capillaries rather than into ducts.

Glucagon
Produced and secreted by the alpha cells of the islets of Langerhans, glucagon increases blood glucose levels via a negative feedback system. Glucagon restores normal blood glucose levels by stimulating hepatic glucose production through glycogenolysis (the breakdown of glycogen into glucose by hepatic enzymes); glucagon sustains these blood levels through gluconeogenesis (the formation of glycogen from free fatty acids and proteins). An increase in circulating amino acid levels—which occurs with high-protein meals, exercise, and sympathetic nerve stimulation—stimulates glucagon secretion. Somatostatin and decreased blood glucose levels inhibit glucagon secretion.

Insulin
Normally, the pancreas releases insulin into the bloodstream in small pulsating increments at a rate of 1 to 2 units (U) per hour; after meals, the rate increases to 4 to 6 U per hour (see *Ups and downs of insulin secretion,* page 6). Insulin levels begin to increase 8 to 10 minutes after a person eats and reach their peak in 30 to 45 minutes. Blood glucose levels quickly decline, returning to baseline 1½ to 2 hours after the initial ingestion of food.

The beta cells of the islets of Langerhans increase insulin secretion when blood glucose levels rise, for example, after a person finishes a meal; when blood levels of amino acids, glucagon, and secretin rise; and when the parasympathetic nervous system stimulates the beta cells. Insulin lowers blood glucose levels by binding to receptors on the surface of cell membranes and promoting the movement of glucose from the bloodstream into the cells. Insulin also promotes the movement of potassium, phosphate, and magnesium into the cells.

Insulin secretion decreases as blood glucose levels fall between meals and overnight when a person doesn't eat. As insulin levels fall, glycogen stores in the liver release glucose. When glycogen stores fall, as with continued fasting, muscle cells release amino acids to be converted to glucose. If energy needs remain unmet, adipose tissue releases fatty acids, which are converted into glucose (this conversion is called lipolysis). Fatty acids then are metabolized to form ketones (this process is called ketogenesis).

The hormones glucagon, epinephrine, growth hormone, and cortisol counteract the effects of insulin by promoting the release of glycogen, which raises blood glucose levels. Normally, insulin and the other hormones provide a system of checks and balances that maintains blood glucose levels in the range of 70 to 120 mg/dl.

Ups and downs of insulin secretion

The pancreas continuously secretes insulin into the bloodstream at a baseline rate of 1 to 2 units (U) per hour. After a meal, the secretion rate increases to 4 to 6 U per hour. The rate peaks 30 to 45 minutes after breakfast, lunch, and dinner, as shown in the illustration. Over 24 hours, the body secretes 40 to 60 U.

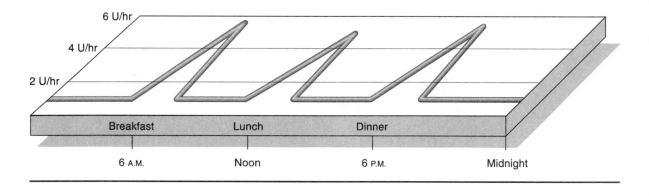

Somatostatin
Somatostatin, also called the growth hormone–inhibiting hormone, is secreted by the delta cells of the islets of Langerhans. Somatostatin regulates alpha and beta cell function and inhibits the secretion of insulin, glucagon, and pancreatic polypeptide.

Pancreatic polypeptide
Produced by the F cells of the islets of Langerhans, pancreatic polypeptides inhibit pancreatic bicarbonate and protein secretion. Pancreatic polypeptides also help to relax the gallbladder, releasing bile to aid in digestion. Somatostatin inhibits the secretion of pancreatic polypeptides.

Hyperglycemic hormones

Three hormones produced outside of the pancreas—epinephrine, growth hormone, and cortisol—all raise blood glucose levels.

A catecholamine produced in the adrenal medulla, epinephrine increases blood glucose levels by stimulating gluconeogenesis and lipolysis, thus aiding in the metabolism of carbohydrates, fats, and proteins. Epinephrine also inhibits the secretion and action of insulin. Stress, exercise, or hypoglycemia can trigger the release of epinephrine. A patient with diabetes may secrete a decreased level of epinephrine—or no epinephrine at all—in response to low blood glucose levels.

The pituitary gland produces and secretes growth hormone, which raises blood glucose levels by increasing protein synthesis and promoting the breakdown of fatty acids in adipose tissue. Stress, exercise, a high-protein diet, and hypoglycemia increase its secretion. Growth hormone prevents hypoglycemia by stimulating the release of glycogen from the liver.

Cortisol, produced in the adrenal cortex, maintains normal liver gluconeogenesis and aids in the conversion of amino acids into glucose in the liver. A potent inhibitor of glucose uptake by tissues, cortisol elevates blood glucose levels and resists the action of insulin. Cortisol levels increase in the early morning and in response to stress and hypoglycemia.

Progression of Type 1 diabetes

A chronic disorder, Type 1 diabetes results from a complete or partial lack of insulin. Without insulin, glucose can't enter the cells. Thus, the cells starve while high levels of glucose remain in the bloodstream. The body, sensing a lack of glucose in the cells, tries to increase its availability by breaking down fat and protein sources and glycogen stores to produce glucose. In another attempt to compensate, the body secretes counterregulatory hormones (glucagon, epinephrine, growth hormone, and cortisol) to increase blood glucose levels. But without insulin, these increases in glucose only contribute further to hyperglycemia.

When the amount of glucose filtered by the kidneys surpasses the amount the kidneys can reabsorb, glucose appears in the urine. The glucose acts as an osmotic diuretic, causing the patient to produce increased amounts of urine. Elevated blood glucose levels also increase the osmotic pull of the blood, which causes water to move from the cells in the tissues into the bloodstream. This intracellular dehydration, along with the dehydration caused by increased urination, produces excessive thirst. Because the cells lack the glucose they need for energy, the person is continually hungry.

As the person burns fat and proteins for energy, fatigue and weight loss result. As body fats continue to break down, toxic levels of ketones are produced. Ketones can't be used efficiently as energy, and as they accumulate in the blood, the pH drops, and metabolic acidosis develops. As the kidneys filter ketones, ketonuria develops. Insulin replacement is necessary to prevent DKA. The signs and symptoms of DKA include nausea, vomiting, electrolyte imbalances, a fruity breath odor, weight loss, and muscle wasting. Without treatment, DKA can progress to coma and death.

After being diagnosed with Type 1 diabetes, many patients experience a remission during which little or no insulin therapy is needed to control blood glucose levels. This honeymoon period can last up to a year, but once it ends, blood glucose levels rise, and insulin requirements increase.

Even when the disease is treated with exogenous insulin, it progresses, producing long-term complications. These complications can be classified as microvascular, macrovascular, and neuropathic. Microvascular complications include retinopathy, which can lead to blindness, and nephropathy, which can lead to renal failure. Macrovascular complications include coronary artery disease, cerebrovascular disease, and peripheral vascular disease. Neuropathies can lead to conditions including impotence and a loss of

RESEARCH UPDATE

Using intensive insulin therapy

One of the biggest concerns for patients with Type 1 diabetes has always been long-term microvascular complications—blindness caused by retinopathy, renal failure caused by nephropathy, and nerve damage caused by neuropathy. In 1993, the Diabetes Control and Complications Trial showed that more frequent insulin injections could better control glucose levels and slow the progression of these complications.

During this 10-year, randomized, controlled study, researchers followed 1,441 people with Type 1 diabetes. The study compared the effects of intensive insulin therapy and conventional insulin therapy on the development and progression of early microvascular complications. People in the control group received the standard treatment of one or two injections of insulin every day. Those in the other group received three or more injections of insulin every day. The results were clear: Intensive therapy does a better job of keeping blood glucose levels as close to normal as possible, which reduces the risk of retinopathy, nephropathy, and neuropathy by about 60%.

Research since this study has shown that most adults and adolescents with Type 1 diabetes can benefit from intensive insulin therapy. In patients with Type 2 diabetes, however, the intensive therapy may exacerbate macrovascular complications, canceling out any benefit.

A patient who uses intensive insulin therapy needs to know that she must rigorously monitor her blood glucose levels and frequently adjust her insulin dose. Doses should change when blood glucose levels fluctuate, when the patient alters her diet or exercise routine, and when she's sick. Be aware that for some patients the expense of intensive therapy may be a burden. Frequent blood glucose monitoring requires more test strips, and the patient must make more visits to her physician, dietitian, and nurse educator.

sensation in the arms and legs. Among patients with Type 1 diabetes, renal disease is the most common cause of death, followed by cardiovascular disease (see *Using intensive insulin therapy*).

Progression of Type 2 diabetes

In a patient with Type 2 diabetes, insulin loses its ability to inhibit glucose production, and beta cells are exposed to elevated blood glucose levels. This constant exposure to insulin leaves the beta cells unable to respond to hyperglycemia.

Peripheral insulin resistance occurs when the number of available insulin receptors in muscle and fat cells decreases. This results in higher blood glucose levels, progressively increasing the person's requirement for insulin secretion. To reverse the process, the person can lose weight, and to reduce blood glucose levels, she can take oral antidiabetic drugs. If these drugs, in conjunction with weight loss, don't work effectively, the person may need insulin. She also may need insulin when she's acutely ill or under stress.

Although the person has high blood glucose levels, she still produces enough insulin to prevent DKA. However, she may lose fluids and electrolytes—losses that can lead to HHNK syndrome.

People with Type 2 diabetes may experience the same long-term complications as those with Type 1 diabetes. However, they're particularly at risk for heart disease—the most common cause of death among patients with Type 2 diabetes. The hyperinsulinemia associated with Type 2 diabetes may be an important risk factor in the development of hypertension, abnormal lipid levels, and atherosclerosis.

Syndrome X is the combination of insulin resistance, hypertension, low high-density lipoprotein cholesterol levels, and increased very-low-density lipoprotein cholesterol levels. By the time most patients are diagnosed with Type 2 diabetes, they've had syndrome X for many years. The combined abnormalities of this syndrome increase the chances of angina, myocardial infarction, cerebrovascular accident, and peripheral vascular disease in patients with Type 2 diabetes.

2

DIABETES MELLITUS

Assessment

You can use a health history and physical examination in two distinct ways to investigate diabetes. When you suspect that a patient has the disorder, you can perform a health history and physical examination to discover the characteristic signs and symptoms and confirm your suspicion. When you already know that a patient has diabetes, you can use a health history and physical examination to help monitor the disease and uncover any complications.

Health history

A health history performed to identify the signs and symptoms of diabetes is similar to any other health history. It should cover your patient's biographical information, chief complaint, history of her present illness, medical history, family history, psychological and social history, and a review of her body systems.

If your patient has already been diagnosed with diabetes, you'll also need to review her treatment plan, the problems she encounters in living with diabetes, and any acute and chronic complications. The health history can also help you uncover problems with treatment compliance and patient concerns.

Biographical information

Begin the health history by gathering biographical information about your patient. If you suspect she has diabetes, make sure you note her age, ethnic group, and living arrangements.

Your patient's age at the time of diagnosis provides a clue to the type of diabetes. Type 1 diabetes usually begins in early adolescence; Type 2, after age 35. Use caution, however; a patient over age 35 can be diagnosed with Type 1 diabetes, and a child can be diagnosed with Type 2 diabetes.

A person's ethnic group may be a risk factor for diabetes. Mexican-Americans, Native Americans, and African-Americans have a higher rate of diabetes than those in other groups. No one knows why.

Whether a person lives alone has nothing to do with the disease process, of course, but it may have a lot to do with disease management. A spouse or partner who cooks for the patient can have a tremendous impact on the dietary aspect of diabetes treatment. And a spouse or partner can also provide much needed emotional support as the patient undergoes lifestyle changes to control her blood glucose levels.

Chief complaint

Common chief complaints include polyuria, polydipsia, polyphagia, and weight loss. With diabetes, the patient feels constantly hungry because the glucose that usually feeds body cells remains in the blood. Excessive urination occurs as the kidneys try to eliminate the glucose from the blood. As glucose leaves the body through urine, the body loses water, which results in dehydration and thirst. Weight loss develops as cells are deprived of their main energy source—glucose.

Polyuria, polydipsia, and polyphagia may be pronounced in patients with Type 1 diabetes because the loss of insulin occurs abruptly. These signs can also develop in Type 2 diabetes, but because the loss of insulin occurs more slowly, they're usually milder and are commonly overlooked. Other symptoms include fatigue and weakness.

In many cases, Type 2 diabetes goes undetected for many years. Therefore, a patient's chief complaint may result from a complication of diabetes rather than the diabetes itself. Complaints of visual disturbances, neurologic impairment, cardiovascular dysfunction, or frequent infections should alert you to question the patient more closely about signs and symptoms of diabetes.

History of present illness

Investigating your patient's present illness adds to the information you've already gathered about her chief complaint. Find out when the present illness started, what the first symptoms were, and if any recent treatments have relieved them.

Medical history

Your patient's medical history may help you uncover risk factors for diabetes, complications of diabetes, and problems that may affect her ability to manage the disease.

Risk factors for diabetes include obesity (especially central or android obesity in which weight accumulates around the abdomen, giving the patient an apple shape), impaired glucose tolerance, previous gestational diabetes, and delivery of a baby weighing more than 9 pounds. Pancreatic surgery or a history of pancreatitis may also increase your patient's risk of diabetes. Medical conditions that may be complications of diabetes include cardiovascular disease such as atherosclerosis, vision loss, neuropathies, and kidney disease.

Although allergies aren't considered a risk factor for diabetes, they may pose a problem in managing the disease. For example, a patient who needs insulin therapy but is allergic to beef or pork can use only human insulin. A patient who's allergic to sulfa will not be able to take sulfonylureas.

Because managing diabetes requires the patient to master several skills, you should ask about injuries and impairments. A patient who

has poor eyesight or a hand injury may not be able to draw up the correct dose of insulin, inject insulin, or monitor her blood glucose levels without help from someone else or the use of assistive devices, such as magnifiers or dose aids. Knowing about your patient's injuries and impairments will help you individualize her treatment plan.

Also, gather information about the patient's diet, medications, level of activity, and use of alcohol and tobacco.

Diet is one of the cornerstones of diabetes management. And noncompliance and lack of knowledge are two key causes of uncontrolled diabetes. To find out about your patient's eating habits, have her do a 3-day diet recall. For variety and accuracy, one of the days should be a non-workday. Explore your patient's likes and dislikes, the types and quantities of food she eats, her mealtimes, and snack habits. Assess her knowledge of nutrition, her attitudes about food, and her understanding of food's relationship to obesity. Eating disorders such as anorexia nervosa and bulimia can make glucose control especially difficult. The following questions may help you uncover these disorders:
• What concerns do you have about your weight?
• Have you ever made yourself vomit or used laxatives to control your weight?
• What do you think of your body when you look in the mirror?

Your patient's current drugs may interact with drugs used to treat diabetes. Or they may cause hyperglycemia or hypoglycemia, making it difficult for her to control her blood glucose levels (see *Drugs that alter blood glucose levels*).

A sedentary lifestyle is also a risk factor for diabetes. Ask your patient about her exercise habits and the activities she performs on workdays and non-workdays. Ask her about exercise likes and dislikes and any exercise programs that she has undertaken in the past. This information will help when you and she plan the exercise portion of her long-term treatment. Your patient is more likely to comply with her exercise program if she gets to choose an activity that she enjoys.

Finally, ask your patient about her use of alcohol and tobacco. Alcohol can alter blood glucose levels in a patient with diabetes and place her at risk for hypoglycemia and hyperglycemic emergencies such as diabetic ketoacidosis (DKA) and hyperglycemic hyperosmolar nonketotic (HHNK) syndrome. Smoking decreases insulin's effectiveness. It also increases the risk of amputation if your patient already has peripheral vascular disease as a result of undiagnosed or poorly managed diabetes.

Family history

A family history of diabetes is a major risk factor. If you uncover such a history, find out which type other family members have. The risk of a child developing Type 1 diabetes if a parent has Type 1 diabetes is considerably lower than the risk of a child developing Type 2 diabetes later in life if a parent has Type 2 diabetes.

A family history of diabetes may influence your patient's feelings and attitudes about the disease. A family member who has had major complications from diabetes or who doesn't comply with the treatment plan can be a source of fear and misunderstanding for your patient. Uncovering a family history of diabetes provides an opportunity for you to explore your patient's attitudes, misconceptions, and fears about the disease.

Psychological and social history

Diabetes has lifelong financial and lifestyle implications for your patient and her family. The financial burden of paying for treatment supplies or obtaining adequate health care coverage can make it difficult for your patient to keep up with other financial responsibilities. In many cases, these adjustments and financial burdens affect the family, and anger and resentment may sow the seeds of future noncompliance.

The psychological and social history portion of the health history should include questions about the patient's strengths and weaknesses, attitudes about health and illness, coping skills, socioeconomic class, cultural background, position and status in the family, level of education, religious background, and hobbies and interests. This information can help you tailor your patient's treatment plan to perhaps improve her compliance. For example, a Jewish patient who doesn't eat pork will be more likely to comply with therapy that includes human insulin instead of pork insulin. A patient who requires insulin but who likes to sleep in on the weekend will need to manage her insulin and dietary intake differently on Saturday and Sunday.

The patient's financial situation can have a major impact on her willingness to purchase the

Drugs that alter blood glucose levels

When taking your patient's health history, be sure to ask which drugs she's taking and to explain that certain drugs can cause fluctuations in her blood glucose levels. The following drugs can increase or decrease blood glucose levels and will probably be withheld by a physician before a blood glucose test.

Drugs that increase blood glucose levels	Drugs that decrease blood glucose levels
• beta-blockers	• alcohol
• caffeine (large doses)	• chloroquine
• corticosteroids	• clofibrate
• diazoxide	• disopyramide
• epinephrine	• monoamine oxidase inhibitors
• niacin	• pentamidine
• nicotine	• phenylbutazone
• oral contraceptives	• salicylates (large doses)
• phenytoin	• sulfonamides
• thiazide and thiazide-like diuretics	

supplies she needs to help control blood glucose levels. If you recognize a patient's financial concerns early on, give her an appropriate referral so that she can get the assistance she needs to manage her diabetes.

Review of body systems

Begin the review of body systems by asking your patient about her general well-being. Commonly, a patient with diabetes will say that she doesn't feel as well as she used to, and she'll attribute her fatigue and weakness to growing older.

Ask your patient about her weight history. A recent weight loss that's not attributed to diet or a recent illness is a typical symptom of diabetes, especially Type 1 diabetes. People with Type 2 diabetes are usually obese. No one is sure why. Some researchers speculate that obesity is a factor in the development of Type 2 diabetes because fat cells require more insulin per cell than nonfat cells do. This leads to substandard insulin production as the pancreas works overtime to meet the obese patient's insulin demands. Other researchers believe that obesity is actually an early sign of Type 2 diabetes.

Ask your patient about any skin conditions. One common symptom is dry, itchy skin, which develops because of mild dehydration associated with hyperglycemia. The itchiness is caused by glucose pooling under the skin. Such pooling also creates an ideal environment for skin infections, another common complaint of patients with diabetes. Patients may also report skin discoloration and chronic skin conditions, such as ulcers that don't heal.

Next, ask your patient about visual disturbances. As glucose levels rise, glucose molecules cause blood vessels in the eyes to become congested and vision to blur. If your patient has prolonged hyperglycemia, she may report that she has trouble reading. She also may tell you that she sees dark spots, rings around lights, or flashing lights. Find out how often she has her eyes examined, when she last had them examined, and whether an ophthalmologist performed the examination. A patient with diabetes requires frequent eye examinations because the disease is one of the major causes of new cases of blindness diagnosed each year. Because of the complexity of diabetic retinopathy, a common complication associated with diabetes, an ophthalmologist should perform all eye examinations on a patient with diabetes.

Ask your patient about any history of periodontal disease or oral infections. These problems are common in patients with diabetes because of glucose pooling in gum tissue, which leads to frequent infections and destruction of delicate oral tissues.

Diabetes is also a major risk factor for arteriosclerosis, so ask your patient if she has any of the signs or symptoms of cardiovascular or peripheral vascular abnormalities: heart problems, chest pain, shortness of breath, hypertension, elevated cholesterol and triglyceride levels, cold feet, pain that occurs with walking, or leg or foot ulcers. Arteriosclerosis that affects the cerebral arteries may cause the patient to report transient ischemic attacks—brief episodes of dizziness, loss of sight, slurred speech, or feelings of numbness or weakness in one arm or leg.

Neuropathy, which may occur because of excessive glucose coating of the nerves, results from prolonged hyperglycemia. History findings that suggest peripheral neuropathy include a pins-and-needles sensation, sharp stabbing pains, and numbness in the hands or feet. Some patients may report leg pain that occurs only at night and is relieved by walking. Complaints that suggest autonomic neuropathy include nausea and vomiting, abdominal bloating, and nocturnal diarrhea, all of which are typical signs and symptoms of gastroparesis.

Some patients may complain of dizziness when changing position (suggesting orthostatic hypotension), an irregular pulse rhythm, or a fixed heart rate despite exercise (suggesting an electrical dysfunction of the heart).

Prolonged hyperglycemia may also lead to diabetic nephropathy, which is usually well advanced before the patient experiences any symptoms. Ask your patient whether she has ever been told that she has protein in her urine. Also, ask her if she has ever had urinary tract or kidney infections. If she has, take a detailed history of the infections including the frequency, signs and symptoms, and treatment.

Ask your patient about reproductive abnormalities. Sexual dysfunction, including loss of libido, commonly develops in patients with diabetes. Impotence may develop in men with diabetes because of both blood vessel disease and neuropathy caused by chronic hyperglycemia. Women with diabetes may report frequent vaginal infections.

Diabetes regimen

If your patient has already been diagnosed with diabetes, you'll need to ask some additional questions about her regimen. Specifically, you should ask about her medication, diet, exercise, and monitoring techniques (see *What to ask your patient about her diabetes regimen*).

Insulin and other drugs used to control diabetes lower blood glucose levels, putting patients at risk for hypoglycemia. Inappropriate diet and

What to ask your patient about her diabetes regimen

When you take the health history of a patient who has diabetes, you need to ask specific questions about her regimen—her medications, diet, exercise program, and glucose monitoring. If your patient uses insulin, ask her to demonstrate her injection technique. And have all patients with diabetes demonstrate their blood glucose monitoring technique.

Based on your patient's regimen, select the appropriate questions from this list:

Insulin
- What type of insulin do you use? How much? When?
- Into which part of your body do you inject the insulin?
- Do you rotate your injection sites?
- Do you inject your insulin or does someone do it for you?
- Have you missed any injections in the last 2 weeks? How many?
- Do you have any problem drawing up the correct amount of insulin?

Oral antidiabetic drugs
- What is the name of your antidiabetic drug?
- How many pills are you supposed to take each day? How many do you actually take?
- Have you missed any pills in the last 2 weeks? How many?

Diet and exercise
- Has your physician recommended that you follow a diet to control your diabetes or to lose weight?
- How many calories are you supposed to have each day? Do you stick to that limit?
- What time do you usually eat your meals? What about snacks?
- Have you skipped any meals in the last 2 weeks? How many? Which meals?
- Who shops for your food? Who prepares your food?
- What's the hardest part of your diet?
- Has your weight changed in the last year? By how much?
- Is exercise part of your regimen?
- What kind of exercise do you do? How often? For how long?

Blood glucose control
- How often have you checked your blood glucose level in the last month?
- In the past 2 weeks, have you felt tired, very thirsty, confused, or shaky? Have you had to go to the bathroom two or more times during the night? Have you had nightmares or bad dreams?
- How do you feel when you have a reaction to low blood glucose levels? How often have you felt that way in the last 2 weeks?
- How do you treat a reaction from low blood glucose levels?

excessive exercise can also cause hypoglycemia. Ask your patient about the frequency of her hypoglycemic episodes and any signs or symptoms. Although hypoglycemic signs and symptoms may vary from patient to patient, the most common ones include headache, tremors, difficulty concentrating, drowsiness, irritability, anxiety, weakness, cold and clammy skin, light-headedness, difficulty talking, and rapid heartbeat. If left uncorrected, hypoglycemia can lead to seizures and coma. Find out what kind of treatment your patient has received for hypoglycemia and how she has responded. Also, ask her if she can identify the cause of each episode (see *What's causing your patient's hypoglycemia?,* page 14). This information will help you evaluate your patient's compliance with her regimen and her understanding of hypoglycemia. It may also lead to a change in the regimen.

Hyperglycemia may develop when your patient encounters stress and unavoidable changes in her daily life. Find out how much she understands about hyperglycemia and its two emergency complications: DKA and HHNK syndrome. Ask her about the frequency and severity of hyperglycemia, the signs or symptoms she experiences, any treatment she has received, and any changes made in her treatment plan. Frequent treatment for hyperglycemia may mean that she isn't complying with her treatment plan or that it's ineffective. To help her, explore the reasons for her hyperglycemia. Also, ask her if she understands sick-day rules and urine ketone testing. Illness is a common cause of hyperglycemic emergencies.

What's causing your patient's hypoglycemia?

Use this checklist of possible causes to help discover why your patient is experiencing hypoglycemic episodes:
• skipped or delayed meals
• small portions of food
• increased physical exertion
• high insulin dose
• incorrect timing of insulin injection and meals
• decreased insulin clearance because of renal disease
• alcohol ingestion
• drug interactions.

Finally, ask your patient if she has any concerns about her treatment plan. Her answers will help you and other members of the health care team identify potential problems and redesign a treatment plan that best fits her needs.

Physical examination

Although the physical examination traditionally follows the health history, you'll actually begin your examination during the history. For example, you'll probably note the patient's general appearance and speech almost immediately. Irritability, difficulty concentrating, and a fruity breath odor are all common signs of hyperglycemia that has progressed to DKA in a patient with undetected Type 1 diabetes.

If you suspect that your patient has diabetes, pay particular attention to her vital signs, height and weight, skin, head and neck, heart and blood vessels, mental status, neurologic function, and kidneys and bladder. If you already know that your patient has diabetes, be sure to assess her for complications of the disease.

Vital signs

After noting your patient's general appearance, take her vital signs. Vital sign abnormalities may or may not appear in diabetes. If hyperglycemia isn't severe, vital signs may be normal. If the patient's hyperglycemia has progressed to DKA or HHNK syndrome, you may detect hypotension, a weak and rapid pulse, Kussmaul's respirations (deep but rapid respirations characteristic of DKA) or shallow and rapid respirations characteristic of HHNK syndrome, and an elevated temperature. Hypotension and a weak, rapid pulse may be caused by dehydration that results from polyuria. Kussmaul's respirations are a compensatory mechanism in which the patient's lungs attempt to alleviate excessive acid buildup in the body caused by ketone formation. Shallow, rapid respirations result from hypovolemic shock caused by extreme polyuria. An elevated temperature may stem from dehydration, but it commonly occurs because of an underlying infection.

Long-standing, undetected diabetes may have caused enough blood vessel damage to result in hypertension or enough nerve damage to result in autonomic neuropathy. Autonomic neuropathy may cause a systolic blood pressure drop of more than 10 mm Hg when the patient changes position or a fixed heart rate that doesn't change with inspiration or exercise.

Height and weight

Next, check your patient's height and weight. Patients with Type 1 diabetes are usually underweight or average weight, whereas patients with Type 2 diabetes are usually overweight at the time of diagnosis. A recent rapid weight loss is a common sign of Type 1 diabetes. Poorly controlled diabetes may cause stunted growth in children.

Skin

Skin abnormalities are common with diabetes (see *Recognizing skin disorders*). With prolonged hyperglycemia, the skin can appear dry and flaky. If the skin is itchy, the patient may have scratch marks. The skin may be flushed and warm in patients with DKA or pale and cool in those with HHNK syndrome, depending on the blood glucose level. A patient with hyperglycemia may have no diaphoresis when she has a fever because of the dehydration caused by polyuria.

When a patient's diabetes goes undetected or is poorly controlled, glucose accumulates under

Recognizing skin disorders

Common in patients with diabetes, skin disorders may result directly from diabetes or indirectly from associated conditions, such as insulin resistance or lipid abnormalities.

Cause	Skin disorder	Characteristics
Diabetes	• diabetic dermopathy	• small atrophic, red-brown lesions • appears in pretibial area in up to 50% of patients • primarily affects men over age 50
	• necrobiosis lipoidica	• asymptomatic, nonulcerated, yellowish sclerotic plaques • appears in about 3% of patients with diabetes • affects more men than women
	• lipodystrophy	• loss of subcutaneous fatty tissue • may be generalized or affect only part of body • leads to overdeveloped muscles
Insulin resistance	• acanthosis nigricans	• hyperpigmented, evenly thickened, and folded skin over joints
Lipid abnormalities	• eruptive xanthomas	• multiple yellow-red and yellow-orange papules over joints, buttocks, and body • corrected with good diabetes control
	• xanthelasma	• irregular plaques over eyelids • begins as small yellow-orange spots that grow together and thicken • most common type of xanthoma
	• xanthochromia	• yellowish skin on sole of foot • accompanied by increased carotene and blood cholesterol • rare

the skin and causes skin infections. Candidiasis, a common infection, may cause redness, maceration, and oozing. The patient also may have small pustular lesions. Infections usually occur in areas that have a lot of moisture, such as under the arms, under the breasts, and in the groin.

Your patient's legs and feet may show signs of peripheral vascular disease caused by prolonged hyperglycemia. The skin may appear shiny and thin and be cool to the touch. You may also see evidence of hair loss. Toenails may appear thick and ridged. And the patient may have leg or foot ulcers. You may note brown spots on your patient's shins—a sign of small internal hemorrhages resulting from minor trauma to the area. The hemorrhages are harmless in themselves, but they do indicate that changes have occurred to peripheral blood vessels as a result of diabetes.

Head and neck

In a person with diabetes, the oral mucous membranes may appear dry because of dehydration. When inspecting the patient's gums, you may find that they bleed easily and appear swollen—an indication of periodontal disease caused by glucose pooling. Patients with diabetes who practice poor oral hygiene and poor blood glucose control commonly have oral infections. For example, white patches on the tongue, palate, and buccal mucosa are signs of oral thrush. Many ulcers covered with a pseudomembrane and thick oral secretions are signs of Vincent's angina (trench mouth).

Hyperglycemia affects the eyes in many ways. It may alter visual acuity, making it difficult for the patient to read a Snellen chart. Ocular neuropathy impairs extraocular eye movements. Pro-

A view of proliferative diabetic retinopathy

This view through an ophthalmoscope shows the characteristics of proliferative diabetic retinopathy. The retinal capillaries are occluded, and new blood vessels have formed—a process called neovascularization. In time, these vessels become fibrous and rupture, causing hemorrhage and vitreous humor contraction. If the occluded capillaries bleed while the vitreous humor contracts, the patient is at risk for tractional retinal detachment. If the macula is involved, she'll lose her vision.

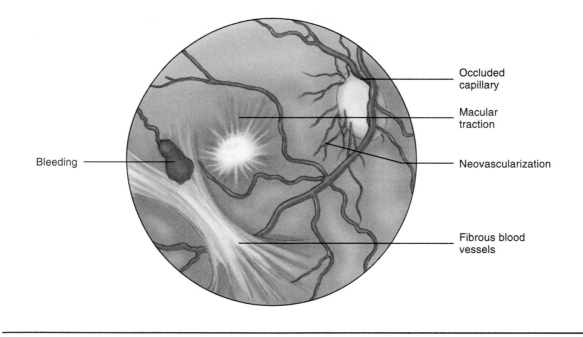

Bleeding

Occluded capillary

Macular traction

Neovascularization

Fibrous blood vessels

longed hyperglycemia may cause eye disorders such as xanthelasma (slightly raised, yellowish, well-defined plaques that appear along the nasal side of the eyelids), cataracts (opacities visible on or in the lens that take on various shapes and colors), and glaucoma (increased intraocular pressure). Prolonged hyperglycemia also may cause diabetic retinopathy—an abnormality of the retina detected by ophthalmoscopic examination (see *A view of proliferative diabetic retinopathy*).

Heart and blood vessels

You may find cardiovascular abnormalities if your patient's diabetes hasn't been diagnosed or if she's having difficulty controlling her blood glucose levels with her prescribed treatment.

Most cardiac abnormalities are detected during the health history and through diagnostic tests rather than during the physical examination. If your patient has peripheral vascular disease, you may find abnormal skin changes, as discussed earlier. When palpating the peripheral pulses, especially the pedal pulse, you may note a decreased or absent pulse.

To check arterial competence, have your patient elevate her legs while she moves her feet up and down. Then have her sit with her legs dangling; normal color should return to her legs in about 10 seconds. A slowly developing dusky color indicates arterial insufficiency.

Mental status and neurologic function

Hypoglycemia caused by diabetes therapy that's too aggressive or by poor management (for example, using insulin without eating) can cause neurologic signs such as tremors, faintness, and difficulty in communicating. If left untreated, hypoglycemia can quickly lead to a loss of consciousness, seizures, and death. Hyperglycemia can cause such abnormalities as slowed thought processes, slurred speech, irritability, and confusion. Hyperglycemia that has progressed to DKA can cause a patient to appear drunk. If the hyperglycemia goes untreated, she'll eventually lapse into a coma.

Extreme hyperglycemia that occurs in HHNK syndrome causes changes in mental status, ranging from mild confusion to coma. Some patients may suffer seizures and transient hemiplegia. Commonly, the patient's neurologic condition is initially thought to result from a stroke; however, a routine blood glucose level quickly identifies diabetes as the source of the problem.

Long-standing hyperglycemia may lead to diabetic neuropathy, which can be further classified as peripheral or autonomic. Carefully examine your patient's arms and legs for peripheral neuropathy. You may find signs of atrophy of the small muscles, which will be most pronounced in the interosseous space between the thumb and first finger. Trauma to the hands caused by cigarette or stove burns may indicate sensory loss.

Peripheral neuropathy that affects the feet and legs is usually bilateral and symmetric, so compare physical findings in both legs. Peripheral neuropathy may also cause deep tendon reflexes to be diminished or absent, and the patient may have leg or foot ulcers. Sensory testing involving pain, temperature, light touch, vibration, position, and discriminative sensations may reveal that sensations are decreased or absent.

Autonomic neuropathy develops when the nerves that lead to various organs are damaged by hyperglycemia. Most abnormalities of autonomic neuropathy can be detected during the health history and through diagnostic tests. Some patients with autonomic neuropathy may experience unpredictable diarrhea (especially at night) or difficulty urinating.

Kidneys and bladder

Abnormalities of the kidneys and bladder are usually detected during the health history and through diagnostic tests. For example, a history of frequent urinary tract infections (UTIs) may be an early sign of kidney disease. When examined, a urine sample may be foul smelling and cloudy, suggesting a UTI. Long-standing diabetes can also cause neurogenic bladder and incontinence.

Complications of diabetes

A physical examination of a patient who has already been diagnosed with diabetes will help you identify the effects of acute and chronic complications. You may also discover body changes that have occurred as a result of therapy, especially insulin injections and blood glucose level monitoring.

Hypoglycemia sometimes causes no signs or symptoms and must be detected by blood glucose monitoring. If hypoglycemia goes undetected, the sudden collapse of a patient may be the first warning sign. Here's what happens: Because the nerves of the autonomic nervous system are coated with glucose for a long time, nerve transmission slows. And because of this slowing, the patient doesn't experience the early signs and symptoms of hypoglycemia. Instead, she experiences unexpected hypoglycemic episodes, such as a collapse.

Because diabetes is commonly treated by tightly controlling blood glucose levels, you should examine your patient for and ask her about signs and symptoms of hypoglycemia. One of the major adverse effects of tight control is an increase in the number and severity of hypoglycemic episodes. If your patient has diabetic retinopathy, tight control may briefly worsen the condition, so immediately report any changes in your patient's visual acuity.

Be sure to examine the sites where your patient has injected insulin and drawn blood for self-monitoring. If she uses pork or beef insulin, you may note skin abnormalities, such as fatty accumulations under the skin or areas of atrophy, which appear as hollow spots. Repeated injections into the same spot cause these abnormalities and can adversely affect insulin absorption.

To find out if your patient is actually performing blood glucose monitoring, examine her fingertips for puncture marks and calluses. A callus may be an ideal area from which to draw blood because the patient will experience less discomfort and be more likely to test her blood regularly.

Diagnostic tests

A physician may order diagnostic tests to diagnose diabetes, detect diabetic complications, or monitor the effectiveness of a patient's therapy. Of course, a patient should also perform self-monitoring to check the effectiveness of her therapy.

Early detection of diabetic complications allows for early treatment, which can minimize their destructive effects. Tests that help diagnose a complication can be repeated to monitor its progress.

Blood tests

Blood tests used to diagnose diabetes include the fasting blood glucose test, the 2-hour oral glucose tolerance test, and the random blood glucose test. The glycosylated hemoglobin test is used to monitor the effectiveness of a patient's therapy.

Blood tests used to detect and monitor the progression of diabetic complications include a fasting lipid profile for cardiovascular disease and serum creatinine and blood urea nitrogen (BUN) tests for renal disease.

Fasting blood glucose test
A fasting blood glucose test evaluates the patient's ability to regulate glucose levels. A blood sample is taken by venipuncture after the patient has fasted for about 8 hours. Although values may vary slightly among laboratories, a finding between 70 and 120 mg/dl is considered normal in nonpregnant adults (see *Reviewing normal glucose levels*). A physician makes a diagnosis of diabetes if the finding is 126 mg/dl or more.

A fasting blood glucose test can also be used to monitor the effectiveness of the patient's treatment. If the glucose level is consistently elevated, the patient's prescribed regimen may need to be changed. However, an elevated fasting blood glucose level in a patient with Type 1 diabetes doesn't always signal a need for more insulin. If the patient

has the Somogyi phenomenon, less insulin may be needed. This phenomenon results from insulin-induced nocturnal hypoglycemia, which causes counterregulatory hormones to raise blood glucose levels through internal compensatory mechanisms. To alleviate the phenomenon, the physician will decrease the patient's insulin dosage to eliminate nocturnal hypoglycemia.

Nursing considerations
Before the test, tell your patient that she must fast for 8 hours. Make sure she understands that during the fast she may eat nothing and drink only water. Instruct her to fast for no more than 16 hours before the test. A fast of more than 16 hours or less than 8 hours can falsely increase glucose levels.

If the patient already uses insulin or an oral antidiabetic drug, her physician will withhold it during the fast. After the test, the patient can go back to her regular medication schedule. Instruct your patient to maintain a normal activity level during the fast. Any increase in activity can lower blood glucose levels and cause a false normal result.

If your patient is hospitalized before the test and her diabetic medication hasn't been withheld during the fast, check her during the night for hypoglycemia. If she appears restless or diaphoretic while sleeping, wake her and check her blood glucose level. Nightmares and a headache in the morning also suggest nocturnal hypoglycemia. If you detect hypoglycemia, break the fast, appropriately treat the patient, and reschedule the test. If the patient isn't hospitalized and her diabetic medication hasn't been withheld, have a family member check her during the night.

If you draw the blood for a fasting blood glucose test to be performed at a laboratory, send the sample immediately. If the sample is left at room temperature, blood glucose levels will decrease. If you can't send it right away, refrigerate it.

To monitor blood glucose levels at home, a patient can perform a fasting blood glucose test, using a fingerstick and a self-monitoring meter. Explain that if the test shows hyperglycemia, she should check the calibration of her meter. If it's correct, she should repeat the test to verify her initial results. Reassure your patient that blood glucose levels fluctuate and an infrequent elevation in the fasting blood glucose level doesn't indicate a loss of diabetic control. Elevated levels are significant only if they persist.

Two-hour oral glucose tolerance test

A 2-hour oral glucose tolerance test determines your patient's ability to adjust to and dispose of a glucose load. The test is especially helpful for detecting diabetes in the following patients:

- those who show signs and symptoms of diabetes but have normal fasting blood glucose levels
- those who have risk factors for diabetes but have normal fasting blood glucose levels
- those who have complications usually associated with diabetes.

After the patient fasts for 8 hours, a blood sample is obtained by venipuncture. Next, the patient drinks 75 to 100 grams of glucose. Then additional blood samples are obtained at 30-minute to 60-minute intervals for 2 hours.

The results of an oral glucose tolerance test are normal if the initial fasting blood glucose level is 70 to 115 mg/dl, the final 2-hour glucose level is less than 125 mg/dl, and all glucose values in between are less than 200 mg/dl. Despite two normal fasting blood glucose test results, a physician can diagnose diabetes in a nonpregnant adult who has an oral glucose tolerance test in which the 2-hour plasma glucose level is 200 mg/dl or more.

The 2-hour oral glucose tolerance test isn't used to monitor a patient's diabetes treatment. However, it can be used to monitor patients who have impaired glucose tolerance and who are at risk for developing diabetes later in life. Despite a normal fasting glucose test result, a physician can diagnose a patient with impaired glucose tolerance if the 2-hour glucose level is 140 to 200 mg/dl.

Nursing considerations

When preparing your patient for a 2-hour oral glucose tolerance test, instruct her to maintain a normal diet and activity level for 3 days before the test. Failure to do so may interfere with the test results. Some drugs such as diuretics, nicotinic acid, and beta-blockers may also interfere with test results. High doses of some hormones can affect the results, as well. When possible, the patient's physician will discontinue these drugs for 3 days before the test.

The patient will need to fast for 8 hours before the test. Try to schedule it for the morning so that most of the fasting time will occur while she's sleeping.

Instruct your patient to drink the glucose solution within 5 minutes. During the 2 hours re-

Reviewing normal glucose levels

A physician may use a fasting blood glucose test, a 2-hour oral glucose tolerance test, or a random blood glucose test to diagnose diabetes. A glycosylated hemoglobin test helps you monitor your patient's blood glucose levels. The following table shows the normal values for each of these tests.

Test	Normal values
Fasting blood glucose	• 70–115 mg/dl
2-hour oral glucose tolerance	• Fasting: 70–115 mg/dl • 1 hour: 190 mg/dl or less • 2 hours: 125 mg/dl or less
Random blood glucose	• Less than 190 mg/dl within 2 hours of eating • Less than 125 mg/dl 2 hours or more after eating
Glycosylated hemoglobin	• A_{1a}: 1.6% of total hemoglobin • A_{1b}: 0.8% of total hemoglobin • A_{1c}: 3%–6% of total hemoglobin

quired for the test, the patient should remain seated and not smoke.

Hypoglycemia probably won't occur after a glucose load has been administered to a patient suspected of having diabetes, but it could occur if the patient has another unsuspected disorder, such as islet cell tumors. If the patient develops signs and symptoms of hypoglycemia, draw a blood sample for confirmation. If the patient is hypoglycemic, stop the test immediately and provide the appropriate treatment.

Send all samples to the laboratory immediately or refrigerate them to prevent altered test results.

Random blood glucose test

A random blood glucose test also can be used to diagnose diabetes. The test requires a blood sample obtained by venipuncture anytime during the day or night. The test results are normal if the level is less than 190 mg/dl within 2 hours of eating and less than 125 mg/dl 2 hours or more after eating. A random blood glucose level that's 200 mg/dl or more and accompanied by the typical signs of diabetes (polydipsia, polyuria, polyphagia, and unexplained weight loss) confirms a diagnosis of diabetes.

A random blood glucose test is commonly used by patients with diabetes to monitor their blood glucose level. The test can also be used to confirm hypoglycemia, especially if its signs and symptoms have become blunted over the years. The patient, a family member, or other caregiver can perform a random blood glucose test with a fingerstick and a self-monitoring meter.

Nursing considerations
Send venipuncture samples to the laboratory immediately or refrigerate them to prevent altered test results.

Interpret self-monitoring and laboratory test results in light of your patient's food intake, activity level, and emotional state during the hours immediately before the test. Always recheck unusual results or sudden deviations from the patient's normal blood glucose pattern.

To encourage frequent self-monitoring, tell your patient that maintaining glucose levels as near to normal as possible can slow the progression of long-term microvascular complications: retinopathy and nephropathy. Periodically check your patient's self-monitoring technique and her meter.

If your patient's blood glucose levels remain abnormally high, she may need more frequent blood glucose measurements. If a pattern emerges, such as abnormally high blood glucose levels before dinner, changes in your patient's daily treatment plan may be necessary.

Glycosylated hemoglobin test
The glycosylated hemoglobin test evaluates your patient's response to diabetes therapy. The test measures the degree to which glucose attaches to hemoglobin (a process called glycosylation). Glycosylation occurs continually during the 120-day life of a red blood cell (RBC). The higher the blood glucose level, the greater the attachment. Once glucose attaches to hemoglobin, the process is nearly irreversible, which

makes the glycosylated hemoglobin test an accurate reflection of your patient's average blood glucose level during the 4 to 8 weeks before the test.

The test values are given as a percentage of the total hemoglobin within an RBC. Three hemoglobins can be measured: A_{1a}, A_{1b}, and A_{1c}. The hemoglobin most commonly measured is A_{1c} because it's normally present in the largest quantity (3% to 6% of total hemoglobin). A_{1a} is typically 1.6%; A_{1b} is 0.8%. The closer to normal the patient can maintain her blood glucose level over an extended period, the closer to normal her glycosylated hemoglobin will be.

Nursing considerations
If your patient uses insulin, she should have a glycosylated hemoglobin test every 3 months. For patients who don't use insulin, the frequency of the test depends on their response to therapy, which is determined by fasting blood glucose levels.

Your patient needs no preparation before the test. If you're collecting the specimen, perform a venipuncture and collect the blood in a 5-ml lavender-top tube. Make sure the tube fills completely. Then gently invert it several times to mix the blood and anticoagulant adequately. If hemolysis occurs, collect a new specimen.

If the glycosylated hemoglobin value is elevated but the patient reports normal blood glucose levels from her self-monitoring tests, perform a second glycosylated hemoglobin test to rule out collection or laboratory error. If the second test is consistent with the first, evaluate the patient's self-monitoring technique and correct any errors. If the patient's technique is correct, the problem may be that she's reporting normal values even though her tests reveal elevated glucose levels. Try to make your patient comfortable enough to express any problems she's encountering in trying to comply with her treatment plan, and emphasize the importance of blood glucose control in delaying the development of long-term complications.

Fasting lipid profile
Diabetes is a risk factor for coronary artery disease (CAD). Thus, an adult who has recently been diagnosed with diabetes should have a fasting lipid profile to detect any lipid abnormalities. Obesity and lipid abnormalities—both risk

factors for CAD—are common in patients with Type 2 diabetes, no matter how well they control their blood glucose levels. Plus, diabetes may eliminate the protective effect premenopausal women usually have against CAD.

Before the test, the patient must fast overnight. You'll obtain blood by venipuncture, and the sample will be used to measure total cholesterol, high-density lipoprotein (HDL) cholesterol, low-density lipoprotein (LDL) cholesterol, and triglyceride levels (see *Figures for a normal lipid profile*).

Lipid profiles of patients with Type 2 diabetes commonly show increased total cholesterol, LDL cholesterol, and triglyceride levels and decreased HDL cholesterol levels. A high LDL cholesterol level increases the risk of CAD, whereas a high HDL cholesterol level decreases the risk. High triglyceride and total cholesterol levels also increase the risk of CAD.

If the test detects a lipid abnormality, teach your patient about the need for lifestyle changes, such as a low-fat diet and an exercise program. Her physician may prescribe an antilipemic drug, such as simvastatin or fluvastatin. Patients taking such drugs should have a fasting lipid profile at least once a year.

Effective therapy should lower LDL cholesterol levels in patients with diabetes to less than 130 mg/dl and raise HDL cholesterol levels to more than 35 mg/dl in men and more than 45 mg/dl in women (normal HDL cholesterol levels are more than 45 mg/dl in men and more than 55 mg/dl in women). If your patient has already been diagnosed with CAD, her LDL cholesterol levels should be lowered to 100 mg/dl, and her triglyceride levels should be lowered to 190 mg/dl.

Nursing considerations

Instruct your patient to fast for 12 hours before the test. She should avoid vigorous exercise the day before the test and shouldn't alter her diet before the fast begins. Also, instruct her to avoid alcohol for 24 hours before the test because it may falsely elevate triglyceride levels. If possible, your patient's physician will withhold drugs that may alter cholesterol or triglyceride levels.

Before drawing blood for a fasting lipid profile, determine if your patient has a fever or has had surgery or trauma recently. These conditions may interfere with the test results. If you note such a condition, reschedule the test.

Figures for a normal lipid profile

Diabetes increases a patient's risk of coronary artery disease (CAD), so after being diagnosed with diabetes, your patient should undergo a fasting lipid profile. This profile detects abnormal lipid levels, a major risk factor for CAD.

Type of lipid	Normal value (mg/dl)
Total cholesterol	< 200
Low-density lipoprotein cholesterol	< 130
High-density lipoprotein cholesterol	Women: > 55 Men: > 45
Trigylcerides	< 190

After collecting the blood, send it immediately to the laboratory or refrigerate it to protect it from spontaneous redistribution of the lipoproteins. If the sample becomes frozen, it should be discarded, and the test should be rescheduled.

Serum creatinine and blood urea nitrogen tests

One complication of diabetes is diabetic nephropathy. A quick and simple way to check renal function is to draw a blood sample for serum creatinine and BUN tests. These tests should be performed when the patient is diagnosed with diabetes.

Although the serum creatinine and BUN tests can quickly reveal the patient's renal function, serum creatinine is the more sensitive indicator. Many extrarenal conditions, such as dehydration, can elevate the BUN level, but serum creatinine changes little except in renal disease. A normal serum creatinine level for an adult ranges between 0.7 and 1.5 mg/dl (0.6 and 1.2 mg/dl for adults over age 65). A normal BUN level for an adult ranges between 4 and 22 mg/dl (8 and 18 mg/dl for adults over age 65). Elevations in your patient's serum creatinine and BUN levels require further testing before a physician can make a diagnosis of diabetic nephropathy.

Nursing considerations

Test results are more accurate if your patient fasts for 8 hours beforehand; therefore, try to schedule the test for first thing in the morning, so that most of the fasting time will occur while she is sleeping. Tell her not to eat breakfast.

If your patient is taking ascorbic acid, a barbiturate, or a diuretic, her physician will probably withhold it until after the test because these drugs can raise serum creatinine levels. Note whether your patient is receiving amphotericin B, an aminoglycoside, methicillin, or chloramphenicol. Any of these nephrotoxic drugs could be the source of her renal impairment.

After drawing the blood, send the sample to the laboratory immediately. To prevent hemolysis, which can alter the test results, handle the blood sample gently.

If the BUN level is elevated but the serum creatinine level isn't, consider possible extrarenal causes before repeating the tests. Also, keep in mind that the amount of creatinine produced in the body is related to muscle mass. Therefore, an athlete with normal renal function may have elevated levels of serum creatinine.

If your patient's serum creatinine and BUN levels are both high, check them frequently to monitor her renal function. Abnormal renal function coupled with diabetes places your patient at increased risk for end-stage renal disease and cardiovascular disease. The frequency of these tests depends on how high the patient's serum creatinine and BUN levels are and whether she exhibits other signs.

Urine tests

When a patient is diagnosed with diabetes, urinalysis should be done to detect the presence of glucose, ketones, and protein in the urine. These tests help a physician diagnose certain diabetic complications, such as DKA and renal failure.

A patient who has already been diagnosed with diabetes should periodically have urine ketone and urine protein tests to check for these complications. Routine urinalysis can be used for such monitoring, but patients typically perform the tests themselves using a kit with a dipstick or enzymatic tablet.

Urine glucose test

The urine glucose test, which detects the presence of glucose in the urine, is no longer used to diagnose diabetes because blood glucose tests provide more accurate results. If routine urinalysis reveals glucose in a patient's urine, she should have a blood glucose test to confirm a diagnosis of diabetes.

The use of urine glucose tests to monitor diabetes treatment has diminished because blood glucose monitors are so convenient, inexpensive, and accurate. These monitors give the precise level of glucose in the blood, whereas urine glucose tests merely detect the presence of glucose in urine. Because glucose appears in the urine of adults with healthy kidneys only when blood glucose levels rise above 180 mg/dl, a normal result from a urine glucose test tells the patient little: She may be hypoglycemic, euglycemic, or mildly to moderately hyperglycemic.

Urine ketone test

The urine ketone test, which detects ketones in the urine, aids in the diagnosis of DKA. Ketones are the end products of fat metabolism, which occurs when glucose isn't available for cell use. When blood cells use fat for energy in place of glucose, fat metabolism is incomplete, and ketones accumulate in the patient's blood. Ketones eventually spill over into the patient's urine and can be detected by urinalysis. Ketones usually appear in the urine when blood glucose levels are consistently above 240 mg/dl.

If your patient has Type 1 diabetes, she's prone to develop DKA. When she experiences acute illness or stress, when her blood glucose levels are consistently above 240 mg/dl, or when she has signs or symptoms of DKA (nausea, vomiting, and abdominal pain), she should test her urine for ketones every 4 hours. A pregnant woman with diabetes should test her urine for ketones to monitor her diabetes control. If they're present, her physician will change her treatment plan.

Urine protein test

The urine protein test detects the presence of protein (albumin) in the urine. Usually, small amounts of protein go undetected in routine urinalysis. When protein is detected, the cause may be renal impairment from diabetes. Or it may just be strenuous exercise, exposure to cold, or emotional stress.

Drugs that affect urine test results

Many drugs can alter the results of a patient's urine test for glucose, ketones, or protein. Before such a test, note which drugs your patient is taking. Then if her test results are abnormal, check with the laboratory to see if one of the drugs could be the problem. This list contains drugs that commonly alter test results, falsely indicating glucosuria, ketonuria, and proteinuria.

Glucosuria
- aminosalicylic acid
- ascorbic acid
- cephalosporins
- chloral hydrate
- chloramphenicol
- isoniazid
- levodopa
- methyldopa
- nalidixic acid
- nitrofurantoin
- penicillin G (large doses)
- phenazopyridine
- probenecid
- salicylates (large doses)
- streptomycin
- tetracyclines

Ketonuria
- levodopa
- phenazopyridine
- phenolsulfonphthalein
- phenothiazines
- salicylates
- sulfobromophthalein

Proteinuria
- acetazolamide
- aminosalicylic acid
- cephalothin (large doses)
- nafcillin
- sodium bicarbonate
- tolbutamide
- tolmetin

When protein is detected in a patient with diabetes, urinalysis should be repeated. If the second test detects protein too, a 24-hour urine protein test should be done to determine the type of renal impairment. Protein levels of 150 mg in urine over 24 hours are normal. Levels higher than 150 mg indicate the need for further testing.

Diabetes can seriously impair kidney function and is one of the leading causes of end-stage renal disease. Even if your patient has no protein in her urine when she's diagnosed with diabetes, encourage her to have her urine monitored periodically. All postpubertal patients who've had diabetes for 5 years or more and all patients with Type 2 diabetes should have their urine tested for protein once a year.

Nursing considerations

Collecting urine for urinalysis requires no preparation on the part of the patient. However, you should obtain a history of recent drug use. Many drugs can alter the results of a routine urinalysis (see *Drugs that affect urine test results*). To prevent inaccurate test results, send the urine sample to the laboratory immediately. If this isn't possible, refrigerate the sample until it's transported.

If you're using a dipstick or enzymatic tablet to test urine, carefully follow the manufacturer's instructions. Recheck abnormal results.

When preparing your patient for a 24-hour urine collection, tell her to save all urine in the special container provided. She should keep the container refrigerated throughout the collection period. Instruct the patient not to contaminate the urine with toilet tissue, vaginal secretions, mucus, or fecal material. She should maintain a normal fluid intake because diluted urine may cause false normal results.

Other tests

Patients with diabetes should periodically have certain tests—such as a filament test, electrocardiogram (ECG), and exercise stress test—to detect complications of diabetes. They should also

Testing sensory loss with a monofilament device

A filament test can help you find out if your patient has a sensory loss in her feet. To perform the test, place the monofilament device on the ten spots shown—nine spots on the bottom of each foot and one spot on the top—and have your patient say *yes* if she can feel pressure. When you touch the skin with the device, make sure the filament bends; this ensures that the device exerts the correct amount of pressure on the skin.

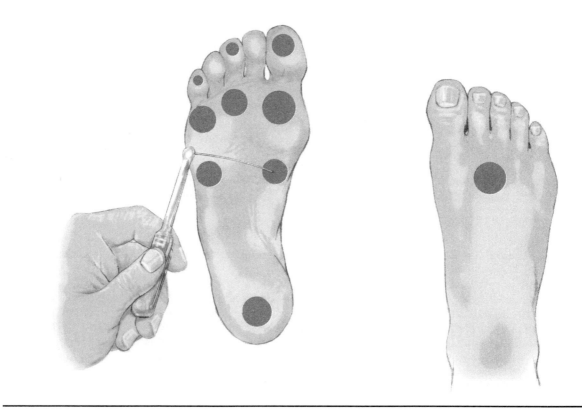

have regular extensive ophthalmic examinations to detect diabetic retinopathy.

Filament test

Peripheral neuropathy, a common complication of diabetes, causes sensory loss in the arms and legs. Such sensory loss in the feet increases the patient's risk of developing foot ulcers that could ultimately lead to amputation.

Usually, sensory loss is diagnosed by an examiner touching different areas of the patient's foot with a pin. Unfortunately, this technique isn't reliable. An examiner may not exert the same amount of pressure on each area, and some examiners are more heavy-handed than others. In

fact, the same examiner may be heavy-handed one day and have a lighter touch the next, making comparisons difficult.

Filament testing with a monofilament device alleviates these problems. The device places exactly 10 grams of force on a small area of the skin (see *Testing sensory loss with a monofilament device*). To assess sensory loss in the feet, an examiner uses the device at 10 sites on each foot.

The test result is normal if the patient feels the filament in all 10 spots on each foot. The result is abnormal if she doesn't feel it in one or more spots.

Filament testing can be used to monitor the progression of a patient's sensory loss and to

HEALTH PROMOTION

Preventing foot ulcers

Foot ulcers are a major cause of foot and leg amputation in patients with diabetes. Yet, almost half of these amputations could be prevented by using a foot ulcer prevention plan.

Before developing such a plan, explain to your patient the role that glucose control plays in preventing and healing foot ulcers. If your patient doesn't have a foot ulcer, tell her that consistently high blood glucose levels increase her risk of developing one. If your patient already has a foot ulcer, tell her that poor glucose control hinders recovery and increases the risk of a recurrence.

Assessing the patient
Begin by assessing your patient's feet for abnormalities such as corns or bunions, which increase the risk of ulceration. Ask her how she cares for her feet.

Next, assess your patient for risk factors. If she has a history of diabetic neuropathy or peripheral vascular disease, she's at greatest risk for developing a foot ulcer. Unfortunately, the development of a foot ulcer may be the first sign that your patient has neuropathy or peripheral vascular disease.

Implementing the plan
If your patient has no history of neuropathy or peripheral vascular disease and her foot assessment reveals no abnormalities, focus on correcting any misconceptions she may have about foot care. Then, instruct her in a daily foot care routine, which should include keeping her feet clean and dry, examining her feet for blisters, and wearing comfortable shoes. Also, advise your patient to have her feet examined by a physician at least once a year.

If your patient has calluses or corns, teach her how to manage the condition with an emery board, callus file, or pumice stone. Tell her that cutting calluses or corns off her feet or using an over-the-counter medicated pad to treat them may cause an ulcer to form. If your patient's calluses or corns are caused by abnormally high or low arches, refer her to a specialist. Other abnormalities, such as hammer toes and metatarsal deformities, may require special shoes, regular care by a podiatrist, or surgical repair of the deformity.

If your patient already has a foot ulcer, your plan of care will include treating the ulcer and determining what caused it. Depending on the type of ulcer and its location, treatment may include the following:
- removal of the cause (for example, poor-fitting shoes)
- a restriction on weight-bearing activities, if the ulcer is on the plantar of the foot
- wound care to heal the ulcer
- infection control, including antibiotic therapy
- follow-up care.

To help prevent another ulcer, you should also review your patient's knowledge and her compliance with routine foot care.

help in tailoring an ulcer prevention program for her.

Nursing considerations
Have the patient lie down on the examination table and instruct her to say *yes* each time she feels the filament. Have her keep her eyes closed to avoid an invalid response. After the test, develop an ulcer prevention program for your patient (see *Preventing foot ulcers*).

Electrocardiogram
As mentioned, diabetes is a major risk factor for CAD, which is the most common cause of death in patients with diabetes. An ECG evaluates the electrical activity of your patient's heart and can detect evidence of myocardial ischemia, myocardial infarction, and arrhythmias caused by ischemia.

An ECG should be performed regularly to monitor the effects of your patient's diabetes on her heart. An annual ECG is sufficient, unless your patient shows symptoms of heart disease or a previous ECG was abnormal.

Nursing considerations
Reassure your patient that an ECG doesn't hurt or cause an electric shock. Some preparation may be needed before applying the electrodes to her skin. For example, if she has been sweating, the sites should be dried. If a patient has a lot of

hair at the electrode sites, you may need to shave them to provide better contact.

Exercise stress test

This test places exercise demands on the heart and can uncover CAD not detected with an ECG. Many patients with diabetes have additional risk factors for CAD, such as obesity, hypertension, and abnormal blood lipid levels. Thus, a physician may have a patient undergo an exercise stress test even if her ECG is normal.

A stress test can also be used to monitor the progression of CAD. A patient may require periodic stress tests, especially if new symptoms of CAD appear or new risk factors are identified.

Nursing considerations

Review your patient's drug history and find out from her physician which drugs should be withheld and which she should take on the day of the stress test. A physician may withhold oral antidiabetic drugs because exercise lowers blood glucose levels. If your patient uses insulin, her physician may prescribe a lower dose to avoid hypoglycemia during the test.

Instruct your patient to rest the day before the test so that she has the energy to perform it. She should also fast for at least 3 hours and avoid smoking for at least 1 hour before the test. Explain to your patient what she can expect during the test and what she should wear. This information may ease her anxiety.

Determine if your patient has autonomic neuropathy, which affects involuntary functions, such as heart rate and blood pressure. During stress testing, patients with such neuropathy may not experience chest pain even though ischemia develops. Also, the blood pressure may go very high or very low when exercising. If your patient has autonomic neuropathy, closely monitor her throughout the test. The physician may even decide that an exercise stress test is inappropriate for such a patient and substitute a dipyridamole-thallium test. With this test, dipyridamole, instead of exercise, is used to put stress on the heart. The thallium acts as a contrast agent.

3

Treatment

Today, patients with diabetes take primary responsibility for their own day-to-day treatment. That commitment requires patients to have a great deal of knowledge about the disease in general and their own status in particular. They have to understand when and how to adjust their medication doses, food intake, and activity level. They must learn how to test their blood glucose levels, plan meals and snacks, read food and medication labels, obtain and test urine specimens for ketones, and manage sick days. Just as important, they must know when to call for help.

As a nurse, you have a paramount role in teaching your patient to manage her own care. She relies on your expertise and your ability to teach her what she needs to know in clear, simple terms. As you teach, be sensitive to your patient's level of comprehension and her ability to perform the necessary tasks. Adjust your teaching to her learning style. You also should be aware of your patient's cultural and health beliefs as well as her fears and concerns about her condition. Create a friendly, relaxed atmosphere to promote an effective exchange of information.

To teach your patient effectively, you also should be aware of scientific breakthroughs, newly approved drugs, new indications for drugs your patient is already taking, and new technology. Ever-improving technology makes it possible for your patient to monitor her blood glucose levels quickly and easily. New oral drugs and forms of insulin continue to reach the market. Insulin-pump therapy is a great help for an increasing number of patients. A nurse who keeps up to date provides a vital service to her patient. Simplifying her self-care even in a small way can make a tremendous difference to her self-confidence and comfort level. Each advance, once learned, can enhance your patient's control of her blood glucose levels, thus improving her quality of life.

Teaching your patient to manage her care may also involve having her meet with a certified diabetes educator. These health care providers have expert knowledge in biology, the social sciences, communication skills, counseling, education, and the care of patients with diabetes. A certified diabetes educator can teach a patient about any of the following topics:
• pathophysiology of diabetes mellitus
• nutritional management and diet
• pharmacologic interventions
• exercise and activity
• self-monitoring for glycemic control
• prevention and management of acute and chronic complications
• psychologic and social issues
• problem-solving skills
• stress management
• use of the health care delivery system.

Nutritional therapy

Nutritional therapy for patients with diabetes has undergone several changes since the first precalculated meal plans and exchange lists were created in the 1950s. These early plans called for a 40% carbohydrate, 20% protein, and 40% fat distribution of calories for all meals. These plans were consistently used until the discovery of a link between high-fat diets and cardiovascular disease. Today, diet plans for diabetes are higher in complex carbohydrates and lower in protein and fat.

With each change, the approach to nutritional therapy has become more individualized and more closely linked to a patient's blood glucose levels, lifestyle, and food preferences. Patients are no longer given standard lists of foods to avoid and sent on their way.

Nutritional therapy today is comprehensive and ongoing, and it involves assessment, goal setting, intervention, and regular reevaluation. Patients learn to monitor their blood glucose levels at home and to make diet, exercise, and medication dosage choices based on those levels. This close monitoring of blood glucose levels postpones the onset and progression of microvascular and macrovascular complications and neuropathy.

Other changes have taken place as well. For years, for example, starches were considered the preferred form of carbohydrates for patients with diabetes, who were instructed to avoid all simple sugars. Studies have shown, however, that blood glucose levels don't respond any better to complex carbohydrates, such as starches, than to simple ones, such as sugars. This finding gives patients far more freedom in selecting foods. Allowing patients with diabetes to include up to 5% of their carbohydrate intake as sugar represents a major change in philosophy that many health care workers may find harder to accept than their patients.

Out of habit, however, many patients and health care practitioners continue to use the more conventional regimens. Patients who have followed conventional nutritional therapy for years may be afraid to learn a new method or may simply be tired of learning new techniques related to diabetes. Those patients need your teaching and encouragement as they strive to adopt a healthier, more flexible way to use their diets to keep their disease under control. You may need the support of colleagues yourself as you become increasingly familiar with new goals and recommendations and begin to use and teach them exclusively.

Because food plays a vital role in every patient's self-care, you'll have a great deal to teach. Don't try to tell your patient everything in one or two sessions; she must understand this information well before she can implement it every day. During your sessions, you'll cover these subjects:
- weight control
- major dietary components, such as carbohydrates, proteins, and fats

- nutritional guidelines for choosing foods, such as how to read food labels
- nutritional plans, including setting goals, adapting plans for cultural and ethnic considerations and for the special needs of elderly and debilitated patients, and planning sick days.

Weight control

Obesity is a major risk factor in the development of Type 2 diabetes. As a patient's weight rises, so do her insulin resistance, glucose intolerance, lipid levels, and blood pressure.

When outlining weight loss goals for your patient, consider her age, physical activity, general health, lifestyle, and current weight. Instruct her to ingest only the number of calories she needs. Children should consume enough calories to permit normal growth and development. For example, girls between ages 11 and 14 should consume 17 calories per pound of body weight per day, and boys between ages 11 and 14 should consume 30 calories per pound of body weight per day. Adults should maintain a reasonable body weight. If your patient is pregnant or breast-feeding, she should eat 300 to 500 more calories than is recommended for her age.

Along with other members of your patient's health care team, devise weight-loss programs that promote healthy eating habits. Tailor each program to your patient's lifestyle. Most people can safely and realistically expect to lose ½ to 3 pounds per week.

If your patient is cutting back on calories, instruct her that fewer calories can cause blood glucose levels to fall. Teach your patient to monitor her blood glucose levels carefully and to adjust her medication as appropriate.

Dietary components

Base your diet recommendations on treatment goals designed specifically for your patient (see *Creating a nutritional plan*). Consider the various roles of proteins, carbohydrates, fats, sweeteners, fiber, sodium, and alcohol in your patient's diet.

Protein
A person needs protein for normal growth and development and maintenance of body protein stores. Proteins are made up of amino acids that

are used for building and rebuilding the body. Proteins also act as enzymes, hormones, and antibodies. Proteins not needed for growth and development are converted into glycogen or fats and stored in the body until they're needed as energy.

The recommended protein intake for a patient with diabetes is 10% to 20% of total daily calories. Eating too much protein increases the glomerular rate, which makes the kidneys work harder. If your patient develops nephropathy, teach her to restrict her protein to 0.8 g/kg of body weight per day. For example, a man who weighs 68 kilograms should consume 54 grams of protein per day. Reducing protein intake decreases proteinuria and eases the work performed by the kidneys.

Large amounts of protein can raise blood glucose levels. Instruct your patient to monitor her blood glucose levels to determine if she should adjust her insulin dose for meals containing large amounts of protein.

Carbohydrates

Carbohydrates supply the body's primary source of energy. The brain and red blood cells use only glucose, the building block of carbohydrates. The American Diabetes Association recommends determining your patient's protein requirements, using the recommended dietary allowance of 0.8 g/kg of body weight for adults, before determining the desired amount of carbohydrates and fat. Also, use your patient's treatment goals, habits, and blood glucose and lipid goals as guides.

When your patient chooses which carbohydrates to consume, instruct her to focus on the glycemic value of a carbohydrate rather than on the type of carbohydrate, such as simple or complex. The glycemic index, created in 1981, provides average glycemic values of certain foods. It can help you predict the rise in blood glucose after your patient has eaten certain carbohydrates. Foods that raise blood glucose levels quickly have a high glycemic value. These include white bread, some cereals, glucose, and root vegetables, such as carrots and potatoes. Foods with a low glycemic value include nuts, legumes, dairy products, fructose, and raw fruits.

Advise your patient to use the index as a guide and to monitor her blood glucose levels after she eats certain foods. Make it clear, however, that the glycemic value of a food is not equivalent to its nutritional value. Although sucrose has a lower glycemic value than a potato, for example,

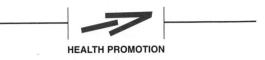

HEALTH PROMOTION

Creating a nutritional plan

As you and your patient develop her nutritional plan, think about how the various components of the diet will affect her blood glucose levels and what she will need to maintain health. The accompanying table lists the dietary components and makes recommendations about their part in your patient's nutritional plan.

Components	Recommendations
Protein	• 10% to 20% of calories ingested per day should be from protein.
Carbohydrates	• Total amount varies with treatment goals. • Percentage determined after total daily fat and protein has been determined. • Total amount of carbohydrates more important than type of carbohydrate.
Fats	• Total amount varies with treatment goals. • Saturated fat should represent < 10% of calories ingested per day (if low-density lipoprotein cholesterol level is high, < 7%). • Monounsaturated fats preferred. • Up to 10% of calories per day may come from polyunsaturated fat.
Sweeteners	• Up to 5% of carbohydrates may be in form of sucrose or fructose. • Nonnutritive sweeteners may be used.
Fiber	• 20 to 35 g/day (same as in general population).
Sodium	• < 3,000 mg/day. • < 2,400 mg/day if hypertensive.
Alcohol	• No more than one alcoholic drink (1 oz of alcohol) per day for women; no more than two alcoholic drinks per day for men.

it provides far less nutritional value. And inform your patient that the glycemic value of a food can rise or fall depending on many factors, including the ripeness of the food, the preparation of the food, and the other foods eaten at the same meal.

If your patient is using regular insulin, she can count grams of carbohydrates to help her make food choices. Instruct her to count the total number of grams of carbohydrate in a meal she's planning to eat. She should then compare that number to the amount of carbohydrate recommended for that particular meal in her meal plan. If she's consuming more than is recommended, she can increase her regular insulin dose by 1 unit for every additional 10 grams of carbohydrate. If she's consuming fewer carbohydrates than is recommended, she can decrease her insulin by 1 unit for every 10 grams less.

Instruct your patient to count grams of carbohydrate by consulting food labels, exchange lists, and carbohydrate-counting books. Counting grams of carbohydrate allows for more accurate insulin dosing and more flexible meal scheduling. It also reduces the number of hypoglycemic and hyperglycemic episodes.

Fats

The primary role of fat in diet is that of an energy source, either for immediate needs or for storage in adipose tissue for later use. However, excessive fat intake causes elevated levels of blood lipids, which consist of cholesterol, lipoproteins, and triglycerides. Lipoproteins are classified as low-density lipoproteins (LDLs), very-low-density lipoproteins (VLDLs), high-density lipoproteins (HDLs), and chylomicrons. Elevated levels of blood lipids put a person at risk for cardiovascular disease. For your patient with diabetes, high lipid levels are particularly dangerous because diabetes itself is a risk factor for cardiovascular disease.

Chylomicrons, which transport fats, break down in the liver and recombine into VLDLs, which consist mainly of triglycerides. Hyperinsulinemia and insulin resistance, common in patients with Type 2 diabetes, can trigger an overproduction of VLDLs, which may in turn trigger hypertriglyceridemia. Because insulin also stimulates the production of VLDLs, patients who use insulin must be particularly careful about eating fats.

LDLs transport cholesterol from the liver to the cells for deposit in peripheral tissues. An elevated LDL cholesterol level is strongly associated with the risk of heart disease. Taking the reverse route, HDLs transport cholesterol from peripheral tissues to the liver for catabolism and excretion. Increased levels of HDL cholesterol protect a person against heart disease.

Because HDL cholesterol levels are inversely related to triglyceride levels, many people with Type 2 diabetes have low levels of HDL cholesterol. This deficiency puts them at increased risk for developing atherosclerosis. As they gain better control over their blood glucose levels, their HDL cholesterol levels rise.

Patients can lower their blood lipid levels by reducing their total fat intake, losing weight, improving blood glucose levels, and changing the types of fat they consume. They should consume less than 300 mg of cholesterol per day. To help reduce cholesterol intake, patients with diabetes should eat no more than four egg yolks, the most concentrated source of cholesterol, per week.

Less than 10% of total daily calories should come from saturated fat. The acceptable amount of total fat per day, however, depends on your patient's needs. Reducing total fat to 20% to 30% of calories reduces the risk of coronary artery disease for most people. This reduction calls for an increase in carbohydrate calories to 50% or more. While such a high-carbohydrate diet is healthy for people with Type 1 diabetes, it could increase blood glucose and triglyceride levels in insulin-resistant patients with Type 2 diabetes.

Saturated fat increases the risk of atherosclerosis by increasing levels of chylomicrons and LDLs. Most saturated fats come from dairy products, red meats, and other animal sources. Coconut oil, palm oil, and cocoa butter also contain saturated fats. Most of the fat in your patient's diet should come from monounsaturated fats. Substituting monounsaturated fats for saturated fats may improve hypertriglyceridemia in patients with Type 2 diabetes without raising their LDL cholesterol levels. Sources of monounsaturated fats include canola, peanut, and olive oils. Your patient can also lower her cholesterol levels by substituting polyunsaturated fats—corn, sunflower, safflower, and soybean oils—for saturated fats.

Sweeteners

Sweeteners are classified as caloric or noncaloric. Sucrose, fructose, and alcohol sugars are the most common caloric sweeteners. Caloric sweeteners are no longer banned from the diets of patients with diabetes. But if your patient consumes sucrose or fructose, she must exchange it for another carbohydrate. Just like other sources of carbohydrate, sucrose and fructose provide 4 calories per gram. However, your patient shouldn't consume more than 5% of her daily carbohydrate calories in the form of caloric sweeteners.

Sugars in alcohol—sorbitol, xylitol, and mannitol—have little effect on blood glucose levels. Your patient shouldn't include them when calculating the carbohydrate content of foods. She also shouldn't use them to treat hypoglycemia.

Patients with diabetes may eat all the noncaloric sweeteners currently approved for use in the United States: aspartame, acesulfame K, and saccharin. They contain virtually no calories and have a negligible effect on blood glucose.

Fiber

Water-insoluble fiber (which includes wheat, bran, and whole grain products) affects mainly the lower gastrointestinal (GI) tract, where it increases fecal bulk, helps to prevent constipation, and may reduce the risk of colon cancer. Water-soluble fiber (which includes guar and pectin) affects the upper GI tract by delaying gastric emptying and increasing the intestinal transport time. It may also lower levels of total cholesterol and LDL cholesterol.

Although fiber's beneficial effect on glucose level control remains unproved, eating 20 to 35 grams of water-insoluble or water-soluble fiber a day does promote evacuation and lower lipid levels. Instruct your patients who are increasing their fiber intake to do so gradually and to drink at least 8 cups of fluid a day to minimize GI discomfort.

Sodium

The American Diabetes Association recommendations for sodium, less than 3,000 mg per day, are no more restrictive than is common for the general population. Patients with diabetes who also have hypertension should ingest no more than 2,400 mg of sodium per day.

Alcohol

Try to convince your patient with diabetes to limit her alcohol consumption. Alcohol is high in calories, tends to be ketogenic, and increases the risk of hypoglycemia. Women should have no more than one drink (1 ounce of alcohol) per day; men, two drinks per day. Patients who are trying to lose weight and those with hypertriglyceridemia should limit their intake to less than two drinks per week.

When you advise your patient about alcohol consumption, take the caloric value of each drink into account. For example, 8 ounces of regular beer contains 100 calories; 3½ ounces of table wine contains 85 calories. Because the caloric value of alcohol is similar to fat, alcohol may be substituted for fat in the diet. One drink is equivalent to two fat exchanges.

Any patient who's using insulin or taking an oral antidiabetic drug should consume alcohol only with a meal. Alcohol and certain sulfonylureas may cause a disulfiram-like reaction: flushing, headache, nausea, and breathlessness. Alcohol and metformin can increase the risk of lactic acidosis.

Because alcohol inhibits gluconeogenesis, a patient with diabetes must watch carefully for hypoglycemia when she consumes alcohol. When she's fasting, or when glycogen stores are depleted, her body can't make glucose from noncarbohydrate sources, such as fat and protein. So, when blood glucose levels begin to drop, the normal compensatory mechanism of converting stored energy into glucose is blocked by the alcohol. The result is hypoglycemia.

Food labels

The Food and Drug Administration's requirements for food labels have made a big difference to patients with diabetes as they shop for food. The information on labels is useful not only for assessing individual products but also for comparing ingredients of similar products and of different brands of the same product (see *Teaching your patient to read food labels,* page 32).

Show your patient several labels of healthful and less healthful foods. Point out that many imported foods lack nutritional information.

Ingredients on food labels are listed in descending order by weight. Determining total sugar content may take some analysis, however, because different forms can be listed separately. Give your patient a list of sugar's many names, including sorghum, sucrose, lactose, and maple syrup. Explain that foods labeled dietetic aren't

HEALTH PROMOTION

Teaching your patient to read food labels

Food facts on labels provide important nutritional information for patients with diabetes. The information makes it easier than ever to choose foods to help control blood glucose and lipid levels. Show your patient how to read labels properly—and how to avoid being fooled by them. This label for a frozen dinner shows what patients should look for.

1. Check the serving size. Note that a ½ cup serving is much less than most adults eat.
2. Check the calories from fat and don't be fooled by the percentage of fat. That number is a percentage of the total daily requirements for fat. The percentage of fat in the particular food can be much higher. To find this percentage, divide the calories from fat (279) by the total calories (320). Using this simple math, you'd find that this food is 87% fat. Remember, the American Heart Association recommends foods with less than 30% fat content.
3. Check the amount of cholesterol. Remember that cholesterol should be limited to less than 300 mg a day.
4. Check the sodium content. The 800 mg here is more than 30% of the daily allowance.
5. Check the chart. Teach your patients to compare the recommended daily amounts on this chart with the amounts in the particular food listed above. Emphasize that the amounts listed here are for the entire day.

Nutrition Facts

Serving Size 1/2 cup (110 g)   ❶
Servings Per Container 2.5

Amount Per Serving

Calories 320	Calories from Fat 279 ❷

	% Daily Value*
Total Fat 31 g	48%
Saturated Fat 17 g	85%
Cholesterol 320 mg	❸
Sodium 800 mg	31% ❹
Total Carbohydrate 82 g	33%
Dietary Fiber 2 g	8%
Sugars 5 g	
Protein 7 g	
Vitamin A 8% •	Vitamin C 32%
Calcium 4% •	Iron 10%

*Percentage Daily Values are based on a 2,000 calorie diet. Your daily values may be higher or lower depending on your calorie needs:

Calories:		2,000	2,500
Total Fat	Less than	65 g	80 g
Sat. Fat	Less than	20 g	25 g
Cholesterol	Less than	300 mg	300 mg
Sodium	Less than	2,400 mg	2,400 mg
Total Carbohydrate		300 g	375 g
Dietary Fiber		25 g	30 g

❺

Calories per gram:
Fat 9   •   Carbohydrate 4   •   Protein 4

necessarily sugar-free and that *natural* doesn't mean *sugar-free*. Cane sugar, for example, is natural. Dietetic foods are usually more expensive, and they're unnecessary for patients who make an effort to choose foods intelligently.

Food labels also list the number of calories, total fat content, and amount of saturated fat per serving. The difference between total fat and saturated fat is the portion that consists of polyunsaturated or monounsaturated fats. The polyunsatu-

rated and monounsaturated fat content should be greater than the saturated fat content. Also listed are levels of cholesterol, sodium, total carbohydrate, fiber, sugar, and protein.

A food label promising no cholesterol can be misleading. Vegetable oils containing no cholesterol, for example, may be high in saturated fats. Also, teach your patient to scrutinize labels claiming that a food is a certain percentage fat free. A product that is 75% fat free contains 25% fat by weight—and even more than 25% of the total calories may come from fat. The total calories from fat, listed next to the total calories on the label, will give your patient a clearer picture of fat content. Teach her to carefully read labels boasting *fewer calories, light,* or *lite.*

Besides ingredients, food labels now list details of nutritional content. This information makes it easier for your patient to choose foods in accordance with her treatment goals.

The information on the food label is based on the serving size, which appears at the top of the food label. Make sure your patient understands that the nutritional content of the entire package isn't being described unless the label states that the container has only one serving. The percent of daily value listed on the label is based on a 2,000-calorie diet; teach patients with a different calorie plan to take this into consideration.

Your patient's nutritional plan

Any rigid plan for managing diabetes is now considered both inadequate and unrealistic. Today, instead of requiring that a patient change her lifestyle to accommodate the plan, a nutritional specialist will adapt a plan to the patient's physiologic needs and lifestyle.

Your patient should learn self-management techniques from a registered dietitian, preferably one who is also a certified diabetes educator. A registered dietitian possesses the tools and techniques for teaching nutritional self-management and counseling patients about making dietary changes. Your role is to reinforce what the dietitian teaches your patient.

The first step in creating a nutritional plan is to assess your patient's needs, compiling the following information:
- height, weight, blood pressure, blood glucose levels, lipid profiles, and glycosylated hemoglobin levels
- diet history, focusing on your patient's current nutritional intake and habits, likes and dislikes, and cultural or ethnic influences
- social history, including lifestyle, daily schedule, finances, and activity level
- current diet, including calories, nutrient distribution, and types of carbohydrate, protein, and fat ingested.

The next step is mutual goal setting, which directly involves your patient in her own care. Nutritional goals are created in light of your patient's preferences and concerns.

Once goals have been set, the patient implements the nutritional plan. For a person with Type 1 diabetes, the plan should stress consistency in daily food intake, maintenance of desirable body weight, and integration of insulin therapy with the type and amount of food eaten. Matching insulin doses with the type and amount of food requires the patient to eat her meals at the same time every day; eat the appropriate amounts of fat, carbohydrates, and protein; and consume the appropriate number of calories.

Your patient should monitor her blood glucose levels before meals. She should also check her blood glucose levels after meals to evaluate the patterns that emerge after she eats certain foods. She can then adjust her insulin when her routine changes—for instance, when she eats out, eats more or less food than usual, exercises, or is sick.

If your patient has Type 2 diabetes, the nutritional plan focuses on the types of foods she eats, the timing of meals, the distribution of calories among a day's meals and snacks, and the number of calories ingested. When the dietitian plans the composition of a patient's meals, she will also consider the patient's medication regimen.

If your patient needs to lose weight, a dietitian will set realistic goals. As your patient loses weight, her carbohydrate tolerance will improve. If hypercholesterolemia, hypertriglyceridemia, and poor glucose control persist, the dietitian will have to reevaluate your patient's calorie intake and make necessary adjustments in her cholesterol, fat, and carbohydrate intake. You'll be in an excellent position to observe the course of treatment and to inform the dietitian when changes are necessary.

Cultural and ethnic considerations
Each patient's cultural and ethnic background strongly influences her food customs, eating rituals, food preparation, and body image. Religion also can affect dietary habits. For example, Hindus are vegetarians, and Orthodox Jews follow kosher dietary laws.

Family traditions may dictate mealtime habits and foods to be eaten or avoided. A patient's finances, social status, and geographic region af-

HEALTH PROMOTION

Teaching your patient sick-day rules

When your patient is ill, she needs to follow sick-day rules to prevent serious complications, such as diabetic ketoacidosis and hyperglycemic hyperosmolar nonketotic syndrome. Make sure your patient knows the rules and understands their importance:

- She should continue to take her usual dose of insulin or oral antidiabetic drug.
- She should monitor her blood glucose level every 2 to 4 hours.
- If she has Type 1 diabetes and her blood glucose level is over 240 mg/dl, she should check her urine for ketones.
- If her blood glucose level is over 250 mg/dl for two or more readings, if she has large amounts of ketones in her urine, or if she has a fever and is vomiting, she should call her physician.
- She should drink at least 8 ounces of calorie-free fluid—water, diet soda, or tea—every hour.
- If she has been vomiting, she should drink clear fluids. When her blood glucose level ranges from 250 to 300 mg/dl, she should drink calorie-free fluids. When her blood glucose is between 180 and 250 mg/dl before a meal, she should substitute easily tolerated foods and beverages that contain the amount of carbohydrate she usually eats.
- If she's unable to follow her normal meal plan, she should eat these easily tolerated foods. Each serving provides 15 grams of carbohydrates.
  ½ cup of unsweetened apple juice
  1 cup of low-fat beef broth
  ½ to ¾ cup of caffeine-free regular soda
  1 cup of Gatorade
  ½ cup of Cream of Wheat
  1 slice of dry toast
  3 squares of Graham crackers
  6 squares of Saltines

fect the type and availability of foods she eats, as well. The health care team performs a thorough nutritional assessment of cultural and ethnic practices and incorporates them into a personalized nutritional plan.

Adaptations for elderly patients

A dietitian adapts a nutritional plan for an elderly patient with diabetes based on her special needs caused by aging. For instance, the poor vision that typically accompanies old age can affect a patient's nutritional status by making it hard for her to read food labels or blood glucose meter results. Also, decreased mobility commonly affects a person's ability to buy and prepare food. And declining mental status may make it difficult for your patient to plan and prepare meals or even remember to eat (or whether she has eaten).

Many older people have limited finances, so they may not purchase a wide variety of fresh foods. They often eat irregularly, skipping meals or eating on a random schedule. A declining sense of taste and poor dentition affect nutrition by making mealtimes seem less pleasurable and more trouble than they're worth. Other elderly people may have a chronic disease, such as kidney or cardiac disease, that increases the challenge of developing a nutritional plan.

Many elderly people take several drugs at the same time, increasing the risk of food-drug and drug-drug interactions, which may affect appetite, taste, and the ability to digest, absorb, metabolize, and excrete nutrients.

Meals delivered to a patient's home may improve mealtime regularity and food variety. But as with meals served in long-term care facilities, home-delivered meals may limit the patient's control over food choices and meal timing. A meal plan that concentrates on eating meals at the same time every day and eating foods that provide good nutrition may be the best way to overcome the obstacles faced by elderly patients.

Sick days

Illness may cause your patient to alter her nutritional, exercise, and medication plans. When she's well, plan and discuss with her and her family how to manage sick days. The goal of a sick-day plan is to prevent serious complications, such as diabetic ketoacidosis (DKA) and hyperglycemic hyperosmolar nonketotic (HHNK) syndrome, from developing and to prevent hospitalization (see *Teaching your patient sick-day rules*).

Exercise

Along with a diet plan and a medication regimen, a patient with diabetes needs an exercise program. Exercise can help her control her blood glucose levels, improve her body's use of insulin and glucose, and control her weight. Your patient with diabetes has much to gain from regular exercise, but inform her of the risks as well. Giving her proper instruction and follow-up can help make exercise more effective and enjoyable.

Physiologic effects of exercise

For the first 5 to 10 minutes of exercise, the main fuel used by a person without diabetes is stored muscle glycogen. But it can be used only to meet the energy needs of the muscle in which it's contained. With prolonged exercise, the body uses glycogen from the liver, fat in the form of triglycerides, and nonesterified fatty acids (NEFA).

As a person continues to exercise, muscle glycogen stores are depleted. Muscle glycogen depletion stimulates liver gluconeogenesis, which begins the replacement of glycogen stores. This happens in two stages. First, immediately after exercise, cell permeability to glucose increases, and muscle glycogen stores are restored rapidly with no need for insulin. In the second stage, muscle glycogen returns to near-normal levels, glucose uptake decreases, and insulin action increases.

In a person who has diabetes, the body's use of muscle glycogen, triglycerides, liver glycogen, and NEFA differs. During short-term exercise, the rate of gluconeogenesis rises to two to three times above her baseline. Her liver's response to brief exercise resembles the response to prolonged exercise in people without diabetes.

In people without diabetes and in those with diabetes who have mildly elevated blood glucose levels, an initial drop in NEFA concentration is followed by a gradual increase as exercise continues. In patients with diabetes who have severe hyperglycemia and ketosis, levels of NEFA are elevated, even at rest. For them, the increase in NEFA during exercise is even greater.

Normally, ketones aren't a major source of fuel for the muscles. The body of a patient with diabetes who has mild ketosis, however, uses ketones for fuel during exercise.

A minimum amount of insulin is needed for glucose uptake by muscles and for the regulation of gluconeogenesis by the liver. An insulin deficiency triggers the abnormal secretion of counterregulatory hormones, which raise blood glucose levels. If exercise fails to lower high blood glucose levels, hyperglycemia results.

In patients with Type 1 diabetes, hypoglycemia rarely occurs during exercise but can occur up to a day later. Possible causes for late-onset hypoglycemia include glycogen depletion in the liver or muscles from intense or prolonged exercise, increases in insulin sensitivity, the use of glucose to replenish glycogen stores, counterregulatory response defect, and inappropriate adjustments of food intake or insulin therapy.

Benefits
Exercise increases the insulin sensitivity of patients with diabetes, reducing their insulin needs. Exercise also improves glucose tolerance. After exercise, blood glucose levels drop. An overall improvement in glucose metabolism may continue for days after an exercise session.

Many of the long-term benefits of exercise for patients with diabetes are the same as for anyone else. These benefits include improved fitness and sense of well-being, better body composition and weight control, and improved physical strength.

Exercise also helps reduce the risk of developing atherosclerosis. In patients with Type 2 diabetes, a regular exercise program lowers the levels of triglycerides and VLDLs. However, HDL levels don't change, possibly because the level of exercise required to raise HDL cholesterol levels is greater than is recommended for patients with diabetes. A combination of exercise and nutritional therapy may reduce blood pressure in people who have Type 2 diabetes with hypertension. This combination may even prevent or delay the development of Type 2 diabetes in those at risk for the disease.

Risks
Before beginning an exercise program, your patient should undergo a thorough physical examination that includes an exercise stress test and a review of her blood glucose control.

Teach your patient how to ensure safe exercise. First, she must bring her blood glucose levels under control. Before each exercise session, she should eat a snack if her blood glucose levels are less than 100 mg/dl. She shouldn't exercise if her fasting blood glucose levels are greater than 250 mg/dl and ketones are present in her urine or if blood glucose levels are greater than 300 mg/dl, whether ketones are present or not.

Teach your patient to coordinate meals and exercise. She should consume 15 grams of carbohydrate for each hour of moderate exercise. A good time to exercise is 1 to 2 hours after a meal. Late-afternoon exercise causes a greater drop in blood glucose levels than exercising before or after breakfast.

Your patient should avoid exercising during peak action times of insulin. She also should avoid injecting insulin into a muscle that will be exercised, because of the risk of hypoglycemia. Patients who have Type 2 diabetes and are taking a sulfonylurea are at risk for developing hypoglycemia during or after exercise. In patients who regulate blood glucose levels by diet alone, mild or moderate exercise is unlikely to induce hypoglycemia.

Your patient's exercise program

The physician will make exercise choices for your patient based on her type of diabetes, diabetic complications, other medical problems, and her exercise preferences.

All exercise plans should spell out the types of exercise to be performed as well as their intensity, duration, and frequency. Exercise should be regular and rhythmic and should use the large muscle groups. Good examples include walking, bicycling, and swimming—isometric exercises that place a safe, steady workload on the heart. Your patient shouldn't use isotonic exercises such as weight lifting because they make the heart rate and blood pressure rise rapidly.

Your patient should begin her exercise program with a warm-up of at least 5 minutes, gradually increasing her heart rate. She should then move on to 5 to 7 minutes of stretching to further increase her heart rate. Stretching also improves the flexibility of muscles that may be impaired by glycated muscle collagen.

Next comes the training period, which consists of 20 to 30 minutes of aerobic activity within your patient's target heart rate. A person who hasn't exercised in some time or who has never exercised may have to start with sessions of 5 to 10 minutes and gradually increase them to 30 minutes.

After aerobic activity, your patient should spend 10 to 15 minutes cooling down. The intensity of exercise is gradually decreased to allow her heart rate and blood pressure to slowly return to baseline. During the cooldown your patient should perform muscle-strengthening exercises for 5 to 10 minutes followed by stretching and relaxation for about 5 minutes.

Glucose tolerance declines after 24 hours without exercise, so your patient should exercise at least 3 days a week. Achieving continuous, improved glucose control requires even more frequent exercise. If your patient is trying to lose weight, she may have to exercise 5 or 6 days a week.

Exercise intensity

The target heart rate, which is 70% to 85% of your patient's maximum heart rate, determines the intensity of exercise. A physician may order an exercise stress test to determine your patient's target heart rate. Some patients with diabetes have silent ischemia. Their maximum heart rates may be 15% to 20% lower than those of people without diabetes.

Another method used to establish the intensity of exercise is the patient's rating of perceived exertion. Using a scale of 0 (no exertion) to 10 (extreme exertion), she rates how hard she is working. If your patient's perceived exertion is 3, instruct her to increase her exertion gradually until her rating reaches 5 (moderate exertion).

Show your patient how to take a pulse so that she can monitor her heart rate during exercise. Advise her that exercise shouldn't cause shortness of breath. Explain other signs and symptoms that indicate a need to stop exercise, including light-headedness and fatigue. Review the signs and symptoms of hypoglycemia and hyperglycemia. Demonstrate how to use feelings of exertion, such as fatigue, to monitor exercise intensity. This is particularly useful for patients with autonomic neuropathy, whose heart rates may not accurately reflect the intensity of exercise.

Instruct your patient to carry medical identification and a readily available source of carbohydrate whenever she exercises.

Blood glucose levels

Instruct your patient with diabetes to monitor her blood glucose levels before and after exercise. When she exercises for more than an hour, she should stop after 1 hour to check her blood glucose levels again before resuming exercise.

Your patient should continue to monitor her blood glucose levels throughout the day because hypoglycemia can occur many hours after exercise. In patients who are controlling Type 2 diabetes with diet alone, however, low to moderate exercise is unlikely to provoke hypoglycemia.

Point out that blood glucose response differs throughout the day. Suggest that your patient keep a log to help integrate meals, insulin therapy, and exercise times into the best daily pattern.

Special considerations

Many people with diabetes aren't physically fit, lead sedentary lives, and have microvascular, macrovascular, or neuropathic complications. However, they can still benefit from exercise that's modified for their needs.

If your patient has peripheral vascular disease, an assessment of arterial circulation is essential. Her exercise regimen may be modified to include interval training, such as walking with frequent rest periods. If your patient has only limited use of her legs because of claudication, chair or upper body exercise is a good alternative.

Your patient with retinopathy should avoid isotonic exercises, which provoke straining and cause blood pressure to rise rapidly, either of which can precipitate a hemorrhage of the vitreous humor. For this patient, aerobic exercises shouldn't jar her head or require a head-down position.

Patients with nephropathy and those receiving hemodialysis tend to have low hemoglobin levels and hematocrit and impaired cardiac function. All these conditions contribute to an extremely low capacity for exercise. These patients should begin exercising slowly for short periods and increase gradually. In patients with renal osteodystrophy, weight-bearing exercise may improve bone density.

Although exercise can't reverse sensorimotor neuropathy, it can improve the effects of disuse. Because patients with sensorimotor neuropathy have decreased sensation, they should perform stretching exercises gently and avoid high-impact exercises. Instead, they should use low-impact exercises such as walking, bicycling, and swimming. Range-of-motion exercises can prevent or minimize joint contractures. Because of her decreased sensation, instruct your patient to inspect her feet daily for blisters, redness, fissures, and ulcerations.

Patients with autonomic neuropathy and those taking beta-blockers may have an impaired counterregulatory response that fixes the heart rate at 80 to 90 beats per minute even when they're exercising. The result is limited exercise tolerance. Explain to your patient that sudden death or a silent myocardial infarction can occur when her heart fails to respond to nerve impulses. If your patient with autonomic neuropathy doesn't have a fixed heart rate, her target heart rate should start low and then gradually increase over several exercise sessions. Advise her to avoid sudden changes in body position and significant changes in heart rate and blood pressure.

Medications

All patients with Type 1 diabetes, and some patients with Type 2 diabetes, need to take medication to control their disease. Type 1 diabetes can be treated with insulin injections; most Type 2 diabetes can be treated with oral antidiabetic drugs. Some patients with Type 2 diabetes require two or three oral antidiabetic drugs or a combination of oral antidiabetic drugs and insulin. During periods of physiologic stress—such as fever, trauma, infection, or surgery—patients with Type 2 diabetes may need temporary insulin therapy. To reverse the effects of a hypoglycemic episode, a patient with either type of diabetes may take glucagon.

Explain to your patient that medication alone can't control diabetes. Instruct her to follow a regular schedule for meals, exercise, and medication. Teach your patient and her family to recognize the signs and symptoms of hypoglycemia and hyperglycemia. Also, teach them how to manage hyperglycemic and hypoglycemic episodes and when to contact a physician. Stress the importance of monitoring blood glucose levels at home and teach your patient proper self-monitoring technique. Also explain that she should have periodic laboratory tests for glycosylated hemoglobin, kidney and liver function, and hematologic profiles.

Advise your patient to contact her physician before taking any over-the-counter drugs. She should also contact her physician before discontinuing her diabetes medication or altering its dosage. Tell your patient to always carry medical identification and a source of glucose for emergencies.

Insulin therapy

All patients with Type 1 diabetes must use insulin. Because the insulin dose is determined by blood glucose levels, you and your patient must monitor those levels with particular care.

People with Type 2 diabetes produce some insulin, but generally not enough to lower their blood glucose levels. If other treatments can't control their blood glucose levels, they may also require insulin. Some patients with Type 2 diabetes may require insulin only temporarily during times of stress.

All insulins are administered subcutaneously. Regular insulin may be administered I.V. Because of its protein nature, insulin must be administered by injection. Given orally, it would be digested and destroyed in the GI tract.

Insulin restores the cells' ability to use glucose as a source of energy, but researchers don't know exactly how. Insulin is involved in cell membrane transport, so it increases cell growth and the metabolism of carbohydrates, proteins, and fats.

Insulin maintains blood glucose levels through several mechanisms. In the liver, insulin decreases the breakdown of glycogen, prevents the formation of new sources of glucose from amino acids, and prevents the formation of ketone bodies. At the same time, insulin increases the synthesis and storage of glycogen and fatty acids and decreases the breakdown of fat in adipose tissue. Insulin also enhances the use of amino acids and decreases the breakdown of protein in muscle tissue.

Types of insulin

Insulin is classified as rapid-acting, intermediate-acting, or long-acting, depending on its onset, peak, and duration of activity (see *Insulin preparations: Onset, peak, and duration*).

Most rapid-acting insulins begin working in 30 minutes and reach their peak in 2 to 5 hours. Their duration of action is 6 to 8 hours. One form of rapid-acting insulin, lispro, begins working in 5 to 15 minutes and reaches its peak in 30 to 90 minutes. Its duration of action is 2 to 4 hours. Rapid-acting insulins compensate for the meals eaten after injection. For some patients, using lispro before a meal improves postprandial glycemic control and reduces the risk of hypoglycemia because of its short duration of action. Other rapid-acting insulins include regular and Semilente insulin.

Intermediate-acting insulin starts working in 1 to 3 hours and reaches its peak in 4 to 15 hours. Its duration of action is 18 to 24 hours. It may be given in split doses, before meals, but the patient must eat at the time of peak action to prevent hypoglycemia. Intermediate-acting insulins include neutral protamine Hagedorn (NPH) and Lente insulins. NPH insulin contains protamine sulfate, a protein derived from fish that can cause an allergic reaction. Lente insulin is a good choice for people sensitive to protamine.

Long-acting insulin starts to work in 4 to 6 hours and reaches its peak in 8 to 20 hours. Its duration of action is 24 to 28 hours. Ultralente, the only long-acting insulin, gives patients a consistent insulin effect.

Some patients need a mixture of insulins: One that's rapid-acting, such as regular insulin, for a fast onset and one that's intermediate-acting, such as NPH, for a longer duration of action. These insulin mixtures are available in premixed bottles. For example, NPH and regular insulin are available in 70/30 and 50/50 mixtures. The premixed bottles are especially useful for elderly patients or patients with vision loss.

Sources of insulin

Extracts of beef and pork pancreas were once the only sources of insulin. Beef insulin is no longer used, except in some beef and pork mixtures, and pork insulin is rarely used. Today, human insulin, which is derived from recombinant deoxyribonucleic acid technology, and the human analog lispro are the two forms most commonly used. Insulin from all sources appears to be equally effective at controlling blood glucose levels. However, human insulin causes less lipoatrophy, less antibody production, and fewer allergic reactions. And it's absorbed faster than pork insulins.

Changing between pork and human sources of insulin can disrupt blood glucose levels and require dosage adjustments. People who need insulin only temporarily—a patient with Type 2 diabetes undergoing surgery, for example—should use human insulin.

Indications and contraindications

Insulin is essential for everyone with Type 1 diabetes. Type 2 patients may need it if diet, exercise, weight control, and oral antidiabetic drugs haven't been effective. They may also need it during periods of stress involving fever, severe trauma, infection, major surgery, DKA, and HHNK syndrome. Insulin therapy is recommended for women with gestational diabetes if diet alone doesn't control blood glucose levels.

Insulin preparations: Onset, peak, and duration

Use this table to review the onset, peak, and duration of various insulin preparations. Remember, however, that the injection site and exercise can cause these times to vary.

Preparation and manufacturer	Species	Onset	Peak (hr)	Duration (hr)
Rapid-acting insulin				
Lispro (Lilly)	human	5–15 min	0.5–1.5	2–4
Humulin R (Lilly)	human	30 min	2–4	6–8
Regular Iletin I (Lilly)	beef and pork mix	30 min	2–4	6–8
Regular Iletin II (Lilly)	pork	30 min	2–4	6–8
Novolin R (Novo Nordisk)	human	30 min	2.5–5	8
Purified Pork Regular (Novo Nordisk)	pork	30 min	2.5–5	8
Velosulin BR Human (Novo Nordisk)	human	30 min	1–3	8
Intermediate-acting insulin				
Humulin N (Lilly)	human	1–2 hr	6–12	18–24
NPH Iletin I (Lilly)	beef and pork mix	1–2 hr	6–12	18–24
NPH Iletin II (Lilly)	pork	1–2 hr	6–12	18–24
Novolin N Human (Novo Nordisk)	human	1.5 hr	4–12	24
Purified Pork NPH Isophane (Novo Nordisk)	pork	1.5 hr	4–12	24
Humulin L (Lilly)	human	1–3 hr	6–12	18–24
Lente Iletin I (Lilly)	beef and pork mix	1–3 hr	6–12	18–24
Lente Iletin II (Lilly)	pork	1–3 hr	6–12	18–24
Novolin L Human (Novo Nordisk)	human	2.5 hr	7–15	22
Purified Pork Lente (Novo Nordisk)	pork	2.5 hr	7–15	22
Long-acting insulin				
Humulin U (Lilly)	human	4–6 hr	8–20	24–28
Combinations				
Humulin 70/30 (Lilly)	human	30 min	2–12	18–24
Humulin 50/50 (Lilly)	human	30 min	2–12	18–24
Novolin 70/30 Human (Novo Nordisk)	human	30 min	2–12	24

RESEARCH UPDATE

Should patients wipe the injection site with alcohol?

Traditionally, patients with diabetes have been taught to wipe the insulin bottle and their injection site with alcohol before injecting insulin. But these steps may not be necessary.

Several Florida nurses noticed that plenty of patients failed to wipe the injection site, yet subsequent inflammation and infection were rare. These nurses then enlisted 50 outpatients with diabetes for a study, and the patients were divided into three groups.

- One group wiped the bottle and the site with an alcohol swab 5 seconds before injections.
- One group wiped the bottle and the site with tap water on a cotton ball before injections.
- One group didn't wipe the bottle or the site before injections.

Each group performed 36 injections. All patients used the abdomen as an injection site. Before and after the injections, physicians examined the site for erythema, tenderness, and edema.

No patient experienced an infection or any other complications at the injection site. Those who wiped the sites with tap water or didn't wipe the sites at all reported that the injection didn't sting.

Adverse effects and interactions

Hypoglycemia is the most common adverse effect of insulin therapy. Other adverse effects include lipodystrophy, insulin resistance, and, in rare cases, insulin allergy.

The two types of lipodystrophy are lipoatrophy and lipohypertrophy. Lipoatrophy, which is caused by animal insulins, results from the breakdown of adipose tissue at the injection site or in areas away from the injection site and causes a loss of fatty tissue. Dimpling may result from an injection with an impure insulin preparation or may be an immune response. Treatment includes injecting human insulin or steroids around the area of breakdown.

Lipohypertrophy occurs after repeated injections into the same site. The skin in the hypertrophied area eventually loses sensation. Because the hypertrophied area is an accumulation of fatty tissue, tell your patient not to use it for additional injections because the insulin will be absorbed erratically.

Insulin resistance results from the formation of antibodies that bind to insulin, making it inactive. Patients with cirrhosis of the liver or a disease of the endocrine glands may also develop insulin resistance. The patient becomes unresponsive to usual doses and may need as much as several hundred units of insulin a day. Changing from animal to human insulin or purified pork insulin may correct the problem. Or a corticosteroid may treat it. For obese patients who have nonimmunologic insulin resistance, the treatment is weight loss.

A patient with an insulin allergy may develop redness, swelling, aching, and pruritus at the injection site 4 to 8 hours after the injection. Or she may develop systemic allergic reactions.

Insulin products derived from animal sources cause allergies in some patients. The physician will probably substitute human insulin.

Some people are allergic to the insulin preparations or to the preservatives in the solution. Other people may be hypersensitive to the skin-cleansing agent used before injection (see *Should patients wipe the injection site with alcohol?*). Some patients are allergic to the latex in the stopper of the vial or in the plunger of the syringe. If any allergic reactions occur, your patient should contact her physician immediately.

Systemic allergic reactions to insulin are uncommon, especially with purified insulin preparations. If an anaphylactic reaction occurs, however, it may be life threatening. The signs and symptoms include rash, shortness of breath, tachycardia, hypotension, diaphoresis, angioedema, and anaphylaxis. Patients with severe systemic reactions should have a skin test before they begin using a new insulin preparation.

Several drugs can increase or decrease the action of insulin (see *Drug interactions with insulin*). No foods interact with insulin. However, to achieve optimal glycemic control, patients should follow their prescribed meal plan in conjunction with their insulin prescription.

Administration

The dosage and number of daily insulin injections depend on each patient's circumstances. Many patients are on an insulin regimen that requires different kinds or mixes of insulin. The physician considers the time of insulin administration, diet, and exercise when determining dosages. After initial insulin dosages have been determined, monitor the effects of the insulin.

Your patient will inject insulin subcutaneously with a short (½ inch), small-bore (27, 28, or 29 gauge) needle (see *Sites for subcutaneous insulin injections,* page 42).

The rate of absorption of insulins other than lispro varies with the injection site. Insulin is absorbed from the abdomen faster than from any other site. The upper arm provides the next most rapid absorption, followed by the thigh and buttock. Instruct your patient not to administer insulin within a 2-inch radius of the umbilicus to prevent injection into a blood vessel. Because the rate of absorption of insulin changes with the injection site, patients should rotate injection sites within one area, such as the abdomen, before moving to another, such as the upper arm.

Body temperature also affects absorption. Increased blood flow from sitting in a sauna, having a fever, or exercising a muscle causes insulin to be absorbed more quickly than usual.

Storage: Tell your patient that she can keep unopened bottles of insulin in the refrigerator for up to 3 months. She shouldn't freeze the insulin because freezing can cause clumping. A bottle in current use can be stored at room temperature, out of direct sunlight and extreme heat, for up to 1 month. Prefilled syringes may be stored in the refrigerator vertically (needle up) for 1 to 2 weeks. Instruct her to check the expiration date on the insulin bottle periodically and to discard the insulin when it expires.

Injection: When teaching your patient how to inject insulin, first instruct her to roll the bottle of insulin suspension gently between her hands so that the contents don't form bubbles or foam. If a bottle of insulin contains granules or clumps after mixing, instruct her to discard the bottle. Because regular insulin is clear, the bottle doesn't have to be rolled before use. Instruct your patient to discard the bottle of regular insulin if it's discolored or cloudy or contains granular material.

Next, instruct your patient to stretch the skin at the injection site and insert the needle at a 90-degree angle (see *Teaching your patient to inject insulin*, page 43).

Several new alternatives to syringes simplify insulin injection. Spring-operated insulin pens,

Drug interactions with insulin

Drugs that increase the hypoglycemic effect	Drugs that decrease the hypoglycemic effect
• alcohol	• corticosteroids
• anabolic steroids	• dextrothyroxine
• beta-blockers	• dobutamine
• clofibrate	• epinephrine
• fenfluramine	• nicotine
• guanethidine	• nicotinic acid
• monoamine oxidase inhibitors	• pentamidine
• oral contraceptives	• phenytoin
• oral antidiabetic drugs	• thiazide diuretics
• pentamidine	• thyroid hormone preparations
• phenylbutazone	
• salicylates	
• sulfinpyrazone	
• tetracyclines	

which are preloaded with bottles of insulin, are convenient and accurate. The cartridges, which don't have to be refrigerated, supply enough insulin for 3 to 5 days. Using the pen, however, requires skill and dexterity. Patients with impaired vision can buy devices that facilitate drawing up and administering insulin with a syringe, including syringe magnifiers, needle guides, bottle stabilizers, and nonvisual insulin measurement systems.

Disposal: Advise your patient to dispose of needles and lancets in a hard plastic container, such as an empty detergent bottle, or a metal container with a tightly secured lid. If the patient uses coffee cans to dispose of needles, caution her to reinforce the plastic lid with several layers

Sites for subcutaneous insulin injections

Your patient can use any of the highlighted body areas to inject her insulin, but you should explain that the abdomen absorbs insulin faster than any other area. The upper arm provides the next most rapid absorption, followed by the thigh and buttock. Many patients choose the thigh over the arm or buttock, however, because it's easier to reach.

Explain that the patient doesn't have to alternate areas but that she should rotate sites within a particular area.

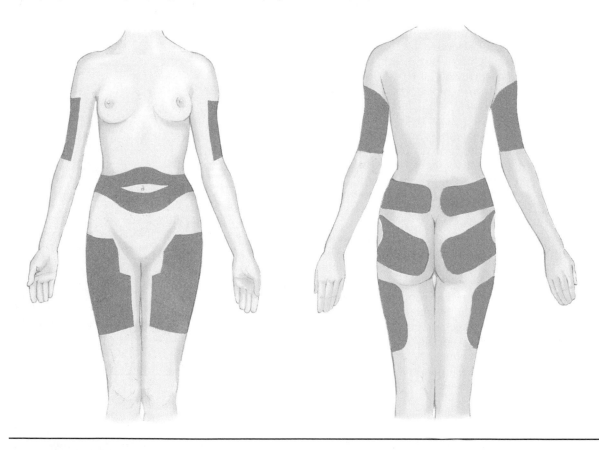

of duct tape. Some drugstores sell commercial containers like the ones used in hospitals.

Tell your patient to put needle containers in the regular trash—never with recyclables. If she lives in an area with a depot system for dropping off used syringes, encourage her to do that.

Insulin pumps: Instead of using subcutaneous injections, some patients can use insulin-pump therapy, a method of insulin administration that more closely mimics the normal function of the pancreas. To be a candidate for the insulin pump, a patient must have Type 1 diabetes, be able to monitor her own blood glucose levels, and be able to operate the pump. Patients using pump therapy also must be highly motivated; they'll have to monitor their blood glucose levels at least four times a day and keep careful records to help evaluate their therapy.

The battery-powered pump contains a syringe and a computer chip that stores information for insulin administration. To administer insulin, the patient attaches an infusion set with a small catheter to the pump. She then inserts the catheter

HOME CARE

Teaching your patient to inject insulin

When teaching your patient how to inject insulin, give her the following instructions:

1. Assemble all equipment. Then wash your hands with warm water and soap.
2. If you're using intermediate-acting or long-acting insulin, gently roll the bottle between your hands. Never shake the bottle. If you're using regular insulin, skip this step.
3. Clean the top of the bottle with alcohol. Let it dry so that you don't inadvertently introduce alcohol into the insulin.
4. Inject an amount of air into the bottle equal to the amount of insulin to be drawn up.
5. If you're mixing more than one type of insulin, draw up the regular insulin first. Be sure to draw up the proper amount of insulin. If you see air bubbles in the syringe, gently tap it with your finger and push lightly on the plunger, as shown.

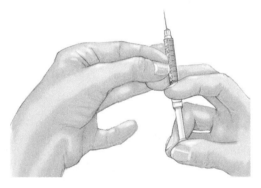

6. Clean the injection site with alcohol or warm water. If you use alcohol, let it dry before injecting the insulin.
7. Spread the skin at the injection site. Smoothly inject the needle at a 90-degree angle.

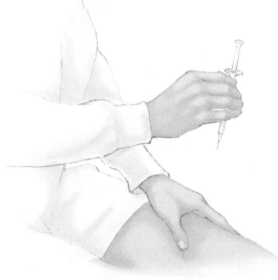

8. Withdraw the needle and immediately apply pressure to the injection site with a cotton ball or alcohol swab. Don't massage the area.
9. Discard the needle in a puncture-resistant container, such as a coffee can.

---

into her abdomen, arm, or thigh. She can wear the pump 24 hours a day but should change the injection site every 72 hours. She should also change the site when it becomes inflamed or painful, or whenever the system leaks or becomes clogged.

Using the pump provides several benefits. Because blood glucose levels can be more tightly controlled, glycosylated hemoglobin levels and the number of hyperglycemic episodes can be reduced. The pump may also help lower the number of congenital birth defects in children who are born to mothers with diabetes. Insulin-pump

therapy also may help delay the progression of microvascular and macrovascular complications and neuropathy.

Blood glucose monitoring

Explain to your patient the importance of monitoring her blood glucose levels at home. Ideally, she should monitor blood glucose four or more times a day—before all meals and before a bedtime snack. Teach her how to use her glucose monitoring equipment (see *Teaching your patient to use a blood glucose meter*, pages 44 and 45). Explain that

HOME CARE

Teaching your patient to use a blood glucose meter

Patients with diabetes face the daily challenge of keeping their blood glucose levels as close to normal as possible through a complex treatment regimen that demands many lifestyle changes. To monitor their blood glucose levels closely, patients need to use a blood glucose meter at least four times a day. Then based on the results, they can adjust their diet and medication dosages accordingly.

Use the following teaching guide to help your patient understand self-monitoring and to promote her comfort.

Preparing for the test

Most patients check their blood glucose levels at specific times during the day, usually before meals and before bedtime. Teach your patient to choose a clean, well-lit location to perform the test, for example, the kitchen table. Then explain that she'll need to assemble the following supplies:
• lancet or self-sticking device
• glucose meter
• test strip
• cotton ball
• pen and paper or logbook to record results.

Remind her to check that the batteries in the meter are fresh and that the test strips aren't outdated. Most meters require calibration on a regular basis. Tell your patient to follow the manufacturer's recommendations for calibration procedures.

Performing the test

1. Instruct your patient to wash her hands with warm soapy water. Doing so will not only help prevent infection but will also promote blood flow to the skin surface so that she can obtain an adequate drop of blood.

2. Tell your patient to turn on the blood glucose meter and insert the test strip before she sticks her finger for blood.

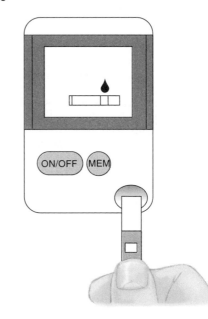

3. Explain that she should choose an injection site along the side or top of her fingertip. Tell her to avoid the center of the finger pad because she has more nerve endings there. Advise her that her fingers may be sore for the first few days and that she can either rotate the sites to help ease the discomfort or use the same site over and over again so that a callus forms, making subsequent fingersticks virtually painless.

4. As she sticks her finger, instruct her to firmly squeeze it with the thumb and forefinger of her other hand. This will help to express the blood and reduce sensation to the site.

errors in technique can lead to inaccurate results, which can in turn lead to poor treatment decisions. Reevaluate her technique regularly.

Encourage your patient to maintain a written log of blood glucose levels even if the meter on her machine stores information. She should also record her activity status and eating patterns. Instruct her to take her log to her regular physician appointments.

Your patient should monitor her urine for ketones when blood glucose levels are more than 250 mg/dl and when she feels unusually stressed. Tablets, strips, and tapes are available for urine ketone testing.

5. After she sticks her finger, instruct her to squeeze it until a full, hanging droplet of blood forms.

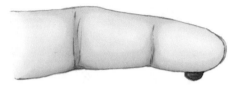

6. Then tell her to drop the blood directly onto the test strip. Caution her not to smear the blood onto the strip or to touch it with her finger. Explain that the natural oils on her skin can interfere with the test results.

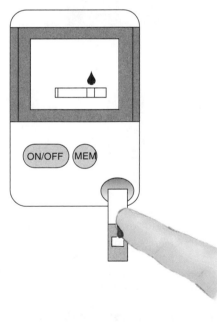

7. Instruct her to cover the target area on the test strip completely.

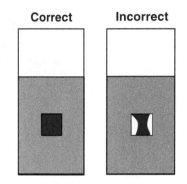

Correct   **Incorrect**

8. Now tell the patient to apply gentle pressure to the puncture site with a cotton ball to stop the bleeding.
9. Blood glucose readings appear on the meter's display window in 45 to 60 seconds. Show your patient how to record the results along with the date, time, and any other appropriate information.

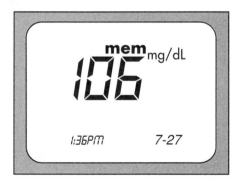

Oral antidiabetic drugs

For people with Type 2 diabetes, the first line of treatment is nutritional therapy coupled with exercise. If diet and exercise don't control blood glucose levels adequately, a physician may prescribe oral antidiabetic drugs. These drugs, which are effective only when the pancreas continues to secrete at least some insulin, aren't effective for patients with Type 1 diabetes.

Sulfonylureas, which have been used to treat Type 2 diabetes since the mid-1950s, enhance the action of insulin. Second-generation sulfonylureas were approved for use in the United States in

Sulfonylureas: Dosage and duration of action

Sulfonylureas are categorized as first-generation, second-generation, and third-generation. All three are effective in treating diabetes. But second-generation drugs are more potent that the first-generation drugs, and the one third-generation drug is more potent than the second-generation drugs.

Drug	Dosage	Duration of action (hr)
First-generation		
acetohexamide	• 0.25–1.5 g/day • single or divided dose	12–24
chlorpropamide	• 0.1–0.75 g/day • single dose	up to 60
tolazamide	• 0.1–0.75 g/day • single or divided dose	12–24
tolbutamide	• 0.5–3 g/day • divided dose	6–12
Second-generation		
glipizide	• 2.5–40 mg/day • divided dose if more than 15 mg/day	12–24
glyburide	• 1.25–20 mg/day	16–24
Third-generation		
glimepiride	• starting dose: 1–2 mg/day • maintenance dose: 1–4 mg/day	24

1984, and one third-generation sulfonylurea was introduced in 1995. Other oral antidiabetic drugs used to treat Type 2 diabetes include metformin and acarbose, which lower blood glucose levels without stimulating the secretion of insulin. The oral antidiabetic drug, troglitazone, promotes the body's sensitivity to insulin.

Sulfonylureas

Sulfonylurea drugs enhance the action of insulin by increasing the number of insulin receptors on the cell membranes and increasing insulin-binding sites on the cells.

Although all three generations of the drug are equally effective in treating diabetes, second-generation sulfonylureas (which include glipizide and glyburide) are 100 times more potent than first-generation sulfonylureas (which include acetohex-

amide and tolbutamide). Plus, they cause less toxicity and have fewer drug interactions. Glimepiride, the only third-generation sulfonylurea, is more potent than the second-generation drugs. It not only enhances the action of insulin but also stimulates the use of glucose in peripheral tissue (see *Sulfonylureas: Dosage and duration of action*).

Indications and contraindications

Oral sulfonylurea drugs are indicated for patients with uncomplicated Type 2 diabetes that can't be controlled with diet and exercise alone. These drugs can be used alone or with insulin or metformin.

Sulfonylureas are contraindicated for patients who are hypersensitive to sulfonamide preparations. Sulfonylureas aren't appropriate for patients who have Type 1 diabetes or ketoacidosis or patients who are in diabetic coma. Severe liver or kidney disease may limit the effectiveness of these drugs because they're metabolized by the liver and excreted by the kidneys.

During periods of psychologic or physiologic stress—including infection, fever, trauma, and surgery—a physician may replace sulfonylureas with insulin. The elderly and patients with thyroid disease or severe hypoglycemic reactions should take sulfonylurea drugs with particular caution because signs of hypoglycemia may be intensified.

Sulfonylureas are contraindicated for patients who are pregnant. A physician will substitute insulin throughout the pregnancy.

Adverse effects and interactions

Hypoglycemia is the most common adverse effect of sulfonylureas. The usual triggers are eating too little food and exercising too much. A drug overdose or drug interactions also may cause hypoglycemia. Elderly patients have increased sensitivity to sulfonylureas (except glimepiride), and hypoglycemia is hard to detect in them. Patients with liver or kidney disease are more prone to developing hypoglycemia because the drugs accumulate in the liver or kidneys.

If a sulfonylurea causes GI tract symptoms—including nausea, epigastric fullness, and heartburn—lowering the dose may ease them. Sulfonylureas may also cause transient allergic skin reactions such as pruritus, eczema, and urticaria. If such reactions persist, the patient must stop taking the drug. Your patient also may develop photosensitivity. If so, encourage her to use sunscreen and to wear protective clothing.

Hematologic reactions, such as agranulocytosis, hemolytic or aplastic anemia, leukopenia, and thrombocytopenia, may also occur. If your patient experiences a hematologic reaction, her physician may discontinue the drug and substitute insulin.

Sulfonylureas stimulate the release of antidiuretic hormone, resulting in water retention and hyponatremia. Patients with heart failure or cirrhosis of the liver are more prone to developing this reaction (see *Heart failure and sulfonylurea therapy*).

Sulfonylureas may be taken with food to prevent GI upset. However, food delays the absorption of glipizide, so advise your patient to take it 30 minutes before a meal. If a physician prescribes twice-a-day dosing for your patient, she

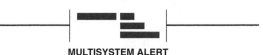

MULTISYSTEM ALERT

Heart failure and sulfonylurea therapy

When a person with diabetes and heart failure takes a sulfonylurea, her body may release antidiuretic hormone—and the resulting water retention and hyponatremia can spell danger.

If you're caring for such a patient, watch for signs and symptoms of the syndrome of inappropriate antidiuretic hormone: weight gain despite anorexia, nausea, and vomiting; muscle weakness; restlessness; and possibly seizures and coma.

If you note these signs and symptoms, begin emergency treatment as prescribed to increase sodium levels and prevent central nervous system injury and death. If the patient experiences hyponatremia associated with increased blood volume, a physician will prescribe normal or hypertonic saline solution and furosemide to induce the excretion of more dilute urine.

should take the first dose at breakfast and the second dose at dinner. Patients who have difficulty swallowing may crush tablets, with the exception of glipizide, and take them with food or fluids.

Many drugs can alter the action of sulfonylureas (see *Drug interactions with sulfonylureas,* page 48). For example, patients who are also taking digitalis glycosides may have increased serum digitalis levels.

Disulfiram-like reactions, especially facial flushing, occur when a person takes sulfonylureas with alcohol or any medication that contains alcohol, such as some cold remedies. Chronic alcohol use may reduce the drug's effectiveness.

Metformin

Metformin, classified as a biguanide, doesn't enhance insulin secretion, so it won't predispose the patient to hypoglycemia or cause the weight gain associated with other glucose-lowering drugs. Metformin lowers blood glucose levels and improves glucose tolerance by decreasing glucose production in the liver and increasing the mus-

Drug interactions with sulfonylureas

Drugs that increase the effects of sulfonylureas	Drugs that decrease the effects of sulfonylureas
• anticoagulants	• corticosteroids
• beta-blockers, including ophthalmic preparations	• diazoxide
• chloramphenicol	• hydantoins
• insulin	• phenothiazines
• magnesium salts	• rifampin
• methyldopa	• sympathomimetic drugs, such as epinephrine
• monoamine oxidase inhibitors	• diuretics
• nonsteroidal anti-inflammatory drugs	• thyroid hormone preparations
• probenecid	
• sulfonamide anti-infectives	
• tricyclic antidepressants	

cles' use of insulin. It also decreases intestinal absorption of glucose.

Metformin increases the binding of insulin to its cellular receptor sites and decreases the potential for insulin resistance. The drug enhances the uptake of glucose by the muscles and adipose tissue. During the day, especially after lunch, the drug lowers postprandial blood glucose levels. This phenomenon may be attributed to delayed glucose absorption or to the time required for metformin to be absorbed and accumulate in the tissues.

Taking the drug also reduces levels of serum triglycerides, total cholesterol, and LDL cholesterol, and increases levels of HDL cholesterol.

The initial dose of metformin is 500 mg twice a day, with morning and evening meals. A physician gradually increases the dose by 500 mg per week until the patient's fasting blood glucose and glycosylated hemoglobin levels are as close to normal as possible. The total recommended dosage is 2,500 mg per day in three doses. Metformin can be used alone or with sulfonylurea therapy.

Indications and contraindications

Patients with Type 2 diabetes whose disease can't be managed satisfactorily by diet and exercise alone take metformin to reduce hyperglycemia. If metformin and diet therapy are ineffective, a physician may add a sulfonylurea.

Before your patient begins metformin therapy, assess her kidney function and verify that her serum creatinine levels are below 1.5 mg/dl to prevent lactic acidosis. If they're above 1.5 mg/dl, her physician will substitute another drug. Instruct your patient to contact her physician immediately if she experiences difficulty breathing, muscle aches, fatigue, unusual sleepiness, or nonspecific symptoms, which may indicate lactic acidosis (see *When metformin therapy leads to lactic acidosis*).

Metformin is contraindicated for patients with kidney dysfunction, cardiopulmonary disease, infection, hypersensitivity to the drug, or ketosis. Patients undergoing radiologic tests such as excretory urography, angiography, and scans that use parenteral iodinated contrast media shouldn't receive metformin within 48 hours of the test. The contrast media can predispose a patient to acute kidney failure and an accumulation of metformin in the kidneys, which can lead to lactic acidosis.

A physician should stop metformin therapy before surgery if food and fluid intake is restricted. The patient shouldn't resume therapy until kidney function has returned to her baseline and she's eating meals.

Usually, insulin and metformin aren't used simultaneously. If a patient needs insulin, metformin should be discontinued.

Adverse effects and interactions

The most common adverse effects of metformin are GI signs and symptoms such as diarrhea, anorexia, nausea, bloating, and a metallic taste in the mouth. Tell your patient that she can prevent GI irritation by taking metformin with food, which also helps to delay rapid drug absorption. Patients who have difficulty swallowing may crush metformin and mix it with food or liquids. If diar-

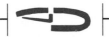

DANGEROUS COMPLICATIONS

When metformin therapy leads to lactic acidosis

Lactic acidosis, a rare metabolic complication that results from the accumulation of metformin, is a life-threatening medical emergency. Diabetes is one of several conditions that can lead to lactic acidosis. Renal insufficiency, cardiac or respiratory insufficiency, severe infection, liver disease, and acute alcohol abuse also may contribute to the accumulation of metformin in the kidneys.

Assessment
Initial symptoms of lactic acidosis may be insidious. A patient may experience malaise, muscle aches, nonspecific abdominal distress, respiratory difficulty, and progressive drowsiness. As the condition worsens, hypothermia, hypotension, and bradyarrhythmias may develop. Suspect lactic acidosis in any patient with metabolic acidosis and no evidence of ketoacidosis (ketonemia and ketonuria).

If a patient has lactic acidosis, laboratory findings will include blood lactate levels above 5 mmol/L, decreased blood pH, electrolyte imbalances with an increased anion gap, and an increased lactate-pyruvate ratio. If metformin is the cause of the lactic acidosis, blood levels of the drug will be greater than 5 mg/ml.

Immediate interventions
With prompt treatment, a patient's signs and symptoms can be reversed. Immediately discontinue metformin therapy and begin hemodialysis. Provide cardiovascular and respiratory support, as needed.

Monitor the patient's electrocardiogram, if indicated. Also, closely monitor her vital signs, fluid intake and output, and kidney function. Start an I.V. infusion to increase tissue perfusion. Then monitor the patient's electrolyte levels and replace electrolytes as necessary. Her condition is potentially critical until the acidosis is reversed and fluids and electrolytes return to normal.

---

rhea or vomiting is severe, your patient's physician may stop metformin therapy temporarily.

Patients who don't get enough vitamin B_{12} or calcium may develop asymptomatic vitamin B_{12} deficiency when taking metformin because the drug interferes with the absorption of the vitamin. Taking vitamin B_{12} supplements or discontinuing metformin therapy rapidly reverses the deficiency.

If your patient is taking a drug for a bacterial infection, angina, thyroid disease, coughing, asthma, a skin condition, or anxiety, it may alter the effects of her metformin therapy. For example, many calcium channel blockers and corticosteroids can decrease the effects of metformin and may seriously undermine blood glucose control (see *Drug interactions with metformin,* page 50).

Acarbose
Acarbose, an intestinal alpha-glucosidase inhibitor, decreases postprandial hyperglycemia by inhibiting the digestion and absorption of carbohydrates. It achieves this by inhibiting the enzymes responsible for the digestion of starches and other carbohydrates in the brush border of the small intestine.

The peak action of acarbose occurs within 1 hour of ingestion. The drug is metabolized by intestinal bacteria and digestive enzymes. Because the half-life for acarbose is only about 2 hours, the drug should be taken three times a day.

A physician will begin acarbose therapy at 25 mg three times a day. She will adjust dosages every 4 to 8 weeks based on 1-hour postprandial blood glucose levels and on tolerance until an effective dose is achieved. The maximum recommended dosage is 50 mg three times a day for patients who weigh 60 kg or less. For those who weigh more than 60 kg, the maximum dosage is 100 mg three times a day.

Indications and contraindications
Acarbose is used with stable Type 2 patients as an adjunct to diet and exercise to reduce blood

Drug interactions with metformin

If your patient is taking metformin, find out if she's also taking any drugs that can increase or decrease its effects. Many of the drugs that decrease metformin's effects may dangerously weaken or even eliminate glycemic control.

Drugs that increase the effects of metformin	Drugs that decrease the effects of metformin
• alcohol	• calcium channel blockers
• amiloride	• corticosteroids (drugs for ear and eye infections, inhalers, medicated skin creams)
• cimetidine	• estrogens
• digoxin	• isoniazid
• furosemide	• nicotinic acid
• iodinated contrast media	• phenothiazines
• morphine	• phenytoin
• nifedipine	• oral contraceptives
• procainamide	• sympathomimetic drugs (many cough and cold preparations)
• quinine	• thyroid hormone preparations
• triamterene	
• trimethoprim	
• vancomycin	

glucose levels. This drug benefits patients who can't achieve near-normal blood glucose levels with sulfonylureas or metformin.

Because acarbose increases gas formation in the intestine, it's contraindicated for anyone with inflammatory bowel disease, ulcerations of the colon, or intestinal obstruction. The drug is also contraindicated for patients with chronic intestinal diseases that alter digestion or absorption. Acarbose is contraindicated during pregnancy or breast-feeding. Patients with kidney dysfunction, DKA, or a hypersensitivity to the drug also shouldn't take it.

Adverse effects and interactions
The most common reactions to acarbose are GI signs and symptoms. Patients may complain of abdominal pain, diarrhea, and flatulence caused by undigested carbohydrates in the intestines. These signs and symptoms tend to subside with time. At doses of 100 mg, acarbose may cause an asymptomatic, reversible increase in serum transaminase levels, especially in women.

The action of acarbose decreases with the concurrent use of charcoal, an intestinal adsorbent, and digestive enzyme preparations that contain carbohydrate-splitting enzymes, such as amylase and pancreatin. Hyperglycemia may result if a patient takes acarbose with thiazide and other diuretic drugs, beta-blockers, corticosteroids, phenothiazines, thyroid preparations, estrogens, oral contraceptives, phenytoin, nicotinic acid, sympathomimetics, calcium channel blockers, or isoniazid. Acarbose can be taken with a sulfonylurea or insulin, but these combinations may cause hypoglycemia. However, acarbose can help to prevent weight gain associated with sulfonylurea therapy.

Advise your patients to take acarbose with meals. Because the goal is to prevent the absorption of intestinal glucose, they should take the drug along with the first bite of food. No food interactions occur.

Glucagon

Glucagon is a drug used to treat hypoglycemia and a polypeptide hormone produced and secreted by the alpha cells of the pancreas in response to hypoglycemia. The action of glucagon opposes the action of insulin. When released, glucagon helps to maintain blood levels of glucose by accelerating liver glycogenolysis and gluconeogenesis and reducing glycogen synthesis.

Glucagon can be administered subcutaneously, intramuscularly (I.M.), or I.V. The onset of action is rapid: 5 to 20 minutes subcutaneously, 8 to 10 minutes I.M., and 1 minute I.V.

However, glucagon isn't the first line of defense against hypoglycemia. At the first sign of hypoglycemia, your patient should eat 10 to 15 grams of carbohydrate. If this doesn't resolve the hypoglycemia or the patient can't take carbohydrates orally, teach the family to inject 0.5 to 1.0 mg of glucagon. Then they should monitor the patient's blood glucose levels. Explain that the patient may experience nausea after a glucagon injection. If the patient doesn't respond to the first dose in 20 minutes, a family member should administer another 0.5 to 1.0 mg of glucagon. Instruct the family to seek emergency treatment if the patient doesn't respond after two glucagon injections.

Instruct the patient and her family to keep a glucagon emergency kit handy. Review with them when and how to use it. Teach them to check the expiration date at least once a month and to replace the kit with a new one when it expires.

Indications and contraindications

Glucagon is used to treat severe hypoglycemia in patients with diabetes. People who are hypersensitive to glucagon shouldn't use it. Pregnant women and nursing mothers should use glucagon cautiously because its effects in them aren't known.

Adverse effects and interactions

Nausea and vomiting are common adverse effects of glucagon. Some patients experience generalized allergic reactions such as rash, urticaria, respiratory distress, or hypotension.

Patients who take oral anticoagulant drugs may be prone to bleeding because glucagon increases their hypoprothrombinemic effects. The interaction occurs several days after therapy begins and appears to be dose related. Monitor the patient's prothrombin time, and adjust her dose accordingly. No food interactions are known.

Pancreas and islet cell transplantation

Pancreas transplantation can improve the quality of life for your patient with Type 1 diabetes by eliminating the need for insulin therapy, decreasing daily blood glucose measurements, and eliminating many diet restrictions. Transplantation also eliminates hypoglycemia.

Pancreas transplantation is usually reserved for patients who will also receive a kidney transplant and immunosuppressive therapy. To be a candidate for pancreas and kidney transplantation, a patient must have a condition requiring kidney transplantation and must have significant complications with insulin therapy, such as frequent and severe hypoglycemia and insulin resistance. At some centers, surgeons transplant the pancreas alone to correct significant complications of diabetes in patients who don't also have kidney disease.

Transplantation of the whole pancreas is the only therapy that reliably achieves euglycemia. However, the procedure is undesirable for most patients with Type 1 diabetes because of the risks of rejection and infection and because it requires lifelong immunosuppressive therapy.

As an alternative, a surgeon may transplant insulin-producing islet cells in a patient who is taking immunosuppressive drugs after receiving a transplanted kidney. In islet cell transplantation, the surgeon injects islet cells from the pancreas of a cadaver into the patient's portal vein. The cells lodge in the liver and produce insulin, functioning as if they were in the pancreas. Before injection, the cells can be treated to destroy antigen-producing cells and reduce the risk of rejection.

Most patients continue to require insulin therapy after undergoing islet cell transplantation. For many, however, glucose control improves, and insulin requirements decrease. Some patients no longer need daily insulin injections.

Complications

Patients who have received both a pancreas and a kidney have had the best results. Acute rejection is more common, however, than in patients who receive a kidney alone. Surgical complications after pancreas-only transplantation are common, occur earlier, and lead to death in more cases.

The most common complications after pancreas transplantation include rejection, infection, venous thrombosis, technical problems with duct anastomosis, and diabetes recurrence. Simultaneous kidney and pancreas transplantation causes more wound complications and a higher incidence of cytomegalovirus infection during the perioperative period than transplantations of the pancreas alone, but simultaneous transplantation poses no other long-term risks.

Hyperglycemia is one indication of rejection, but it doesn't develop until 90% of the islet cell mass has become compromised, at which point rejection is usually irreversible. One benefit of simultaneous transplantation is that the condition of the transplanted kidney can help the physician predict the likelihood of pancreas rejection.

Up to 30% of transplant patients develop thrombosis of the vessels that supply the pancreas. Sites of surgical anastomosis can leak. After surgery, watch for hematuria related to the kidney vessels and irritation of the duodenal portion of the pancreas graft.

Infection from opportunistic organisms may occur as a complication of immunosuppressive therapy. Fever is a sign of both acute rejection and infection, so if your postoperative patient develops a fever, perform a thorough assessment. Unrecognized rejection can mean the loss of the transplanted organ. Unrecognized infection can lead to systemic inflammatory response syndrome and death.

Immunosuppressive drugs

Usually, transplant patients take immunosuppressive drugs to prevent the transplanted organ from being rejected over the long term or to treat incipient rejection. They may start to take these drugs before surgery and continue throughout the life of the organ. Methylprednisolone and azathioprine are usually administered I.V. during surgery. As kidney function improves, the patient takes cyclosporine. Maintenance immunosuppressive therapy usually combines prednisone, azathioprine, and cyclosporine. Patients receiving tacrolimus have less risk of organ rejection and new-onset Type 1 diabetes (see *Teaching your patient about immunosuppressive drugs*).

Nursing considerations

When caring for a patient after a kidney and pancreas transplant, repeatedly assess the function of both organs.

Assess your patient for hypovolemia and dehydration, which may damage the kidney tubules and increase the risk of thrombosis of the pancreatic vessels. Monitor the patient's intake and output, vital signs, skin turgor, blood urea nitrogen (BUN) level, creatinine level, and hematocrit. Elevated BUN and creatinine levels may indicate kidney dysfunction and rejection. A steadily declining hematocrit may reflect bleeding.

For the first 24 hours after surgery, adjust I.V. fluids every hour in response to your patient's urine and nasogastric (NG) output. If she has an indwelling urinary catheter, you can monitor urine output accurately. The catheter also decompresses the bladder, allowing the suture line within to heal. After the NG tube and urinary catheter are removed, continue to monitor your patient's intake and output.

Monitor blood glucose levels every 30 minutes to 1 hour for the first 24 hours after surgery and administer insulin or fluids containing dextrose as necessary. A patient may require insulin for 1 to 2 days after surgery because the function of the transplanted pancreas may be delayed. She may also require insulin if she's receiving steroid therapy.

Review your patient's daily laboratory test results, including electrolytes, complete blood count, hemoglobin level, and serum and urine amylase measurements. Collect urine specimens for cumulative amylase determinations taken at 12-hour or 24-hour intervals. Assess insulin, glucagon, and human C peptide levels three or four times per week. Pancreas scans and ultrasound examinations may be performed on the first day after surgery, then once a week until discharge. Ultrasounds examine the function of the new organs and enable the physician to determine the size of the graft and the patency of the veins.

Check your patient's abdominal dressing and incision for blood and urinary drainage and for signs of infection. To decrease postoperative complications, have your patient sit on the side of her bed within 24 hours of surgery. She can begin sitting in a chair and taking short walks the day after surgery. Encourage her to cough, breathe deeply, and change positions frequently.

Patient teaching

A transplant patient may feel overwhelmed at the prospect of going home. Explain to her that she

HOME CARE

Teaching your patient about immunosuppressive drugs

If your patient with diabetes undergoes pancreas and kidney transplantation, you'll need to teach her about immunosuppressive drugs before she's discharged. She'll need to learn the drug's mechanism of action, route of administration, dosage, and any special considerations.

Drug and mechanism of action	Route of administration	Recommended dosage	Special considerations
prednisone • suppresses B and T cells and reduces circulating lymphocytes	• Taken orally; available in scored tablets. • May be given I.V. in the form of methylprednisolone.	• Initial dosage is large (30–40 mg/day or more). • Dosage is tapered over time to 10–20 mg/day or less.	• Advise patient to take drug with food; may cause gastrointestinal (GI) distress. • Unless contraindicated, instruct patient to eat calcium-rich diet because drug may cause osteoporosis. • Warn patient about adverse effects such as hirsutism, cushingoid appearance, and mood swings. • Explain that drug often induces hyperglycemia and that patient's blood glucose levels may be abnormally high when taking large dose.
azathioprine • suppresses humorally-mediated antibody production and cellular hypersensitivity responses	• Taken orally; available in scored tablets.	• 1–3 mg/kg/day	• Advise patient that drug may cause GI distress. • Tell patient that drug may cause bone marrow suppression, so blood counts will be monitored closely.
cyclosporine • prevents cytotoxic T cell proliferation by blocking Interleukin II	• Taken orally; available in gel caps or liquid microemulsion.	• 5–10 mg/kg/day	• Tell patient to take exact amount at same time each day to keep drug blood levels constant. • Instruct patient to keep drug in a cool, dark environment because heat and light break it down. • If patient is taking liquid form, instruct her to use only glass or the medicine cup that comes with the liquid. The drug sticks to plastic, so using a plastic cup will prevent her from receiving the full dose. • Advise patient to avoid grapefruit juice unless same amount is ingested at same time every day because grapefruit juice increases drug's bioavailability.
tacrolimus • prevents cytotoxic T cell proliferation	• Taken orally; available in capsules.	• 0.15–0.30 mg/kg/day	• Instruct patient to take exact amount at same time each day to keep drug blood levels constant. • Explain that drug may cause elevated creatinine and potassium levels and that blood levels will be measured regularly. • Advise patient that drug may cause GI upset.

will have a home care nurse who will continue her care. The home care nurse will assess blood glucose levels, daily intake and output, daily weight, diet (low protein, low sodium, no concentrated sweets), stool for occult blood, and urine for blood, protein, and glucose.

Show your patient how to monitor her blood pressure and temperature. Reinforce the name and action of each drug and review the dosages, times of administration, and possible adverse effects.

Instruct your patient and her family to notify her physician immediately if signs or symptoms of rejection or infection develop or if they can't obtain the prescribed drug. Make sure they know the signs and symptoms of rejection: temperature over 100° F, weight gain of 2 to 3 pounds in 1 day, increased blood pressure, pain, swelling or tenderness over either graft site, and hyperglycemia.

4

Acute Complications

An acute complication of diabetes can quickly deteriorate into a metabolic crisis. Hypoglycemia, for instance, can make your patient's mental status decrease quickly. Left untreated, she can become comatose and suffer permanent brain damage. Acute hyperglycemia can also trigger dangerous consequences.

As a nurse, you're in an excellent position to detect the early signs and symptoms of hypoglycemia, hyperglycemia, and other acute complications such as diabetic ketoacidosis (DKA), and hyperglycemic hyperosmolar nonketotic (HHNK) syndrome (see *Hypoglycemia and hyperglycemia: Signs and symptoms,* page 56). You can also identify findings that suggest the Somogyi phenomenon, an acute complication of treatment, and the dawn phenomenon, another problem related to diabetes. And your quick detection can lead to swift interventions that save your patient from life-threatening consequences.

Hypoglycemia

Hypoglycemia, the most common acute complication of diabetes, occurs when the blood glucose level falls below 60 mg/dl. As you know, glucose is the primary fuel source for the central nervous system (CNS), and the brain requires a continuous supply. When the blood glucose level falls, so does the amount of glucose transported across the blood-brain barrier. When the blood glucose level drops below 40 mg/dl, the brain begins metabolizing glucose at about half the normal rate. This results in signs and symptoms that range from weakness and fatigue to coma.

Compensatory mechanisms

The body responds to hypoglycemia by producing and releasing counterregulatory hormones, such as glucagon and epinephrine. Usually, this process begins when the glucose level falls below 60 mg/dl.

Glucagon, a hormone secreted by the alpha cells of the islets of Langerhans, plays an important role in restoring the blood glucose level to normal. It stimulates the liver to produce glucose through glycogenolysis. The beneficial effect is sustained by gluconeogenesis, in which glucagon forms new glycogen from fatty acids and proteins.

Epinephrine, a catecholamine secreted by the adrenal medulla, increases gluconeogenesis and lipolysis (fat breakdown) by stimulating beta-adrenergic receptors. This process inhibits insulin secretion, causing the blood glucose level to rise, and decreases glucose use by peripheral and visceral tissues.

During prolonged hypoglycemia, other counterregulatory hormones also kick in. Cortisol and growth hormone (GH) help indirectly by reducing insulin's uptake of glucose at peripheral cell receptor sites.

If glucagon or epinephrine secretion is impaired, recovery from insulin-induced hypoglycemia may be delayed. For example, in Type 1 diabetes, the alpha cells commonly become impaired after 4 to 5 years and no longer secrete glucagon in response to a low blood glucose level. Autonomic neuropathy, a chronic complication of diabetes, and beta-blocker therapy also can impair glucagon secretion. When this happens, epinephrine becomes the primary counterregulatory hormone.

Hypoglycemia and hyperglycemia: Signs and symptoms

Body system	Hypoglycemia	Hyperglycemia
Cardiovascular system	• normal hematocrit • tachycardia	• increased hematocrit • tachycardia
Central nervous system	• confusion • convulsions • difficulty concentrating • dizziness • drowsiness • fatigue • headache • nervousness • unconsciousness • weakness	• drowsiness • fatigue • irritability • weakness
Eyes	• vision disturbances, such as blurred vision	• blurred vision • decreased visual acuity • soft eyeballs
Mouth and gastrointestinal system	• hunger • nausea • oral numbness and tingling	• abdominal pain • anorexia • fruity breath odor • hunger • nausea • unusual thirst • vomiting
Renal system	• no significant change	• increased urine output
Skin	• cold sweat • pallor	• dry, flushed skin

However, if long-standing diabetes impairs or eliminates epinephrine secretion, the patient will develop hypoglycemia unawareness. This condition leaves the patient defenseless against hypoglycemic episodes. She won't experience the early warning signs, such as tremors and diaphoresis. Eventually, the lack of cerebral glucose will cause her to develop more advanced symptoms, such as confusion and profound lethargy.

The patient's age and the frequency of hypoglycemic episodes also can affect the body's compensatory response to hypoglycemia. The amount of epinephrine secreted in response to hypoglycemia diminishes with age. And frequent episodes of hypoglycemia progressively slow the secretion of counterregulatory hormones. Patients who follow a regimen of tight glucose control tend to have frequent episodes and are at greater risk for developing profound hypoglycemia.

Risk factors

Although anyone with diabetes can experience hypoglycemia, some patients are at greater risk than others. Risk factors include age, exercise, skipped meals, and alcohol. Women are also at increased risk at the beginning of each menstrual period and immediately after childbirth.

Age

Elderly patients commonly develop liver or kidney insufficiency, which can interfere with the metabolism and excretion of drugs, including oral antidiabetic drugs. Acarbose and metformin, which may be prescribed for elderly diabetic patients, can contribute to hypoglycemia when combined with sulfonylureas.

Many elderly patients live alone, and many consume an inadequate diet because they can't afford to buy nutritious foods. These factors can lead to an unrecognized hypoglycemic episode with potentially fatal results. For example, an elderly patient who eats poorly may develop signs and symptoms of hypoglycemia. If she lives alone and doesn't recognize the signs and symptoms, no one else is available to notice them and provide care. And if she doesn't receive care, she can lapse into a coma and die.

Also, in elderly patients, confusion and other signs of hypoglycemia commonly are mistaken for senile dementia. As a result, hypoglycemia may not be recognized and treated.

Exercise

Exercise can increase the risk of developing hypoglycemia because the skeletal muscles need more glucose for fuel. In patients with Type 2 diabetes, exercise increases the amount of circulating insulin, allowing more glucose to enter the cells. In patients with Type 1 diabetes, exercise causes subcutaneous insulin to enter the bloodstream faster, especially if the injection site is near the muscles being exercised. This sudden release of insulin causes the liver to stop producing glucose, resulting in hypoglycemia.

Prolonged strenuous exercise, which depletes glycogen stores in the muscles and liver, can cause hypoglycemia for up to 24 hours. If a patient is more active than usual or if she exercises strenuously during the day, she may experience hypoglycemia while sleeping.

Skipped meals and alcohol consumption

Delaying or skipping meals, eating too little, or eating a low-carbohydrate meal can lead to hypoglycemia. Alcohol can cause hypoglycemia by inhibiting glucose production in the liver.

Menstruation and pregnancy

Women with diabetes may experience more hypoglycemic episodes at the beginning of menses each month. That's when the progesterone level drops, causing insulin resistance to diminish and the blood glucose level to fall.

Childbirth also puts patients at risk for hypoglycemia. During pregnancy, high levels of estrogen, progesterone, and lactogen increase insulin resistance. Immediately after delivery, these placental hormone levels drop so that insulin resistance—and the blood glucose level—quickly drop as well.

Autonomic and neuroglycopenic signs and symptoms

The early signs and symptoms of hypoglycemia tend to be autonomic. Neuroglycopenic signs and symptoms generally appear later.

Autonomic signs and symptoms
- nervousness
- tremors
- palpitations
- diaphoresis
- anxiety
- pallor
- irritability
- hunger
- paresthesia

Neuroglycopenic signs and symptoms
- dizziness
- headache
- lack of coordination
- difficulty concentrating
- mental dullness
- severe lethargy
- slurred speech
- blurred vision
- mood changes
- seizures
- coma

Signs and symptoms

Some patients with diabetes report signs and symptoms of hypoglycemia at normal blood glucose levels. Usually, this happens when the level drops rapidly and steeply—for instance, from 250 to 100 mg/dl. Other patients experience no signs or symptoms until the level falls as low as 45 mg/dl. These variations may be affected by how tightly a patient controls her blood glucose level. A patient with poor glucose control is likely to experience hypoglycemic signs and symptoms at a much higher glucose level than a patient who uses intensive therapy to achieve tight control.

Typically, the early signs and symptoms of hypoglycemia are classified as autonomic, and the later signs and symptoms are classified as neuroglycopenic (see *Autonomic and neuroglycopenic signs and symptoms*).

Autonomic signs and symptoms

Autonomic signs and symptoms, which occur with early or mild hypoglycemia, are part of the autonomic nervous system's response to increased epinephrine levels. Typically, these signs and symptoms begin to appear when the blood glucose level reaches 60 mg/dl.

Autonomic signs and symptoms include nervousness, tremors, palpitations, tachycardia, diaphoresis, anxiety, and pallor. Tremors and palpitations result from the adrenergic response of the autonomic nervous system; diaphoresis, from the cholinergic response of the autonomic nervous system. The intensity of autonomic signs and symptoms varies greatly, not only from patient to patient but also with each hypoglycemic episode. In elderly patients, age-related changes commonly lead to a loss of autonomic signs and symptoms. For example, sweat gland atrophy may eliminate diaphoresis as a sign of hypoglycemia.

Neuroglycopenic signs and symptoms

Neuroglycopenic signs and symptoms, which result from a diminished supply of glucose to the CNS, develop with moderate to severe hypoglycemia. These signs and symptoms usually don't appear until the blood glucose level falls below 50 mg/dl. Commonly, they occur at night when the patient is asleep.

Early neuroglycopenic signs and symptoms include dizziness, light-headedness, lack of coordination, difficulty concentrating, and slowed thinking. As neuroglycopenia worsens, the patient may experience sleepiness, slurred speech, blurred vision, and mood changes such as irritability, stubbornness, giddiness, and sadness. Ultimately, if hypoglycemia becomes severe, the patient may have seizures—which are more common in children—or slip into a coma. A less common sign, hemiplegia may be mistakenly attributed to a cerebrovascular accident, especially in an elderly patient.

Treatment

The treatment of hypoglycemia depends on your patient's mental status, her ability to swallow, and the severity of her signs and symptoms. If possible, check your patient's blood glucose level to verify that she has hypoglycemia before starting treatment. A sudden drop in the glucose level can trigger the adrenergic response and produce such signs as tremors and diaphoresis without producing hypoglycemia. However, if your patient has signs and symptoms of hypoglycemia but glucose monitoring isn't readily available, don't delay treatment. You're better off treating a normal or high blood glucose level than risking not treating a low level.

If your patient has hypoglycemia and can swallow, give her 15 grams of a rapidly absorbed carbohydrate, such as orange juice, to alleviate symptoms and prevent the blood glucose level from falling further. If symptoms persist after 15 minutes, give her another 15 grams of the rapidly absorbed carbohydrate (see *Treating hypoglycemia with carbohydrates*).

As your patient's symptoms subside and her blood glucose level rises above 70 mg/dl, prevent hypoglycemia from recurring by giving her a snack of complex carbohydrates and protein if she's not scheduled to eat a meal within the hour. A typical snack is six peanut butter crackers or a slice of bread with 1 ounce of meat or cheese. Instruct the patient not to exercise or engage in other strenuous activity for about 1 hour.

If your patient isn't allowed to eat or drink, gently rub 15 grams of glucose gel (or an equivalent dose) between her cheek and gum. Recheck her blood glucose level after 15 minutes. Repeat this treatment if signs and symptoms of hyperglycemia persist.

If your patient loses consciousness or her symptoms worsen, the physician may prescribe an I.V. bolus of 25 to 50 grams of 50% dextrose solution. If she doesn't have an I.V. line in place, the physician may prescribe a subcutaneous or intramuscular glucagon injection, in a dosage of 0.5 mg for a child or 1 mg for an adult. Check her blood glucose level in 10 to 15 minutes. If she doesn't respond to the first glucagon injection, she'll need a second one.

When your patient responds, give her 15 grams of a rapidly absorbed carbohydrate, such as a nondiet soft drink, followed by a snack, as described above. Because glucagon therapy commonly causes nausea and vomiting, use caution when giving your patient food. To prevent her from aspirating vomit, turn her on her left side until the nausea subsides.

If your patient's hypoglycemia results from an excessive dose of an oral antidiabetic drug, she may require hospitalization. The physician may prescribe an initial I.V. bolus of 50% dextrose solution, followed by a continuous infusion of a dextrose solution, such as 10% dextrose in water.

Check your patient's blood glucose level at least every 15 minutes until it returns to normal. Then recheck it every 1 to 2 hours. If the glucose level doesn't respond to dextrose alone, the physician may prescribe glucagon.

Overtreatment

Overtreating hypoglycemia with excess carbohydrates is fairly common. When patients treat themselves at home, they sometimes eat until their symptoms subside instead of eating the recommended amount of a rapidly absorbed carbohydrate and waiting 15 minutes for symptoms to resolve. Other patients overtreat themselves out of fear of losing control or going into a coma—especially if they've experienced moderate or severe symptoms before.

If you're treating your patient with I.V. dextrose, wait 5 to 10 minutes to see if symptoms improve. Remember, overtreating hypoglycemia can lead to rebounding hyperglycemia. Giving the patient extra regular insulin to treat rebounding hyperglycemia can then cause her blood glucose level to fall sharply.

Nursing considerations

Review the onset, peak, and duration of action of the insulin your patient uses. When her insulin is at peak effect, check her for signs and symptoms of hypoglycemia. Be familiar with oral antidiabetic drugs that can cause hypoglycemia, such as sulfonylureas. Whether she uses insulin or oral antidiabetic drugs, monitor her blood glucose level before meals and at bedtime and tell her to do the same at home.

Advise your patient to administer her insulin and oral antidiabetic drugs on time. Patients should eat 5 to 30 minutes after insulin administration, depending on the type of insulin. For example, a patient should eat within 5 minutes after taking Humalog or 30 minutes after taking regular insulin. If your patient leaves the hospital unit temporarily, make sure she takes her insulin and eats her meals on schedule. If a meal will be delayed, give her a snack. Also, provide between-meal and bedtime snacks, if needed, at the time of insulin's peak activity.

If your patient isn't allowed anything by mouth before a procedure, contact her physician to obtain changes in orders for her insulin and oral antidiabetic drugs.

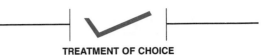

TREATMENT OF CHOICE

Treating hypoglycemia with carbohydrates

Each of the foods listed below supplies 15 grams of carbohydrate, the amount needed to treat hypoglycemia.
- ½ cup of fruit juice
- ½ cup of nondiet soda
- five hard candies
- 1 cup of skim milk
- three 5-gram glucose tablets
- one application of glucose gel, as marked on container

Patient teaching

Teach your patient and her family how to prevent, recognize, and manage hypoglycemia (see *Teaching your patient about hypoglycemia,* page 60). Making your patient an active participant in her care will help her counter feelings of helplessness and loss of control. Enlist her family's help and ease their fears by teaching them about hypoglycemia as well.

If your patient experiences hypoglycemia, help her identify what may have caused it. Even mild hypoglycemia will disrupt her daily routine if it occurs frequently. Anticipating hypoglycemia without understanding its causes and treatment may affect her compliance with her regimen. For example, she may be afraid to inject insulin for fear of another hypoglycemic episode.

Assess your patient for administration problems, such as administering too much insulin or too high a dose of an oral antidiabetic drug. Ask her to demonstrate how she administers insulin. Also, discuss the timing, quantity, and content of her meals as well as the extent and timing of exercise.

Encourage your patient to monitor her blood glucose level regularly and whenever she experiences hypoglycemic symptoms. Such monitoring will help her learn her threshold for hypoglycemia and recognize her typical symptoms at various glucose levels. Then when she experiences hypoglycemia, she can treat it appropriately.

HOME CARE

Teaching your patient about hypoglycemia

Whether your patient recently learned that she has diabetes or she has been treating herself for years, during her hospitalization you should teach—or reinforce—certain essential information about hypoglycemia. Be sure you cover the following areas:

• Explore the possible causes of hypoglycemia.
• Discuss the signs and symptoms of hypoglycemia.
• Discuss how to recognize and treat hypoglycemia promptly.
• Remind her to carry a simple carbohydrate snack, such as peanut butter crackers, at all times to treat hypoglycemia.
• Explain the importance of wearing a bracelet or necklace or carrying a card that indicates she has diabetes.
• Discuss the importance of telling family and friends about her diabetes in case she has a hypoglycemic episode.
• If your patient uses insulin, recommend that she obtain a glucagon kit and teach her family and friends when and how to use it.
• Teach her to monitor her blood glucose level frequently.
• Explain the importance of a regular pattern for eating meals and administering insulin or oral antidiabetic drugs.
• Explain the need to adjust the amount of food, the timing of meals and snacks, or the times of insulin administration when she engages in strenuous physical activity.
• Explain the importance of checking with the physician before taking a new prescription or over-the-counter drug.
• Instruct her to tell her health care providers that she has diabetes and that she uses insulin or oral antidiabetic drugs, as appropriate.

Teach your patient to recheck her blood glucose level 15 minutes after taking a rapidly absorbed carbohydrate. Encourage her to keep rapidly absorbed carbohydrates, such as hard candies or glucose tablets, available at home and to carry them with her when she goes out. Also, advise the patient to carry a nonperishable snack, such as a package of peanut butter crackers, to eat in case a meal isn't available within 1 hour after a hyperglycemic episode.

Identify a family member or friend who can help your patient if she develops hypoglycemia. Teach this person how to prepare and administer glucagon if hypoglycemia hinders the patient's ability to swallow. Warn the patient that nausea is a common adverse effect of glucagon; she may need to take small sips of a carbonated, uncaffeinated soft drink until her nausea subsides.

For an elderly patient who lives alone, identify someone who's willing to learn about hypoglycemia and check on her regularly. Encourage your elderly patient to contact the physician if she experiences frequent hypoglycemia. Also, instruct her to notify the physician if her blood glucose level falls below the target level more often than prescribed guidelines permit. The patient's drug dosage may need to be adjusted.

Advise your patient to buy a medical alert bracelet or necklace that describes her condition and lists the physician's phone number—especially if she's prone to severe hypoglycemia.

When your patient leaves the hospital, give her written discharge instructions about diet, exercise, drugs, blood glucose monitoring, and signs, symptoms, and treatment of hypoglycemia.

Hyperglycemia

Chronic hyperglycemia results from untreated or poorly controlled diabetes. But acute hyperglycemia results from factors that interfere with glucose control—an acute infection, for instance. If hyperglycemia becomes severe enough, the patient may develop a serious condition, such as DKA and HHNK syndrome.

In Type 1 and Type 2 diabetes, hyperglycemia results when an abundance of blood glucose can't enter the cells. As the glucose level in the bloodstream rises, the glucose-rich blood becomes hyperosmolar, drawing fluid from the interstitial and intracellular spaces. Because the body's cells then lack glucose and water, they signal the brain to trigger the patient's thirst mechanism.

As intravascular fluid and the glucose level rise, the body tries to excrete the excess water and glucose through urination. As more urine is produced and excreted, more fluid is drawn from the interstitial and intracellular spaces, resulting in profound dehydration and weight loss.

Risk factors

Physiologic stress caused by illness, infection, injury, emotional trauma, or surgery may upset metabolic homeostasis and result in hyperglycemia by increasing the secretion of counterregulatory hormones, including epinephrine, cortisol, GH, and glucagon.

Epinephrine decreases the uptake of glucose by muscle tissue and inhibits the release of endogenous insulin. Epinephrine also stimulates glycogenolysis, the breakdown of hepatic glycogen into glucose in the bloodstream. Cortisol increases glucose production by the liver and inhibits insulin uptake by muscle tissue. GH and glucagon work to raise the blood glucose level. The resulting hyperglycemia creates an osmotic diuretic effect that increases urine output and fluid requirements.

Certain drugs such as glucocorticosteroids also can cause hyperglycemia. In many cases, however, adjustments in a patient's antidiabetic drug, diet, and exercise regimens can counteract the hyperglycemic effect of such drugs.

Many over-the-counter drugs, including cough and cold remedies that contain sucrose or sugar, and anti-inflammatory drugs can raise the blood glucose level. Also, treatment with hormones, such as oral contraceptives and thyroid preparations, may raise the blood glucose level by increasing insulin resistance (see *Drugs that can worsen hyperglycemia*).

Signs and symptoms

If your patient with diabetes has mild, transient hyperglycemia, she may not have obvious signs and symptoms. If her blood glucose level rises further and remains high, however, she will develop polydipsia, polyphagia, and polyuria.

Remember though, not all patients recognize these signs and symptoms. For example, age-related changes may have impaired an elderly patient's thirst mechanism. And urinary frequency, especially when coupled with incontinence, is commonly mistaken as an expected part of aging.

Drugs that can worsen hyperglycemia

Many drugs can exacerbate hyperglycemia in patients with diabetes. If your patient is taking any of the following, notify her physician:
- alpha and beta agonists
- anticonvulsants
- beta-blockers
- carbonic anhydrase inhibitors
- decongestants
- diet pills
- estrogen and progesterone therapy
- glucagon
- glucocorticoids
- growth hormone
- immunosuppressants
- loop diuretics
- thiazide diuretics
- thyroid preparations.

The weight loss from cellular starvation and dehydration may be rapid and profound, especially in a patient with Type 1 diabetes. Reassure your patient that she'll regain weight quickly after her blood glucose level returns to normal.

Other signs and symptoms of hyperglycemia include fatigue, oral and vaginal yeast infections, constipation, and blurred vision. Be sure to ask your patient about these signs and symptoms. Otherwise, she may attribute them to another cause and not report them.

Diagnostic tests

If your patient's blood glucose level exceeds 125 mg/dl when fasting or 200 mg/dl 2 hours or more after a meal, she's having a hyperglycemic episode. To find out if she's had frequent or severe episodes in the past 2 months, the physician may order a glycosylated hemoglobin (hemoglobin A_{1c}) test. A hemoglobin A_{1c} value of 7% or less suggests that such episodes are uncommon. A value greater than 8% indicates that the patient has had frequent hyperglycemic episodes. A value greater than 13% indicates that her blood glucose level is above normal more often than not. In ei-

What's causing your patient's hyperglycemia?

If acute illness or infection isn't the cause of your patient's hyperglycemia, it may be her diet, exercise level, or drugs. Or she may not be hyperglycemic, but may appear to be because she uses an incorrect technique for self-monitoring or an inaccurate glucose meter.

- Review your patient's recent dietary intake. Did she exceed her allocated food intake? Ask her about mealtimes and eating habits, especially if her blood glucose level is consistently elevated at a particular time of day.
- Ask your patient if she has changed her exercise program. A decrease in exercise or a change in the type of exercise can cause her blood glucose level to fluctuate.
- Review your patient's drugs. Have any dosages been changed recently? Has she stopped taking any drugs? Is she taking a drug that raises the blood glucose level?
- If your patient injects insulin, find out if she uses insulin that's beyond its expiration date. Ask her to demonstrate her administration technique. Does she gently roll cloudy insulin? Is she drawing up the prescribed amount? Do you see large air bubbles in the syringe that might cause her to inject a dose that's smaller than prescribed?
- Examine your patient's glucose meter. Has it been coded correctly for the test strips she uses? If not, glucose values may be inaccurate. Ask her to demonstrate her blood testing technique; improper technique can affect test results. Review her glucose test records. Look for patterns that indicate the need to alter her drug therapy.

ther case, the patient's treatment regimen should be re-evaluated.

Treatment

First, determine what caused your patient's hyperglycemia. Assess her for illness and infection and identify other factors that may be contributing to the hyperglycemia (see *What's causing your patient's hyperglycemia?*). Expect to adjust her diet and exercise regimens as well as her drug therapy, if needed. Administering insulin can lower the blood glucose level temporarily. Keep in mind that a patient with Type 2 diabetes may require temporary treatment with insulin, until an acute infection or illness passes. Nevertheless, eliminating the cause will improve hyperglycemia over time.

Several days after adjusting the patient's treatment regimen, contact her and evaluate the effect of the adjustments. Advise her to take her log of blood glucose measurements and drug administration the next time she visits her physician.

Patient teaching

Make sure your patient knows how to keep a diary of the food she eats and the exercise she performs. Instruct her to weigh herself daily and report a loss or gain of more than 5 pounds in a week.

Teach your patient to recognize the signs and symptoms of common infections, such as urinary tract, periodontal, and superficial staphylococcal infections. Encourage her to visit her dentist and podiatrist routinely to prevent or detect and treat periodontal and foot infections. Also, urge her to have routine gynecologic examinations. Tell your patient that even a seemingly innocuous illness, such as a common cold, can place her at risk for hyperglycemia. And if undetected and untreated, it can lead to DKA or HHNK syndrome. Be sure to review guidelines for sick-day management with your patient and her family.

Help your patient and her family learn to recognize blood glucose levels that signal hyperglycemia and to identify patterns of glucose levels that call for an adjustment in her diabetes treatment regimen. Help the patient identify potential causes of hyperglycemia and explain which actions to take.

Diabetic ketoacidosis

An acute complication, DKA requires rapid intervention to prevent cellular starvation and profound dehydration. Although DKA usually occurs in patients with Type 1 diabetes, it can strike a patient with Type 2 diabetes.

The three major causes of DKA are undiagnosed diabetes, insufficient insulin therapy, and physical or emotional stress.

How diabetic ketoacidosis develops

Without sufficient insulin, the cells can't use glucose for energy. The body, sensing this energy decrease, begins to release and break down its stores of fat. Lipolysis creates glycerol and fatty acids. Glycerol is converted into glucose, and the liver converts fatty acids to ketone bodies. As ketone bodies accumulate, metabolic acidosis develops.

As a last resort, the body begins breaking down protein to create glucose for energy. This increases circulating glucose and nitrogen. In the ongoing absence of available insulin, however, glucose can't enter the cells, and the blood glucose level continues to rise. Eventually, the blood glucose level rises to between 300 and 800 mg/dl.

The increase in blood glucose level and ketone bodies leads to a severe loss of water and electrolytes. The kidneys respond to the increase in circulating glucose by increasing the glomerular filtration rate. As the body tries to remove the excess glucose, urine output climbs. In many cases, it reaches 5 to 8 liters a day (see *Understanding fluid and electrolyte loss in diabetic ketoacidosis,* page 64).

This excessive diuresis results in a loss of sodium, potassium, chloride, bicarbonate and, to a lesser degree, magnesium and phosphate. As sodium and bicarbonate are lost because of osmotic diuresis, acidosis develops. Acidosis leaves the rising level of carbonic acid (a by-product of ketosis) unchallenged. To compensate, the patient develops Kussmaul's respirations (deep rapid breathing) to blow off the carbonic acid.

Signs and symptoms

Signs and symptoms usually begin within 24 hours of the insulin deficiency and may persist for several days before the patient seeks medical attention. Eventually, as her level of consciousness decreases and her polyuria, polydipsia, polyphagia, and weakness become intolerable, she or a family member realizes that she's in crisis.

An acute infection is the most common cause of DKA, so be sure to check for such signs and symptoms as fever, purulent drainage from wounds, tenderness, and localized erythema. Also, check for signs of systemic infection, including urinary tract, pulmonary, and gastrointestinal (GI) infections.

DKA affects the GI system in many ways. At first, as the cellular fuel supply diminishes, hyperglycemia may cause hunger. As dehydration sets in and DKA progresses, the patient experiences anorexia, nausea, vomiting, and abdominal pain. Profound dehydration may lead to constipation. During an abdominal examination, you may note diminished or absent bowel sounds and abdominal tenderness.

The extreme dehydration and hypovolemia that result from DKA cause tachycardia, orthostatic hypotension, dry mucous membranes, poor skin turgor, and flushed, dry skin. The patient reports weakness and fatigue. And as her condition declines, so does her level of consciousness. Typically, she becomes confused, stuporous, and eventually comatose.

When electrolytes, such as potassium, are lost along with fluids, the patient begins to develop signs and symptoms of an electrolyte imbalance, such as hypokalemia. At first, she experiences general malaise and fatigue along with muscle weakness. Eventually, as the potassium level sinks, she develops flaccid muscle paralysis and arrhythmias.

As ketosis sets in, the body tries to rid itself of excess carbonic acid through Kussmaul's respirations. You may note a fruity acetone odor—a sure sign of ketosis—on the patient's breath. As the kidneys filter ketones, ketonuria develops.

Diagnostic tests

To help confirm a diagnosis of DKA and guide treatment, the physician may order laboratory measurements of:
- blood glucose
- blood bicarbonate
- blood urea nitrogen (BUN)
- hematocrit
- urine specific gravity
- blood osmolality
- white blood cell (WBC) count
- blood phosphate
- blood potassium and sodium
- pH.

The blood glucose level may range from 300 to 800 mg/dl. The blood bicarbonate level may drop below 15 mEq/L. Dehydration causes BUN levels,

Understanding fluid and electrolyte loss in diabetic ketoacidosis

When the blood glucose level exceeds the renal threshold, the kidneys try to compensate by excreting excess glucose in urine. However, glucose pulls water and electrolytes, such as potassium and magnesium, along with it. The result is profound dehydration and electrolyte loss.

As shown, glucose moves from the renal vessels into the glomerulus (1) and the proximal tubule (2).

As glucose moves through the descending and ascending loop of Henle, it pulls in water (3). When the glucose-rich water passes through the distal tubule, electrolytes such as potassium and magnesium move in (4). The fluid carrying glucose, water, and electrolytes then passes out of the distal tubule and is excreted in urine (5).

Nephron

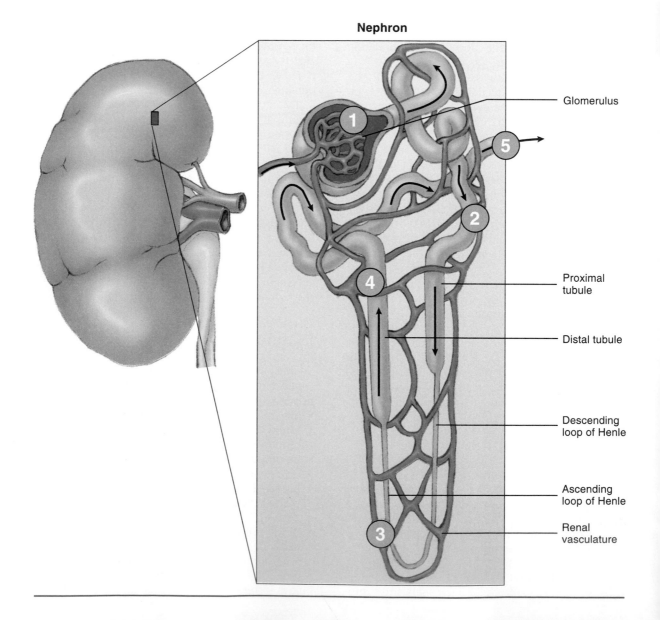

hematocrit, and urine specific gravity to rise. Blood osmolality may soar as high as 330 mOsm/L.

The WBC count may be high from hemoconcentration or infection. If the WBC count remains high after DKA has been treated, the patient probably has an infection. The blood phosphate level may be low. Blood potassium and sodium levels may be high, normal, or low, reflecting shifts between intracellular and extracellular fluid. The total body potassium generally is depleted. As ketones accumulate in the blood, the patient's pH drops below 7.3.

Treatment

The treatment goals for DKA are to replace fluid and electrolytes, provide enough insulin to maintain normal glucose metabolism, and prevent complications (see *Caring for a patient with diabetic ketoacidosis,* pages 66 and 67).

Replacing fluids and electrolytes
Your patient with DKA needs fluid therapy to increase her circulating blood volume and to enhance glucose excretion through the kidneys. The fluid of choice is usually I.V. 0.9% normal saline solution (an isotonic solution) infused at a rate of 1 L/hour for the first hour of therapy. Normal saline solution prevents a rapid fall in extracellular osmolality, reducing the risk of cerebral edema. After the first hour, adjust the infusion rate based on your patient's blood pressure and any persistent fluid loss caused by vomiting and diuresis.

When the patient's blood glucose level drops to between 250 and 300 mg/dl, expect to change the I.V. solution to 5% dextrose mixed with 0.45% normal saline solution to prevent hypoglycemia.

In a patient with DKA, significant diuresis usually leads to a profound electrolyte imbalance. Administering insulin promotes potassium movement into the cells, lowering the blood potassium level even further. Therefore, unless your patient has renal failure and her blood potassium level is too high, expect to replace her potassium, usually 4 to 8 hours after fluid therapy has begun. If her potassium level is below 2.5 mEq/L, however, don't delay potassium replacement: Add 30 to 40 mEq/L of potassium chloride to the first bag of I.V. fluid, as ordered.

If your patient's blood pH is below 7.1, the physician may prescribe sodium bicarbonate. If so, be sure to infuse it slowly—at a rate of 1 to 2 mEq/kg over 2 hours—because sodium bicarbonate can cause metabolic alkalosis if infused to rapidly.

Administering insulin
The goal of insulin therapy is to reverse hyperglycemia and ketoacidosis without causing hypoglycemia.

The physician may prescribe a low-dose continuous I.V. infusion of regular insulin because its rapid action allows fast changes in titration. Anticipate starting with a bolus of 0.1 to 0.15 U/kg. This initial treatment will saturate the insulin receptors in the tissues. After the bolus, the physician may prescribe 0.1 U/kg/hour until the blood glucose level returns to normal. For most patients, this dosage decreases the blood glucose level by 80 to 100 mg/dl/hour. While insulin is being infused, monitor your patient's blood glucose level every hour to assess the treatment's effectiveness. Adjust the infusion rate as needed.

Eventually, your patient can resume subcutaneous insulin therapy. But keep the insulin infusion going for 30 minutes after the first subcutaneous injection.

Preventing complications
Preventing complications is an integral part of DKA treatment. The most common complications are electrolyte imbalances, hypoglycemia, heart failure, and cerebral edema. You can reduce the likelihood of these complications by carefully replacing fluids and electrolytes and closely monitoring laboratory values.

Cerebral edema, a potentially fatal complication, may result from correcting osmolality, acidosis, or hyperglycemia too quickly. Signs and symptoms include headache, lethargy, and loss of consciousness. On physical examination, your patient's pupils will be fixed, unequal, and dilated, and she'll have papilledema. She'll also have bradycardia and hypertension.

Nursing considerations

Providing nursing care to a patient with DKA presents a multisystem challenge. To prevent serious complications, think critically and act quickly.

During fluid replacement, assess your patient's fluid balance to ensure adequate hydration without the complications of fluid overload. Evaluate her vi-

Caring for a patient with diabetic ketoacidosis

	History and physical examination	Diagnostic tests	Discharge planning	
Day 1	• amount of insulin used in past 48 hours • recent history of stress and infections • vital signs every 30–60 minutes • urine output every hour • systems review every 2–4 hours	• complete blood count (CBC) on admission • blood glucose level every hour • electrolytes every hour • arterial blood gases (ABGs) every 1–2 hours • blood urea nitrogen (BUN) and creatinine every 2–4 hours • plasma and urine ketones every 4–8 hours • cultures, as needed	• Determine cause of diabetic ketoacidosis (DKA). • Identify support systems.	
Day 2	• vital signs every 2–4 hours • urine output every 2–4 hours • systems review once per shift	• blood glucose level every 2–4 hours • electrolytes every 2–4 hours • BUN and creatinine every 8–12 hours • plasma and urine ketones once per shift • ABGs, as needed • CBC	• Begin review of diabetes management. • Consult dietitian and exercise physiologist, as needed.	
Day 3	• vital signs every 4–8 hours • systems review and urine output once per shift	• blood glucose level every 4–8 hours • electrolytes, BUN, creatinine, and urine ketones once per shift	• Participate in interdisciplinary review of patient's anticipated home needs.	
Day 4	• vital signs, systems review, and urine output once per shift	• blood glucose level once per shift or as ordered • urine ketones once per shift	• Provide resource options for continued needs. • Schedule follow-up care.	

tal signs, level of consciousness, body weight, intake and output, urine specific gravity, and blood osmolality. And assess her skin turgor and mucous membranes for signs of improved hydration.

Frequently check the I.V. site for signs of infiltration or infection. If your patient has a central line, check all connections.

During rapid fluid replacement, monitor your patient for signs and symptoms of fluid over-load—especially if she's elderly, a child, or at risk for heart failure. Signs and symptoms of heart failure include pulmonary crackles, labored respirations, hypotension, tachycardia, and S_3 or S_4 heart sounds.

Monitor your patient's blood sodium, potassium, bicarbonate, magnesium, and phosphate levels closely. And evaluate her electrocardiogram (ECG) tracings to detect arrhythmias or charac-

Drugs	Interventions	Patient teaching
• regular insulin intramuscularly (I.M.) or I.V. every hour or continuous I.V. drip • potassium replacement therapy, as needed • bicarbonate therapy if pH is below 7.0 • antibiotic therapy, if indicated	• I.V. fluid replacement therapy (typical regimen: 1–2 liters first hour, then 1 liter over 2–3 hours, then 500 ml/hr) • seizure precautions • mouth care every 2 hours • fluid intake when gastrointestinal symptoms abate • bed rest	• Orient to hospital unit. • Explain diagnostic tests and medical therapy. • Include family, as appropriate.
• dosage of regular insulin reduced gradually • potassium replacement therapy, as needed • antibiotic therapy, if indicated	• I.V. therapy slowed or discontinued • liquid diet • bed rest with bathroom privileges	• Teach patient and family about causes and early recognition of signs and symptoms of DKA.
• I.V. or I.M. regular insulin replaced with subcutaneous injections or precrisis insulin regimen • antibiotic therapy, if indicated	• resumption of prescribed precrisis diet plan • fluid intake • limited activity	• Review blood glucose and ketone testing procedures. • Review insulin therapy. • Teach sick-day rules.
• precrisis insulin regimen with adjustments, as needed • antibiotic therapy, if needed	• continued dietary plan • fluid intake • activity as desired	• Review diet, exercise, and stress management. • Ensure understanding of need for follow up and blood glucose control.

teristic changes from abnormally high or low potassium levels (see *Recognizing electrocardiogram changes in hyperkalemia and hypokalemia,* page 68).

Before starting the insulin infusion, flush the tubing with 50 ml of insulin solution to saturate the tubing with insulin. Remember, insulin adheres to I.V. tubing, so if you don't saturate it with insulin, your patient won't receive the full insulin dose. Use an infusion pump to ensure insulin delivery at the prescribed rate.

Monitor the blood glucose level hourly. As the level falls, monitor your patient closely for signs and symptoms of hypoglycemia.

Your patient also requires basic nursing interventions for comfort and hygiene. Although she's dehydrated and thirsty, she may not be able to eat or drink anything until she's no longer feeling

Recognizing electrocardiogram changes in hyperkalemia and hypokalemia

During rapid fluid replacement, always monitor your patient's electrocardiogram (ECG) for changes that indicate too much or too little potassium. The following ECG tracings reflect a normal potassium level, increasing hyperkalemia, and increasing hypokalemia.

Normal potassium level

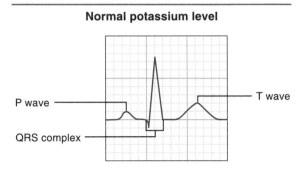

When the potassium level is normal, the QRS complex is less than 0.12 second, and the U wave isn't discernible.

Mild hyperkalemia

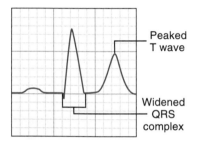

When the potassium level rises to between 6 and 6.5 mEq/L, the QRS complex begins to widen, and the T wave peaks.

Moderate hyperkalemia

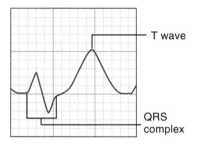

When the potassium level exceeds 7 mEq/L, the QRS complex and T wave lose their defining characteristics.

Severe hyperkalemia

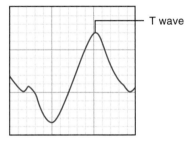

When the potassium level exceeds 10 mEq/L, the QRS complex becomes so wide that it merges with the T wave.

Mild hypokalemia

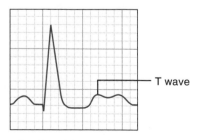

When the potassium level falls to 3 mEq/L, the T wave begins to flatten.

Moderate hypokalemia

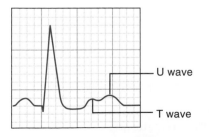

When the potassium level falls below 2 mEq/L, the T wave continues to flatten, and the U wave rises higher than the T wave.

Severe hypokalemia

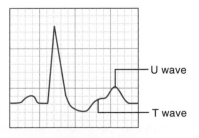

When the potassium level falls to 1 mEq/L, the U wave peaks and merges with the smaller T wave.

Distinguishing between diabetic ketoacidosis and hyperglycemic hyperosmolar nonketotic syndrome

An abnormally high blood glucose level in a patient with diabetes may signal diabetic ketoacidosis (DKA) or hyperglycemic hyperosmolar nonketotic (HHNK) syndrome. This table can help you tell the difference between the two conditions.

Feature	DKA	HHNK syndrome
Type of diabetes	Type 1	Type 2
Blood glucose levels	Usually 300–800 mg/dl	Frequently > 1,000 mg/dl
Dehydration	Yes	Profound
Ketosis	Yes	No
Acidosis	Yes	Mild
Serum osmolality	< 330 mOsm/L	> 330 mOsm/L
Acetone breath	Yes	No
Level of consciousness	Varies, may be sluggish or comatose	Usually impaired, lethargic to comatose

nauseated, vomiting, or complaining of abdominal pain. Providing frequent oral care helps moisten dry lips and mucous membranes, increasing her comfort and giving you an opportunity to assess her hydration.

Skin care is especially important because dehydration and poor tissue perfusion from DKA increase the risk of skin breakdown. Turn and reposition your patient every 2 hours. Use an emollient to keep her skin from becoming scaly, flaky, and vulnerable to breakdown. As you provide skin care, check your patient's skin turgor, color, temperature, and perfusion.

Patient teaching

During acute DKA, the patient probably can't grasp educational information very well, so don't overwhelm her or her family with information right away. Keep your explanations simple and brief; you may have to repeat them several times. Explain care little by little, as you provide it. Tell her why it's important to replace fluids and electrolytes, administer insulin, and continuously monitor vital signs, intake and output,

and blood values. After your patient's condition stabilizes, provide more information.

If DKA is your patient's first indication that she has diabetes, you may be the first health care provider to teach her about the disease and its management. Remember, your hospital's certified diabetes educator can supply vital information and psychological support.

Hyperglycemic hyperosmolar nonketotic syndrome

A medical emergency, HHNK syndrome usually occurs in elderly patients with Type 2 diabetes. A patient who develops HHNK can produce enough insulin to prevent ketoacidosis, but not enough to prevent severe hyperglycemia, diuresis, and loss of extracellular fluid. Some 40% to 60% of patients who develop HHNK syndrome die of severe dehydration and electrolyte loss (see *Distinguishing between diabetic ketoacidosis and hyperglycemic hyperosmolar nonketotic syndrome*).

How hyperglycemic hyperosmolar nonketotic syndrome progresses

Commonly triggered by a stressor such as infection, hyperglycemic hyperosmolar nonketotic syndrome begins with insufficient insulin or insulin resistance and can end in coma or death.

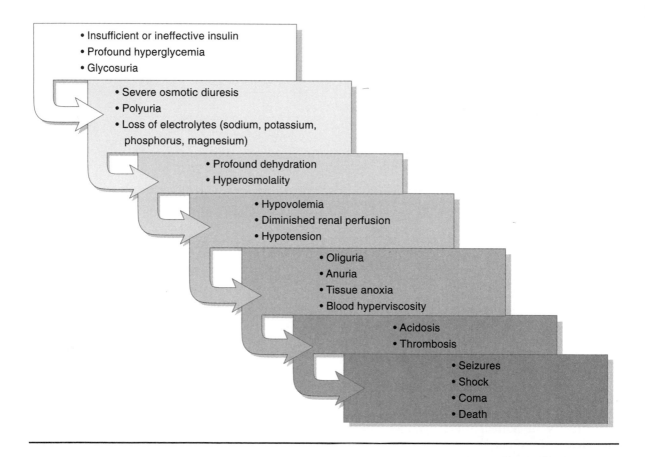

- Insufficient or ineffective insulin
- Profound hyperglycemia
- Glycosuria

- Severe osmotic diuresis
- Polyuria
- Loss of electrolytes (sodium, potassium, phosphorus, magnesium)

- Profound dehydration
- Hyperosmolality

- Hypovolemia
- Diminished renal perfusion
- Hypotension

- Oliguria
- Anuria
- Tissue anoxia
- Blood hyperviscosity

- Acidosis
- Thrombosis

- Seizures
- Shock
- Coma
- Death

This syndrome may appear in a patient who has already been diagnosed with Type 2 diabetes, or it may be the first indication that she has diabetes. Precipitating factors include certain acute and chronic conditions, procedures, and drugs. Acute and chronic conditions include infection, severe emotional stress, myocardial infarction, acute pancreatitis, cerebrovascular accident, GI bleeding, severe burns, uremia, hypothermia, and alcohol intoxication. Procedures that can put a person with Type 2 diabetes at risk for HHNK syndrome include surgery, invasive procedures, dialysis, I.V. hyperali-

mentation, and nasogastric tube feedings. Drugs that can precipitate this syndrome include glucocorticoids, diphenylhydantoin, immunosuppressants, beta-blockers, L-asparaginase, chlorpromazine, diuretics, and diazoxide.

How hyperglycemic hyperosmolar nonketotic syndrome develops

Although the development of HHNK syndrome is similar to that of DKA, the insulin deficiency in

HHNK syndrome isn't absolute. Thus, with some glucose available for energy, lipolysis doesn't occur. Consequently, ketosis and acidosis don't develop.

In HHNK syndrome, as the blood glucose level rises, blood osmolality increases. Intracellular fluid moves into the bloodstream and is excreted by the kidneys. As fluids are lost, the body excretes electrolytes, such as potassium, sodium, and phosphate, causing severe electrolyte imbalances.

The sympathetic nervous system, sensing the body's stress, releases epinephrine, which stimulates gluconeogenesis, further compounding the hyperglycemia. Intracellular dehydration becomes so profound that fluid and oxygen transport to the CNS becomes impaired. Eventually, the result is coma. Dehydration concentrates the blood, increasing the risk of clot formation, thromboemboli, and cardiac, cerebral, and pulmonary infarctions (see *How hyperglycemic hyperosmolar nonketotic syndrome progresses*).

Signs and symptoms

Typically, HHNK syndrome starts slowly. Over days or weeks, the patient experiences extreme thirst and excessive urination. Because these early signs and symptoms may be mistakenly attributed to another cause, appropriate medical care may not begin until after she becomes stuporous or comatose.

Other common signs and symptoms include weight loss, weakness, anorexia, nausea, vomiting, tachycardia, hypotension, orthostatic hypotension, dry skin and mucous membranes, and poor skin turgor. Many patients with HHNK syndrome develop progressive neurologic deterioration, including decreased responsiveness, confusion, lethargy, seizures, focal deficits, paralysis, and hemiparesis or hemisensory loss.

Diagnostic tests

Laboratory tests commonly used to diagnose HHNK syndrome include blood glucose level, urinalysis, arterial blood gas analysis, serum osmolality, BUN level, electrolyte measurements, and hematocrit (see *Testing for hyperglycemic hyperosmolar nonketotic syndrome*).

Testing for hyperglycemic hyperosmolar nonketotic syndrome

If your diabetic patient's laboratory values resemble those shown below, she may have hyperglycemic hyperosmolar nonketotic syndrome.

Laboratory test	Value
Blood glucose level	• > 1,000 mg/dl (may be as high as 2,000 mg/dl)
Urinalysis	• no ketones • glucose present
Arterial blood gas analysis	• slight acidosis
Serum osmolality	• > 330 mOsm/kg
Blood urea nitrogen level	• typically > 60 mg/dl
Serum sodium level	• normal or mildly elevated (typically 145 mEq/L)
Serum potassium level	• varies, may be low, normal, or high
Hematocrit	• commonly high (> 54%)

Treatment

Medical treatment includes rapidly correcting fluid and electrolyte imbalances and hyperglycemia as well as treating the underlying cause.

To replace the patient's fluid volume, the physician may prescribe an isotonic solution, such as 0.9% normal saline solution at a rate of 1 L/hour. After the patient's blood pressure stabilizes (usually, when her systolic pressure exceeds 100 mm Hg), replace the solution with 0.45% normal saline solution, as prescribed. As her blood glucose level drops to between 250 and 300 mg/dl, the physician may add 5% dextrose to the replacement fluid to avoid hypoglycemia.

Add electrolytes, such as potassium and phosphate, to the I.V. fluid, as prescribed. Because profound hypokalemia commonly results from the massive osmotic diuresis, begin replacing potassium within several hours after starting fluid replacement therapy. Before you do, however, ensure that your patient is producing at least 30 ml of urine per hour and that her blood potassium level isn't elevated. The physician may prescribe 20 to 40 mEq of potassium chloride for each liter of fluid. If large doses of potassium replacement are ordered, be sure to monitor your patient's ECG tracings.

To reverse hyperglycemia, the physician may prescribe an infusion of regular insulin at 0.1 units/kg/hour. Stop the infusion when the patient's blood glucose level falls to between 200 to 250 mg/dl, as ordered. Then begin subcutaneous injections, as prescribed. Expect to discontinue insulin therapy when the blood glucose level is under control.

Nursing considerations

As you begin your care, focus on stabilizing your patient's condition, ensuring adequate ventilation, and treating shock, as appropriate. In most cases, your nursing activities and plan of care will revolve around fluid and electrolyte replacement, administering insulin, and preventing such complications as fluid overload.

During fluid replacement, assess your patient's vital signs, intake and output, breath sounds, skin turgor, and mucous membranes. Also, assess her for signs of central venous overload, including jugular vein distention, S_3 heart sounds, tachycardia, increased central venous pressure, dyspnea, and pulmonary crackles. Monitor her electrolyte levels—especially her potassium, sodium, phosphate, and magnesium levels—and assess her for signs and symptoms of electrolyte imbalances.

Assess your patient's neurologic status hourly. If she has a seizure, take seizure precautions: Ensure a patent airway and protect the patient from injury.

If your patient is vomiting, you may have to insert a nasogastric tube. Assess her for bowel sounds and abdominal tenderness. Some patients with autonomic neuropathy develop gastroparesis, which delays gastric emptying. Provide frequent oral care to help moisten her dry lips and mucous membranes and to provide comfort.

Before starting the insulin infusion, flush the tubing with 50 ml of insulin solution to saturate it with insulin. Remember, insulin adheres to I.V. tubing, so if you don't saturate it with insulin, your patient won't receive the full insulin dose. Use an infusion pump to ensure insulin delivery at the prescribed rate.

Monitor the blood glucose level hourly. As it falls, monitor your patient closely for signs and symptoms of hypoglycemia.

Patient teaching

If your patient is confused or unconscious, address your early teaching to her family. During the acute phase of treatment, provide information on the need for fluid and electrolyte replacement, invasive lines, and frequent monitoring.

After your patient's condition stabilizes, teach her about the causes of HHNK syndrome, the signs and symptoms of hyperglycemia, and strategies for preventing HHNK syndrome. Give her complete instructions on using oral antidiabetic drugs and insulin, as appropriate. Explain their expected effects and possible adverse effects. If insulin has been prescribed, observe the patient's administration technique and comment on how she can improve it. Also, be sure she knows how to properly use glucose monitoring equipment.

Reinforce the importance of following the prescribed diet and being aware of the signs and symptoms of hyperglycemia and hypoglycemia. Instruct your patient and her family on emergency care for both conditions.

For an elderly patient with diabetes, help prevent episodes of HHNK syndrome by providing the addresses and telephone numbers of community resources. Many organizations can supply the services of a caregiver or companion to make sure the patient adheres to the drug regimen and prescribed diet.

Somogyi phenomenon

The Somogyi phenomenon is a rebounding of the blood glucose level after an episode of nocturnal hypoglycemia. It results from taking too much insulin late in the day. This uncommon condition primarily affects patients with Type 1 diabetes who inject evening or bedtime doses of insulin (see *Understanding the Somogyi phenomenon*).

Understanding the Somogyi phenomenon

Typically, the Somogyi phenomenon begins when a patient injects an excessive insulin dose late in the day, perhaps at bedtime. At first, the insulin causes nocturnal hypoglycemia, of course. But eventually, the hypoglycemia triggers the release of counterregulatory hormones, which causes rebound hyperglycemia.

If the patient wakes up and discovers that she has fasting hyperglycemia but doesn't know why, she may actually increase her morning insulin dose. Instead of correcting the problem, this action causes the cycle to repeat.

Rather than increasing her morning insulin dose, the patient probably needs to decrease her evening or bedtime insulin dose. She also should check her blood glucose level at 3 A.M. to detect hypoglycemia.

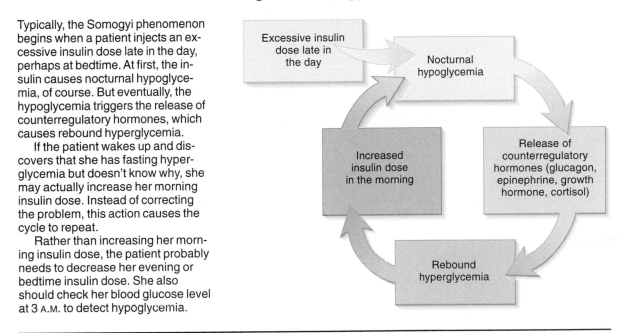

In this phenomenon, the blood glucose level first falls far below normal during the night. When counterregulatory hormones—glucagon, epinephrine, GH, and cortisol—are released, the blood glucose level swings far above normal in the morning, resulting in fasting hyperglycemia.

Signs and symptoms

The Somogyi phenomenon usually produces few signs and symptoms. Typically, if a patient experiences nocturnal hypoglycemia, her blood glucose level will drop at about 3 A.M. If she's asleep, she may toss and turn, perspire more than usual, and have nightmares. If she's awake, she'll notice the characteristic symptoms of hypoglycemia, including irritability, tremors, and hunger. When she awakens the next morning, she may have a headache.

Diagnostic tests

If you suspect the Somogyi phenomenon, check your patient's blood glucose level at 3 A.M. and 7 A.M., using a venipuncture or fingerstick specimen. If she's experiencing the Somogyi phenomenon, the 3 A.M. blood glucose level will be less than 60 mg/dl. By 7 A.M., it will exceed 125 mg/dl.

Treatment

The goal of treatment is to prevent the initial episode of hypoglycemia. The physician may reduce the dosage of the insulin injected before dinner or at bedtime. Also, your patient may need a bedtime snack.

After these changes are made, check her blood glucose level at bedtime, 3 A.M., and 7 A.M. to determine if treatment has been effective.

Patient teaching

Explain to your patient why she needs to lower her evening or bedtime insulin dosage and eat a small bedtime snack. Caution her against eating a large snack, which could contribute to nocturnal and morning hyperglycemia.

Discuss the signs and symptoms of nocturnal hypoglycemia with your patient and her family. Instruct her to report any tremors, night sweats, nightmares, restlessness, or early morning headaches to the physician. Instruct her to check her blood glucose level at 3 A.M. when her insulin doses are being adjusted or when symptoms of hypoglycemia strike.

Dawn phenomenon

The dawn phenomenon is characterized by a rise in the blood glucose level between 4 A.M. and 8 A.M. It is thought to result from the release of GH into the bloodstream in the early morning. This release makes body tissues resistant to insulin, causing the blood glucose level to rise.

Signs and symptoms

The dawn phenomenon produces the typical signs and symptoms of hyperglycemia. However, they usually are not severe because the rise in blood glucose level averages only 30 to 50 mg/dl.

Diagnostic tests

A morning, fasting blood glucose level reveals hyperglycemia. After you determine that your patient has early morning, fasting hyperglycemia, check her blood glucose level at 3 A.M. If she's experiencing the dawn phenomenon, her blood glucose level will begin to rise around 4 A.M.

Treatment

The physician first may advise your patient to reduce or eliminate her evening snack. If this doesn't solve the problem, the physician may prescribe an intermediate-acting dose of insulin at bedtime. If your patient is already administering intermediate-acting insulin at bedtime, the physician may increase the dosage.

Patient teaching

Tell your patient that the morning rise in her blood glucose level probably is caused by her body's release of GH. Emphasize the importance of not eating before bedtime and of administering the bedtime dose of insulin exactly as prescribed.

Explain how occasional monitoring of 3 A.M. and fasting 7 A.M. blood glucose levels can help guide insulin therapy. Make it clear that when she goes home, she should monitor her pre-breakfast blood glucose level and comply with her prescribed drug, diet, and exercise regimens. Instruct her to inform the physician of any abnormal blood glucose level.

5

DIABETES MELLITUS

Chronic Complications

A patient with diabetes mellitus has a high risk of developing chronic complications that can affect just about every body system. If untreated or improperly managed, many of these complications can lead to painful, debilitating, or life-threatening conditions.

Along with other members of the health care team, you're responsible for helping your patient understand that she's at risk for developing microvascular, macrovascular, and neuropathic complications and for teaching her how to prevent them or to slow their progress. If your patient is hospitalized because of chronic complications, you'll need to provide her with thorough teaching about self-care after discharge. To help ensure that she follows through, include family members in your teaching. If your patient will have a home care nurse, she'll evaluate the plan of care continually to determine whether or not the patient is meeting her goals.

Your teaching and plan of care should focus on helping your patient better control her diabetes to postpone or help prevent the onset of complications, detecting signs and symptoms that indicate the onset of complications, and intervening appropriately.

Types of chronic complications

The chronic complications of diabetes are typically classified as microvascular, macrovascular, or neuropathic.

Microvascular complications result from the thickening of capillary and arteriole basement membranes. Although these changes occur in the small blood vessels throughout the body, they most commonly affect the eyes and kidneys, resulting in retinopathy and nephropathy, respectively.

Macrovascular complications of diabetes include coronary artery disease (CAD) and peripheral vascular disease. They result from accelerated atherosclerotic changes in the walls of the coronary arteries and the large and medium blood vessels in the legs and feet.

Diabetic neuropathy, the most common type of chronic complication, can be classified as peripheral (affecting the nerves of the legs and feet), autonomic (affecting involuntary nerves of the internal organs, such as the nerves that innervate the bladder muscles or cardiovascular system), or focal (affecting a single nerve or group of nerves). About 12% of patients have neuropathy when they're diagnosed with diabetes. After 25 years, that number increases to about 60%. If your patient has Type 2 diabetes, she may have sensory and autonomic dysfunction at the time of diagnosis because Type 2 diabetes is commonly diagnosed long after it begins.

As with many other chronic complications of diabetes, the cause of diabetic neuropathy is poorly understood. However, several theories offer possible explanations. In one theory, vascular changes that occur with diabetes may account for many pathophysiologic changes. For example, because many patients with diabetes also have cardiovascular disease, the blood flow to the capillaries that supply nerve tissue may become impaired, resulting in tissue ischemia or necrosis. In another theory, metabolic changes are the culprit. For example, sorbitol and fructose accumulate in the diabetic patient's nerve tissue, and the concentration of *myo*-inositol decreases in the Schwann cells of nerve tissue. Because less *myo*-inositol is available, the myelin sheathes have less protection, and nerve impulses can't be conducted.

Diabetic retinopathy

Diabetic retinopathy, the leading cause of new cases of blindness in the United States, develops more rapidly in patients with Type 1 diabetes than in those with Type 2 diabetes. You're likely to encounter diabetic retinopathy because about 50% of patients have some degree of the disease after they've had diabetes for 10 years. And after having diabetes for 15 years, about 80% of patients have diabetic retinopathy. However, your patient can have diabetic retinopathy and still have unimpaired vision.

Although the underlying cause of diabetic retinopathy isn't fully understood, chronic hyperglycemia, blood platelet abnormalities, and blood vessel narrowing are thought to cause retinal capillary damage. The disease usually occurs in both eyes, but the severity may differ in each eye. Diabetic retinopathy is classified by stage as nonproliferative, preproliferative, or proliferative.

You'll see nonproliferative (or background) retinopathy more commonly than any other stage of the disease. In this stage, the retinal capillaries undergo several changes that impair their ability to transport essential oxygen and nutrients to the retina (see *Inside the eye*). This is what happens: The retinal capillary walls thicken, and capillary fluid leaks through them into the interstitial spaces, causing retinal edema. Eventually, this fluid forms thick yellow deposits, or hard exudates, which can be seen on ophthalmoscopic examination. Also, the retinal capillaries begin to become occluded, and microaneurysms form in the capillary walls. All of these changes cause the capillary walls to bleed easily, resulting in blot hemorrhages in the retina, which are visible on ophthalmoscopic examination.

If the microaneurysms leak into or near the macular area of the retina, macular edema may result. This may cause blurred vision because the macula is the part of the retina that provides the most acute vision. Macular edema, which can occur at any stage of retinopathy, is the most common cause of decreased vision in nonproliferative retinopathy.

Preproliferative retinopathy involves further deterioration and obstruction of the retinal capillaries. Poor capillary perfusion may lead to retinal ischemia and infarction. More hemorrhages occur during this stage, but patients may have no symptoms.

Proliferative retinopathy, the most severe stage of diabetic retinopathy, involves the retina and vitreous cavity. As retinal capillaries become occluded, new blood vessels form to supply blood to the retina (a process called neovascularization). Over time, these new capillaries become fibrous and rupture easily, producing bleeding into the vitreous humor and contraction of the vitreous cavity wall. When blood enters the vitreous humor, light can't reach the retina. Your patient may report seeing red or black spots or lines.

The new fibrous tissue may stick to the cell layer surrounding the vitreous humor. Then the contraction of the fibrous tissue may pull on the vitreous cell layer and the retina, causing your patient to develop tractional retinal detachment. And if the macula is involved, she'll have a complete vision loss.

Signs and symptoms

Your patient may experience no symptoms of diabetic retinopathy, especially in the nonproliferative and preproliferative stages. Symptoms—such as floaters, blurred vision despite corrective lenses, or flashing lights—are generally late indicators of diabetic retinopathy. A diabetic patient should report them immediately to her physician.

Diagnostic tests

To diagnose diabetic retinopathy, an ophthalmologist uses an ophthalmoscopic examination or fluorescein angiography. During an ophthalmoscopic examination, the ophthalmologist dilates the patient's eyes with a mydriatic drug, such as atropine. This dilation permits viewing of the retina, retinal blood vessels, optic disc, macula, and other structures.

The ophthalmologist uses fluorescein angiography to evaluate leaking or occluded retinal vessels. In this outpatient procedure, fluorescein dye is injected into an arm vein. Then the dye travels through the blood to different parts of the body, including the retinal capillaries. By using fluores-

Inside the eye

This cross section shows you the internal structures of the eye. The sclera—the white, opaque outside coat of the eye—helps maintain the eye's shape. The transparent cornea—the anterior, avascular portion of the sclera—permits light to enter the eye. The cornea lies over the pupil and the iris, the colored part of the eye. The aqueous humor, a clear liquid, fills the anterior chamber. The canal of Schlemm, a ring-shaped venous sinus located at the base of the cornea, drains the aqueous humor away from the anterior chamber and into the blood-stream. The avascular lens refracts and focuses images onto the retina.

The choroid, or middle coat, is made up of many arteries and veins. The retina, the innermost coat of the eyeball, is rich in neurons, including the rods and cones, which serve as visual receptors. The retina is connected to the optic nerve, which conducts visual information to the brain. The vitreous humor—a thick, gelatinous material—fills the space behind the lens. It maintains the shape of the eyeball and placement of the retina.

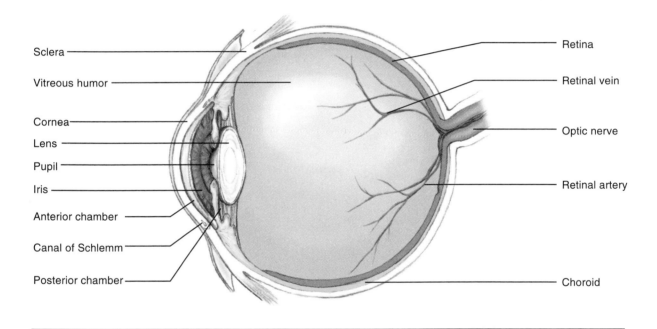

Sclera • Vitreous humor • Cornea • Lens • Pupil • Iris • Anterior chamber • Canal of Schlemm • Posterior chamber • Retina • Retinal vein • Optic nerve • Retinal artery • Choroid

cein dye and a fundus camera with filters, the ophthalmologist can better see the retinal blood vessels and determine if the patient has retinopathy and, if so, to what extent.

Treatment

The treatment of diabetic retinopathy depends on the extent of retinal damage and may include laser photocoagulation or vitrectomy.

With laser photocoagulation, the ophthalmologist uses laser beams to seal microaneurysms and thus reduce their risk of bleeding. Laser photocoagulation can also be used to control new blood vessel growth (see *Understanding laser photocoagulation,* page 78).

The ophthalmologist uses vitrectomy, a surgical procedure, to treat advanced complications of proliferative retinopathy, such as vitreous hemorrhage and tractional retinal detachment.

Vitrectomy requires the use of local or general anesthesia. To begin the procedure, the ophthalmologist makes a small incision behind the cornea. Then he removes blood and fibrous tissue from the vitreous humor and replaces them with

Understanding laser photocoagulation

An ophthalmologist uses laser photocoagulation to seal microaneurysms so that they don't hemorrhage; control the growth of new blood vessels, which may eventually rupture and hemorrhage; and destroy capillaries responsible for plasma and lipid leakage into the retina.

Argon laser photocoagulation, the most common procedure for diabetic retinopathy, uses laser beams to destroy specific aneurysms and new and leaking blood vessels. *Panretinal photocoagulation,* which controls widespread retinal changes, is used to treat patients who have already experienced some bleeding and vision loss and who

have a high risk of more vision loss. In this procedure, the ophthalmologist scatters laser beams across the retina, producing as many as 2,000 burns. These burns reduce the retina's demand for oxygen, which, in turn, reduces new blood vessel growth. In both procedures, the ophthalmologist avoids the macula to protect the patient's visual acuity.

Complications of laser therapy depend on the type and number of treatments. Some patients experience discomfort. Others complain of a slight loss of vision, a decrease in peripheral vision, or impaired night vision.

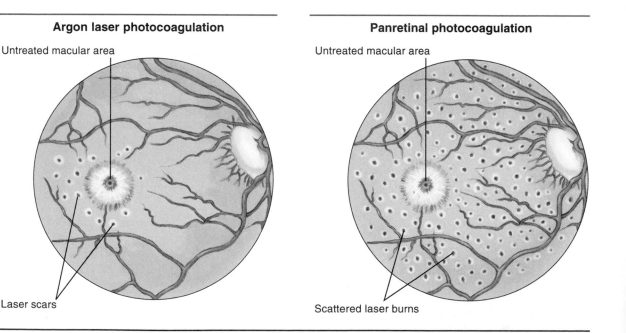

Argon laser photocoagulation

Untreated macular area

Laser scars

Panretinal photocoagulation

Untreated macular area

Scattered laser burns

another fluid, such as normal saline. A silicone oil or gas can be used to hold the retina in place.

Riskier than laser photocoagulation, vitrectomy can result in total vision loss. Because of this, vitrectomy is typically performed on patients with a high risk of complete vision loss—for example, those with bleeding into the vitreous humor and some vision loss that hasn't resolved after 6 months.

Patient teaching

Teach your patient that diabetic retinopathy is a common complication of diabetes and that she may have the disease without experiencing any symptoms.

If your patient has hypertension, explain the relationship between diabetic retinopathy and hypertension, which also damages capillary walls and increases the risk of capillary rupture. Stress the importance of controlling blood pressure and review specific measures she should take, such as controlling her weight and eating a low-sodium diet.

Explain to your patient that uncontrolled hyperglycemia can cause diabetic retinopathy or speed its progression. Encourage her to closely monitor her blood glucose levels at home so that she can keep them as close to normal as possible. Also, encourage her to adjust her diet and exercise in response to her blood glucose levels.

Recommend that all diabetic patients have yearly eye examinations to detect retinopathy early or to monitor its progress. If your patient is pregnant, recommend that she have an examination during the first trimester and then one every 3 months until delivery.

Tell your patient that a routine eye examination includes a history of eye or eye-related symptoms, vision testing, measurement of intraocular pressure, and an ophthalmoscopic examination. Explain to her that the ophthalmoscopic examination is painless but that she may experience minor discomfort when the ophthalmologist administers eyedrops to dilate the pupils. Also, tell her that the eyedrops may cause blurred near-vision and light sensitivity for a short time. Suggest that she arrange for someone to drive her home, and instruct her to wear sunglasses until the effects of the eyedrops wear off.

Tell your patient that if her ophthalmologist suspects diabetic retinopathy but can't confirm it by ophthalmoscopic examination, she may undergo fluorescein angiography. Explain that this procedure is safe and generally painless, that fluorescein is not a radioactive substance, and that the test does not require X-rays. Tell her that she may experience some nausea while the dye is injected. Explain that the fluorescein dye may cause her skin and urine to become yellow for up to 24 hours. Tell her to contact her physician immediately if she experiences an allergic reaction, such as hives or itching.

If your patient has diabetic retinopathy, the ophthalmologist may perform laser photocoagulation therapy. Explain the procedure to your patient and tell her that she may lose some visual acuity, peripheral vision, or night vision. Inform her that during the treatment, she'll see hundreds of bright flashing lights, which may make her feel tired. Although the treatment isn't usually painful, it may be uncomfortable because some parts of the retina are highly sensitive to light. Assure your patient that

she'll receive anesthetic eyedrops to control her discomfort. Explain that the procedure is usually done on an outpatient basis and that she'll have to restrict her activities the following day. She may be required to avoid activities that require the Valsalva maneuver, such as weight lifting, because this will increase her intraocular pressure, which can interfere with healing and cause further retinal damage.

If your patient is undergoing vitrectomy, explain that she may be required to stay overnight in the hospital. Tell her that after surgery she'll wear a pressure patch and eye shield over the treated eye. If a silicone gas or oil is used to hold the retina in place, inform your patient that she may have to lie in a position that keeps the surgical wound toward the back, with the gas or oil above it. She may need to remain in this position for about half of each day for a week after surgery. If indicated, tell her to avoid activities that increase intraocular pressure and to keep her head above her stomach. Explain that her affected eye may be red and sensitive for a short time. Demonstrate how to administer the prescribed eyedrops (see *Teaching your patient to administer eyedrops,* page 80).

If your patient lives alone, assess her ability to prepare her meals and travel to her appointments. If needed, refer her to a home care or other community agency. Also, assess whether impaired vision affects her ability to test her blood glucose levels or to administer the proper dose of insulin. Tell your patient about adaptive tools for blood glucose monitoring that are available for visually impaired patients.

Diabetic nephropathy

In the United States, diabetes is the most common cause of end-stage renal disease, the final stage of nephropathy. Diabetic nephropathy occurs in Type 1 and Type 2 diabetes. About 35% of patients who've had Type 1 diabetes for more than 20 years develop end-stage renal disease. Among those with Type 2 diabetes, the risk of end-stage renal disease may be higher or lower, depending on the patient's ethnic group. African-Americans, Native Americans, and Mexican-Americans are at higher risk than whites. Other risk factors for diabetic nephropathy include hypertension, poor blood glucose control, genetic predisposition, and high protein intake.

Diabetic nephropathy develops over many years. Typically, diabetic nephropathy in patients

HOME CARE

Teaching your patient to administer eyedrops

For your patient with diabetic retinopathy, a physician may prescribe eyedrops to lubricate the eyes, control postoperative pain, or fight infection. To make sure the patient administers the drops correctly, give her these instructions:

1. Wash your hands. Then check the drops for discoloration or sediment. If you see either, return the eyedrops to the pharmacy for a replacement.
2. Warm the eyedrops container by rolling it between your hands for several minutes.
3. Wipe any drainage from your eye with a clean cotton ball or a tissue moistened with water. Always wipe away from your eye, not toward it.
4. Tilt your head back slightly, look up at the ceiling, and pull down your lower eyelid.

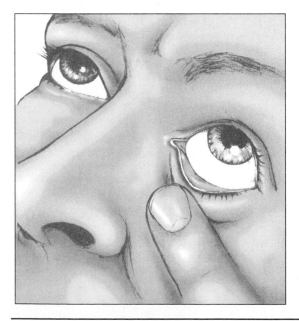

5. Hold the container over the exposed lower part of your eye and place the prescribed number of drops onto the eye. Don't touch the sterile part of the container.

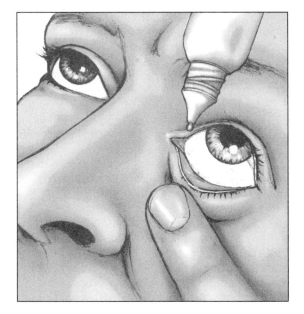

6. Release the lower lid and gently close your eye. Then wipe away excess drops with a clean cotton ball or tissue.
7. Open your eye and keep it open for about 30 seconds. To prevent the eyedrops from being absorbed into your tear duct, gently press on the area where your eyelids join your nose.

with Type 1 diabetes progresses through five stages (see *Stages of diabetic nephropathy*). However, patients with Type 2 diabetes may not progress through these five stages in the same manner as patients with Type 1 diabetes.

The exact cause of kidney destruction in diabetic nephropathy isn't known. What's known is that kidney damage occurs in the glomerulus, which consists of tufts of capillaries in the renal corpuscle, which is surrounded by Bowman's capsule. The glomerular capillaries are made up of three layers of cells: the endothelium, basement membrane, and visceral epithelium. Mesangial cells lie between and support the capillaries.

Stages of diabetic nephropathy

In a patient with Type 1 diabetes, diabetic nephropathy typically progress through five stages.

Stage I
Stage I, which occurs soon after the onset of diabetes, is characterized by renal hypertrophy, an increased glomerular filtration rate (GFR), and an increased glomerular capillary surface area. With tight blood glucose control, the GFR may return to normal. Microalbuminuria may develop, but it can also be reversed with tight blood glucose control.

Stage II
Stage II occurs about 5 years after the onset of diabetes. During this stage, the glomerular capillary basement membrane thickens, and mesangial matrix material accumulates. This reduces the filtration surface area and results in scarring. The GFR remains elevated.

Stage III
Also known as incipient nephropathy, stage III occurs 10 to 15 years after the onset of diabetes. Characteristic signs include persistent microalbuminuria, a high GFR, and increased blood pressure.

Stage IV
Stage IV develops 15 to 25 years after the onset of diabetes. Signs and symptoms include hypertension, retinopathy, and proteinuria that can be detected by a urine dipstick test. The GFR steadily decreases. Intensive treatment at this stage can help slow the progression of the disease to stage V.

Stage V
In stage V, renal failure progresses to the point that the patient needs dialysis or a kidney transplant. This stage generally occurs 20 to 30 years after the onset of diabetes. Signs include elevated blood urea nitrogen and creatinine levels and a rapid decline in the GFR.

Normally, blood enters the glomerulus through the afferent arteriole and exits by the efferent arteriole. As blood passes through the glomerulus, water, electrolytes, creatinine, urea nitrogen, and glucose filter across the capillary basement membrane into Bowman's capsule. This filtrate is similar to blood plasma, but it doesn't normally contain proteins. After the filtrate enters Bowman's capsule, it flows through the tubules of the kidney and is eventually excreted from the body.

In diabetic nephropathy, kidney destruction results from gradual structural changes in the glomerulus. First, the glomerulus enlarges. Then glomerulosclerosis—the replacement of normal glomerular tissue with fibrous scar tissue—occurs. In diffuse glomerulosclerosis, the more common type, the basement membrane of the glomerular capillaries thickens and eventually leaks capillary fluid. Also, the mesangial matrix (the spongy network surrounding the mesangial cells) thickens. In nodular glomerulosclerosis, hyaline nodules (hard masses of glassy, eosinophilic substances) form in the mesangial part of the glomerulus. In both types of glomerulosclerosis, the sclerotic changes disrupt the function of increasing numbers of glomeruli, slowly impairing the patient's renal function.

Signs and symptoms

In the early stages of diabetic nephropathy, a patient usually doesn't experience symptoms. Typically, symptoms occur when her glomerular filtration rate (GFR) is 20% to 30% of normal. The GFR reflects the amount of plasma that passes through the glomerulus per minute. When signs and symptoms develop, they may affect virtually every body system and include:
- polyuria, nocturia, proteinuria, oliguria progressing to anuria
- hypertension, heart failure, pulmonary edema, peripheral edema, arrhythmias, pericarditis
- crackles, shortness of breath, dyspnea, Kussmaul's respirations, pleural effusion, depressed cough reflex, thick sputum, pneumonitis
- anorexia, constipation or diarrhea, hiccups, nausea, vomiting, stomatitis, unpleasant or metallic taste in the mouth

- altered level of consciousness, behavior changes, cognitive changes, lethargy, seizures, coma
- muscle cramps, bone fractures, footdrop
- anemia, increased risk of bleeding, infection
- decreased perspiration; dry, brittle hair; dry, flaky skin; yellow-brown skin; petechiae; pruritus; thin, brittle, ridged nails; uremic frost (urea crystals that form on the skin)
- infertility; decreased libido; anovulation, amenorrhea, anorgasmy in women; impotence in men.

Diagnostic tests

Usually, when a patient is diagnosed with diabetes, the physician orders a complete urinalysis to check for glucose and ketones, but the focus of diagnostic testing is early detection of microalbuminuria. Albumin, one of the most important blood proteins, starts to leak into the urine early in diabetic nephropathy, causing microalbuminuria. If albumin is detected in a routine urinalysis, your patient will need to provide a 24-hour urine sample. Normally, a person excretes 30 mg of albumin in 24 hours. The physician will diagnose microalbuminuria—and diabetic nephropathy— if your patient excretes albumin at a rate of 31 to 299 mg/day or 20 to 199 µ/minute, measured on three different occasions over 6 months.

If your diabetic patient has a normal urine albumin excretion level, then urine albumin and renal function tests should be performed annually. Keep in mind that a urine dipstick test for protein can't detect mild to moderate increases in albumin.

Serum creatinine and blood urea nitrogen (BUN) levels may be used as indirect measurements of the GFR. Normally, the GFR ranges from 100 to 125 ml/minute. Serum creatinine and BUN levels increase as kidney function deteriorates. A doubling of the creatinine level may reflect a 50% reduction in the GFR.

However, these tests aren't always reliable at detecting early nephropathy, and they're not reliable in patients with diminished muscle mass, such as elderly or malnourished individuals, or in those who have protein restrictions, such as patients with advanced renal disease. Also, BUN levels vary based on your patient's hydration or the presence of other disorders, such as liver disease.

Creatinine clearance also measures the GFR. If your patient has diabetic nephropathy, creatinine clearance will be decreased because her glomeruli can't adequately filter the blood.

Treatment

Although diabetic nephropathy has no cure, certain interventions can slow its progress. These interventions include closely controlling blood glucose levels, using antihypertensive therapy, restricting protein intake, treating urinary tract infections (UTIs), withholding nephrotoxic drugs and dyes, and using dialysis and transplantation.

Glucose control
Tight blood glucose control—maintaining glucose levels as close to normal as possible without increasing the frequency or severity of hypoglycemic episodes—can help delay the onset and slow the progression of nephropathy. Tight blood glucose control also can reverse microalbuminuria in some patients. However, tight blood glucose control doesn't affect the course of advanced nephropathy.

Antihypertensive drug therapy
Aggressive antihypertensive therapy may slow the progression of diabetic nephropathy. Certain antihypertensive drugs, such as angiotensin-converting enzyme (ACE) inhibitors and calcium channel blockers, may be used to treat hypertension. They also inhibit diabetic nephropathy in hypertensive patients and in normotensive patients with microalbuminuria.

However, ACE inhibitors may cause hyperkalemia and should be used cautiously if your patient has renal failure. Expect to avoid thiazide diuretics and beta-blockers because thiazide diuretics may worsen hyperlipidemia and hyperglycemia, and beta-blockers may mask or alter the symptoms of hypoglycemia.

Protein restriction
Restricting your patient's protein intake can reduce the rate of urine albumin excretion and kidney deterioration. The typical dietary protein intake in the United States is 1.2 to 1.4 g/kg/day. The physician may prescribe a diet that limits protein intake to 0.8 g/kg/day or less. For exam-

ple, if your patient weighs 143 lb (65 kg), she may be limited to 52 grams of protein per day.

Therapy for urinary tract infections

If your patient develops a UTI, her risk of renal dysfunction increases. If she has signs and symptoms of a UTI, such as dysuria (burning on urination), urinary frequency or urgency, or foul-smelling urine, the physician may request a urine sample for culture and sensitivity testing. And if your patient has an infection, the physician will prescribe an antibiotic. Before administering the antibiotic, however, check a current drug reference to determine if the drug is contraindicated or requires cautious use in a patient with a kidney disease, such as nephropathy.

Nephrotoxic drug and dye restrictions

Your patient may be taking nephrotoxic drugs, such as an aminoglycoside or a nonsteroidal anti-inflammatory drug (NSAID). If so, the physician will monitor her kidney function by testing her serum creatinine levels. If your patient has impaired kidney function, the physician may adjust her drug dosage based on her GFR or creatinine clearance or prescribe a less nephrotoxic drug.

Radiographic dyes also are nephrotoxic. If your patient must undergo a test that requires radiographic dye, the physician may prescribe I.V. mannitol to be given 1 hour before the test to induce osmotic diuresis and minimize nephrotoxic effects.

Dialysis and transplantation

A patient with end-stage renal disease may need hemodialysis or peritoneal dialysis, or she may be a candidate for a kidney transplant. Many patients who undergo hemodialysis develop sclerotic blood vessels from the numerous needle punctures at the dialysis access site. Eventually, they may have no more access sites to continue hemodialysis. These patients may be good candidates for peritoneal dialysis or kidney transplant (see *Understanding dialysis,* pages 84 and 85).

A donor kidney for a transplant can be obtained from a living relative, a living unrelated person, or a cadaver. A transplanted kidney has a 75% to 80% chance of functioning for at least 5 years. However, kidney transplants have many drawbacks:

- Donor kidneys are in short supply. Depending on your patient's blood type and whether she has certain proteins or antibodies, she may never be offered a kidney.
- The risk of organ rejection is high, especially in the first year after the transplant.
- Expensive, long-term therapy with immunosuppressants is needed to help prevent organ rejection.
- Immunosuppression may lead to infection or malignancy.
- Immunosuppression makes tight glucose control more difficult.

Patients who test positive for the human immunodeficiency virus or who have a malignancy aren't candidates for kidney transplant. Those with psychosis, active infection, severe neuropathies, or inoperable cardiovascular disease may not be approved for the procedure. Transplant complications include thrombosis, infection, anastomotic leaks (usually at the ureters), bleeding, and adverse effects of immunosuppression.

Nursing considerations

Monitor your patient's blood glucose levels frequently. As her kidney function deteriorates, she may need less insulin or oral hypoglycemic drugs. That's because one-third of insulin is metabolized and excreted by the kidneys, and as her kidney function deteriorates, insulin is available in the bloodstream for a longer time. Monitor her for signs and symptoms of hypoglycemia, such as diaphoresis, nausea, or vomiting. If she shows signs of hypoglycemia, the physician may reduce her insulin dosage. Or, if your patient takes an oral antidiabetic drug, the physician may prescribe glipizide, which has a shorter half-life than other drugs and is metabolized by the liver to inactive metabolites for excretion by the kidneys.

If your patient has hypertension, assess her for factors, such as obesity or alcohol consumption, that may contribute to hypertension. Also, review her current drug use. Many drugs can increase blood pressure, including corticosteroids, NSAIDs, nasal decongestants, appetite suppressants, and tricyclic antidepressants. During physical examinations, monitor your patient's blood pressure and compare the readings to those in her medical record.

Understanding dialysis

If your patient develops end-stage renal disease, she may require hemodialysis or peritoneal dialysis to prolong her life. The physician probably won't recommend dialysis until your patient's serum creatinine level is about 6 mg/dl.

Hemodialysis

For hemodialysis, the surgeon creates an arteriovenous (AV) access site, usually in the patient's arm, as shown. With each hemodialysis treatment, a needle is inserted into this AV access site. Blood is withdrawn through the arterial line and pumped through a semipermeable membrane in the hemo-

dialysis machine. As the blood is pumped, dialysate moves through the membrane in the opposite direction, allowing body wastes to move by diffusion from an area of high concentration to an area of low concentration.

The pores in the membrane allow electrolytes, blood urea nitrogen, and creatinine to be filtered out, but they prevent larger particles such as blood cells and protein from passing through. The filtered blood is then returned to the patient through the venous line.

Hemodialysis can be performed in your patient's home or in a medical facility. Treatments average 3 to 4 hours, three times each week.

Arteriovenous access for hemodialysis

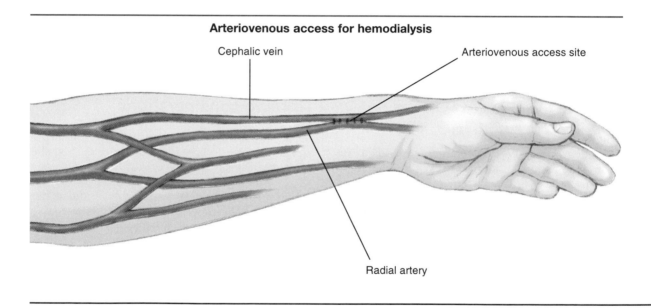

Cephalic vein

Arteriovenous access site

Radial artery

Assess your patient for signs and symptoms of UTI. Frequent infections can speed the progression of nephropathy. If diabetic neuropathy affects her bladder, she may not be able to empty it completely. This may result in urinary stasis, which can increase the risk of infection. To help prevent UTIs, encourage your patient to empty her bladder at least every 2 hours.

Determine whether your patient is taking any nephrotoxic drugs. If she is, inform her physician. If she must undergo a procedure that requires the use of radiographic dye, administer

mannitol as prescribed to induce osmotic diuresis and minimize the dye's nephrotoxic effects. Also, make sure your patient drinks all prescribed fluids after the procedure to dilute her urine, which may decrease the chance of nephrotoxicity from the dye.

If your patient is receiving hemodialysis or peritoneal dialysis, help her adhere to the prescribed diet and fluid restrictions. If she must follow a low-protein diet, advise her to minimize her intake of eggs, meat, and milk products and to eat more starchy food, fats, fruits, and veg-

Peritoneal dialysis

In this closed-drainage procedure, a catheter is placed through an opening in the abdominal wall. At regular intervals, dialysate is instilled into the peritoneal cavity. Through osmosis and diffusion, fluid, electrolytes, and waste products are drawn from the blood, across the peritoneum, and into the dialysate. The peritoneum, which lines the peritoneal cavity, acts as a semipermeable membrane. The dialysate is drained regularly and replaced.

Most patients tolerate peritoneal dialysis better than hemodialysis. The patient's blood pressure usually remains stable, and she experiences less cardiovascular stress and better control of her blood glucose levels. She'll also have a decreased risk of retinal hemorrhage because she won't need the higher doses of heparin that are used with hemodialysis. However, peritoneal dialysis places the patient at higher risk for developing an infection, such as peritonitis.

Catheter placement for peritoneal dialysis

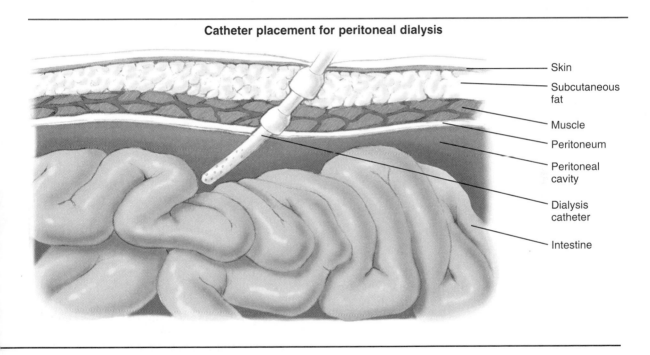

Skin

Subcutaneous fat

Muscle

Peritoneum

Peritoneal cavity

Dialysis catheter

Intestine

etables. If she has difficulty consuming sufficient calories to maintain her weight, suggest that she use a high-calorie nutritional supplement. Keep in mind, however, that peritoneal dialysis can increase calorie absorption from the dialysate as it sits in the peritoneum. If this causes your patient to gain excess weight, urge her to reduce her total calorie intake but not her protein intake. Monitor your patient's fluid and electrolyte status by checking her weight every day.

During each dialysis treatment, assess your patient's arteriovenous (AV) or peritoneal access site for signs and symptoms of infection, such as redness, tenderness, or purulent drainage. Also, assess circulation at the AV shunt or fistula by checking for a palpable thrill; auscultating for a bruit, which should be present; and feeling for warmth over the access site. Don't take a blood pressure reading in the arm that has the AV access site because you may occlude it.

Remember that treatment options for end-stage renal disease may involve difficult choices for your patient and her family. Provide your patient with the information she'll need to make an

Patient teaching: Collecting a 24-hour urine sample

If your patient needs to collect a 24-hour urine sample, teach her these key points to ensure the accuracy of the test results:
- Advise her to post the hours for the timed collection in a conspicuous place, such as over the toilet, so that she doesn't forget.
- Instruct her to write on the urine container the dates and times she starts and stops the urine collection.
- Tell her to keep the urine container in the refrigerator or to store it on ice. If she stores it on ice, she should replace the ice as it melts.
- Instruct the patient to begin the 24-hour collection period by urinating directly into the toilet and then collecting her urine in the container the next time she urinates. Tell her to save all her urine over the next 24 hours.
- Advise your patient to urinate before—not immediately after—a bowel movement to avoid contaminating the sample. Also, remind her not to put toilet paper in the urine sample.
- Tell her to urinate at the end of the 24 hours and to include this urine sample in the timed collection.

informed choice. Keep in mind, however, that her ability to concentrate and think clearly may be affected by uremia. Therefore, if appropriate, delay important decisions about treatment options until after a dialysis treatment.

Provide support and encourage your patient to talk about her feelings and concerns. People respond in various ways when they hear the diagnosis of kidney disease. Your patient may develop depression, anxiety, or stress. So include meetings with a mental health professional, such as a psychiatric clinical nurse specialist or psychologist, as part of your treatment plan. If appropriate, refer your patient and her family to support groups.

If your patient is waiting for a kidney transplant, keep in mind that finding a suitable organ donor takes a long time and places a significant strain on the patient and her family. After your patient undergoes the transplant, her physician will prescribe immunosuppressant drugs. The patient will need to take them for the rest of her life, and they can have serious adverse effects, such as increased risk of infection, weight gain, hallucinations, and increased kidney damage.

The physician will probably adjust your patient's insulin dosage after a kidney transplant because of improved kidney function. And your patient will be taking drugs, such as glucocorticosteroids and cyclosporine, that will increase her blood glucose levels.

Patient teaching

Discuss potential kidney complications of diabetes with your patient and her family. Emphasize the relationship between tight blood glucose control and the onset and progression of kidney disease. Explain the importance of achieving and maintaining a healthy weight, following a safe exercise plan, stopping smoking, and controlling blood cholesterol levels. Explain dietary restrictions, including protein limitation, and refer your patient to a dietitian.

Inform your patient about the association between hypertension and renal disease. Explain that she'll need to have her blood pressure checked regularly, and emphasize the importance of treating her hypertension. Encourage her to report any adverse effects of antihypertensive drugs to her physician. Remind her not to stop antihypertensive therapy without notifying her physician.

Review the signs and symptoms of UTI and the importance of prompt and thorough treatment. Explain the importance of providing a follow-up urine sample for culture and sensitivity testing, if prescribed. Review the procedure for collecting a 24-hour urine sample (see *Patient teaching: Collecting a 24-hour urine sample*). Advise your patient to delay or reschedule screening for urine albumin excretion if she recently participated in strenuous exercise or had an acute febrile illness or a UTI. These factors can temporarily increase urine albumin excretion. Ask your patient if she's taking drugs, such as NSAIDs and ACE inhibitors. These drugs can alter urine protein excretion and should be avoided during testing.

If the patient is receiving hemodialysis or peritoneal dialysis at home, a home care nurse can provide the support and education she needs to perform the procedure independently. In some cases, a family member may need to be taught how to perform it. Or the home care nurse may have to do it.

Coronary artery disease

The most common cause of death in patients with Type 2 diabetes, CAD also develops in many patients with Type 1 diabetes. Patients who have had diabetes for 20 years or longer, are over age 40, or have many cardiovascular risk factors, such as hypertension, obesity, or lipid abnormalities, have a high risk of developing CAD. Men and women with diabetes develop CAD at about the same age.

The development of atherosclerotic changes in the coronary arteries is closely related to the duration and severity of diabetes. The prolonged high levels of blood glucose, free fatty acids, and cholesterol damage the endothelial layer of the arteries. Monocytes adhere to the damaged arteries, and macrophages migrate to these areas. If your patient also has hypertension, the high pressure of blood flowing through the vessels increases the endothelial damage.

This all contributes to lipid accumulation and the development of atherosclerotic plaque. The macrophages release growth factor, which stimulates smooth-muscle cells to enlarge, multiply, and migrate through the layers of the arteries. This further narrows the lumen of the arteries. At the same time, increased numbers of platelets adhere to the damaged endothelium, which causes thrombus formation. If your patient has hyperglycemia, platelets are more likely to adhere to the artery wall. The combination of endothelial damage and increased platelet aggregation leads to accelerated thickening of the lumen, which results in vasoconstriction.

If your patient has insulin resistance, her triglyceride and lipoprotein levels will be elevated, which can damage the endothelial lining even further. Her pancreas produces excessive amounts of substandard insulin to overcome the body's resistance to insulin. So, her body does not have sufficient, effective insulin, which is required to produce lipoprotein lipase, the enzyme that regulates cholesterol.

Progressive atherosclerosis, of course, reduces coronary artery blood flow, which increases the risk of developing myocardial ischemia and infarction.

If your patient has a myocardial infarction (MI), she's at risk for developing diabetic ketoacidosis (DKA). The stress of an MI causes the release of adrenal corticosteroids and catecholamines, which inhibit insulin action and stimulate glucose production. As the glucose level rises, the heart and other vital organs are deprived of their main energy source. As a protective mechanism, the body begins to break down fat to use as a substitute energy source. Fat breakdown is incomplete, causing excessive amounts of ketones to be released into the bloodstream. Because the kidneys can't adequately excrete the ketones, DKA develops. This condition results in electrolyte disturbances, which can lead to life-threatening cardiac arrhythmias.

Signs and symptoms

Your patient may be admitted with the typical signs and symptoms of myocardial ischemia or an MI: chest pain or heaviness with exertion, shortness of breath, diaphoresis, nausea, or vomiting. However, if your diabetic patient has autonomic neuropathy, she may not experience the typical warning signs or symptoms and may have what's commonly called a silent MI.

Diagnostic tests

Tests commonly used to diagnose CAD include electrocardiography, echocardiography, exercise stress testing, coronary angiography, and radionuclide imaging.

Electrocardiography
The electrocardiogram (ECG), which reflects the heart's electrical activity, can detect signs of ischemia, injury, and infarction as well as abnormalities in heart rate and rhythm. However, it doesn't always detect ischemia, injury, and infarction. For example, a patient who has had a transmural MI (an infarction that extends through the entire myocardial wall) usually has a characteristic abnormal Q wave on her ECG. But if the MI only extends through the subendocardial layer, the remaining healthy tissue can still conduct electrical

impulses, and an abnormal Q wave won't appear on the ECG. In general, patients with diabetes are more likely to have this type of an MI.

Echocardiography

An echocardiogram, which records ultrasonic waves reflected off the heart, evaluates the heart's size, shape, and motion. This test can detect changes caused by CAD, such as an increase in the mass of the left ventricular wall, which is more common in patients with diabetes and may by worsened by hypertension. In this way, it identifies patients who are at risk for other cardiac problems, such as an MI and heart failure.

Exercise stress test

Exercise stress testing is a variation of the standard ECG. During this test, the patient's heart rate, heart rhythm, and blood pressure are monitored while she rides a stationary bicycle, walks on a treadmill, or climbs stairs. As the patient's activity level increases, her ECG tracing may show changes if her myocardium doesn't receive enough oxygen and nutrients.

If your patient has CAD or is suspected of having it, exercise stress testing can assess the effects of physical stress on her heart. If she is recovering from an MI or coronary artery bypass surgery, this test can also help predict her response to rehabilitation.

Coronary angiography

A radiographic test, coronary angiography is used to detect coronary artery stenosis or occlusion and to assess the condition of blood vessels beyond the occlusion. In some cases, angiography may be used to guide coronary angioplasty or atherectomy, which may be performed to remove the occlusion. However, angiography should only be used in patients for whom the test will provide vital diagnostic data because its radiographic contrast medium can cause renal impairment, especially in patients who already have nephropathy.

Radionuclide imaging

A patient who has had an MI may undergo radionuclide imaging, which can evaluate the location and extent of myocardial damage. Radionuclide imaging involves the injection of a radioactive substance, such as thallium or technetium Tc 99m pyrophosphate, into the patient's bloodstream. Depending on the specific test, the degree to which the radioactive substance concentrates in the myocardial tissue helps distinguish between normal and abnormal tissue. It can also show the extent and size of an MI.

Treatment

If your patient has CAD, teach her to reduce her risk of developing complications, such as angina and an MI, by eliminating or reducing these modifiable risk factors:
- hyperglycemia
- hypertension
- hypercholesterolemia
- obesity
- cigarette smoking.

Also, teach her about any prescribed drugs or invasive treatments for managing CAD.

Risk factor management

Hyperglycemia, a risk factor for cardiovascular disease, is always your diabetic patient's first priority. A combination of diet, exercise, drugs, and stress reduction can help your patient keep her blood glucose levels as close to normal as possible. Encourage her to monitor her blood glucose levels at home so that she can adjust different aspects of her treatment as needed. Keep in mind, however, that the physician may modify your patient's treatment after a severe cardiac problem to achieve stricter blood glucose control. That's because avoidance of severe hypoglycemia is crucial to preventing arrhythmias, which can lead to more serious cardiac problems, such as an MI.

Hypertension accelerates the vascular changes of already compromised coronary arteries. Monitor your patient's blood pressure frequently. If her blood pressure exceeds 140/85 mm Hg on two separate occasions, she's considered hypertensive. The physician may prescribe lifestyle modifications, such as a low-sodium diet, alcohol restriction, and regular exercise. If 3 months of nonpharmacologic therapy don't reduce your patient's diastolic blood pressure below 90 mm Hg, the physician may prescribe an antihypertensive drug, such as an ACE inhibitor. If your patient's diastolic pressure exceeds 110 mm Hg or if she has microalbuminuria, the physician may prescribe an antihypertensive drug immediately in conjunction with lifestyle modifications.

Many patients with diabetes are at risk for CAD because they have hypercholesterolemia.

HEALTH PROMOTION

Helping your patient stop smoking

If your patient is a smoker, chances are she has been smoking for a long time and may not be willing to give it up just because you tell her she has to. So you'll need to explain how cigarette smoking puts her at high risk for developing serious, life-threatening complications, including coronary artery disease (CAD) and myocardial infarction (MI).

How smoking affects the arteries
The chemicals in cigarette smoke cause damage to the coronary artery endothelium, which has already been damaged by diabetes. These chemicals also increase total cholesterol and triglyceride levels and reduce high-density lipoprotein levels. All of these changes lead to coronary artery occlusion and myocardial ischemia or MI. Nicotine, a powerful vasoconstrictor, causes vasospasm and increases blood pressure, blood viscosity, and clotting factor concentrations, further reducing coronary artery blood flow.

Nursing interventions
- If your patient doesn't smoke but lives with someone who does, explain the dangers of passive smoke, which can be as harmful as smoking itself. Encourage the family member to quit smoking. If he can't quit, instruct him not to smoke around the patient.
- If your patient does smoke, find out how much she smokes and how motivated she is to quit.
- If your patient has tried to quit but hasn't been successful, encourage her to try again. Ask which methods she has tried and ask her why she thinks they didn't work.
- Address her concerns about quitting. For instance, your patient may be afraid that she'll gain weight. If so, encourage her to seek support from her family and an appropriate weight-control support group.
- Discuss with the patient's physician the possibility of using a transdermal nicotine delivery system or nicotine chewing gum. However, remember that these nicotine products, just like cigarettes, may be contraindicated in patients who have CAD or arrhythmias because nicotine causes vasoconstriction, tachycardia, and increased blood pressure. In patients with diabetes, nicotine causes the release of catecholamines from the adrenal medulla, which can cause arrhythmias and other cardiovascular complications.
- Refer your patient to a support group or smoking cessation program. Even if the physician prescribes a nicotine product to offset withdrawal, she may need additional support to help change her behavior.

Even those with normal or near-normal total cholesterol levels may be at risk because their heart-protective, high-density lipoprotein (HDL) levels are abnormally low, and their low-density lipoprotein (LDL) levels are abnormally high. Typically, a low-cholesterol, low-fat diet is recommended for patients whose total cholesterol level exceeds 200 mg/dl and whose LDL level exceeds 130 mg/dl. Encourage your patient to reduce her total fat intake to less than 30% of her total calories and her saturated fat intake to less than 10% of her total calories. If 6 months of diet therapy and exercise don't reduce your patient's LDL level to 160 mg/dl or less, the physician may prescribe a lipid-lowering agent, such as lovastatin.

To help your patient reduce her weight, the physician may prescribe an individualized diet and exercise plan. The goals of the weight-loss program are to help improve your patient's blood glucose levels and better control her blood pressure. She can achieve these goals with even a modest weight loss of 10 to 15 pounds. Help your patient understand that a large weight loss followed by a weight gain is stressful to her body. Instead, encourage her to maintain her weight and blood glucose levels by controlling her food portions, eating balanced nutritious meals, and eating her meals at the same time each day.

If your diabetic patient smokes, she should stop. To help ease her withdrawal symptoms, her physician may prescribe nicotine in a dermal delivery system or a chewing gum. The physician may also encourage her to attend a support group (see *Helping your patient stop smoking*).

Drug therapy

Your patient's physician may prescribe one or more drugs to manage CAD and help prevent its complications.

To treat coronary artery insufficiency, the physician may prescribe a beta-blocker, such as propranolol. But if your patient is using insulin, she may not be able to take beta-blockers because these drugs can impair insulin secretion and alter or mask the signs and symptoms of hypoglycemia. Without the typical warning signs and symptoms of hypoglycemia—such as dizziness, diaphoresis, or nausea—your patient may not realize that her blood glucose level has fallen dangerously low. However, some patients who use insulin can tolerate low doses of cardioselective beta-blockers, such as atenolol, metoprolol, or acebutolol.

If your patient has had an MI, the physician may prescribe aspirin to reduce the risk of further complications of CAD.

If she has angina, the physician may prescribe a nitrate, such as a nitroglycerin patch. Although the nitrate won't interfere with blood glucose control, it can produce severe hypotension. So monitor your patient's blood pressure and teach her about the signs and symptoms of hypotension, such as light-headedness when changing from a lying position to a standing one.

If your diabetic patient has heart failure and hypertension, drug therapy may pose problems. If she also has autonomic neuropathy and orthostatic hypotension, calcium channel blockers may be inappropriate. Although ACE inhibitors have been used successfully in patients with diabetes, they can increase serum potassium levels, requiring close monitoring for signs of hyperkalemia. Thiazide diuretics can raise blood glucose levels and reduce potassium levels, requiring close monitoring for signs of hypoglycemia and hypokalemia. They may also cause impotence or orthostatic hypotension, especially in a patient with autonomic neuropathy.

Invasive treatments

Patients with CAD may also benefit from invasive treatments. In those with coronary ischemia or MI, percutaneous transluminal coronary angioplasty can restore blood flow in blocked coronary arteries. However, if a patient with nephropathy receives radiographic dye during this nonsurgical invasive procedure, she may develop further kidney problems. Coronary artery bypass surgery may also be performed in diabetic patients. However, high glucose levels during surgery can increase the risk of postoperative complications and death.

Patient teaching

Before your patient is discharged, review with her any necessary lifestyle changes, such as lowering her blood pressure or controlling hyperglycemia. Explain that lifestyle changes can control CAD, but they can't cure it. Also, review her prescribed diet and drugs and the signs and symptoms of complications.

Instruct your patient with diabetes to reduce her saturated fat intake to less than 10% of her total calories. If she also has hypertension, urge her to reduce her dietary sodium intake to 2,400 mg per day. If your patient's LDL level is elevated, suggest that she reduce her saturated fat intake to less than 7% of total calories and her cholesterol intake to less than 300 mg per day. Refer your patient to a dietitian who will review the prescribed diet with her and her family.

If your patient is taking prescribed drugs, go over their names, dosages, actions, and adverse effects. If she's taking a beta-blocker, tell her to check her blood glucose levels frequently because the drug may mask the symptoms of hypoglycemia. If blood glucose control is ineffective, tell her to contact the physician immediately. Also, review the procedure for blood glucose monitoring, and observe as the patient demonstrates her technique.

Explain that she may be unable to distinguish the symptoms of angina from those of hypoglycemia. Instruct her to treat hypoglycemia first as she normally would. Then advise her to take sublingual nitroglycerin. If symptoms persist, tell your patient to take two more nitroglycerin tablets, 5 minutes apart. If after taking the third tablet she doesn't experience relief, she should seek emergency medical help.

Explain that patients with diabetes and CAD may have recurring complications. If she experiences any respiratory changes (such as dyspnea or a cough), urinary frequency, or edema in her feet or legs, instruct her to contact the physician immediately. If your patient has a home care nurse, explain that the nurse will carefully assess her for subtle changes that suggest her condition is deteriorating.

If your patient is beginning a cardiac rehabilitation exercise program, tell her to monitor her blood glucose levels frequently and eat several small snacks to reduce the likelihood of developing hypoglycemia. For example, if she exercises for 30 minutes, she may need a snack that has about 15 grams of carbohydrate, which equals one starch or fruit serving. Her blood glucose level should be her guide.

Peripheral vascular disease

Peripheral vascular disease is more common and occurs at a younger age in people with diabetes than in the general population. Among nondiabetic patients, far more men than women develop peripheral vascular disease. However, among those with diabetes, almost as many women as men develop it.

Nondiabetic patients with peripheral vascular disease usually develop a single arterial occlusion in one leg and have normal collateral blood vessels. However, patients with diabetes usually develop several occlusions in both legs and have poor collateral circulation.

In patients who have diabetes and peripheral vascular disease, hyperglycemia, uncontrolled hypertension, or other factors can lead to atherosclerotic changes in the peripheral arteries. These changes may include capillary basement membrane thickening and increased platelet adhesion. They may lead to arterial occlusion, which diminishes the oxygen supply to the tissues, and subsequent muscle tissue ischemia and pain. Unfortunately, the diabetic patient's poor tissue perfusion and impaired small vessels may reduce her ability to develop good collateral circulation to bypass the occlusion (see *Understanding impaired collateral circulation,* pages 92 and 93).

If your diabetic patient has hyperlipidemia, she's at even greater risk for developing peripheral vascular disease. If she smokes, she'll experience further compromised circulation. Smoking increases the progression of atherosclerosis by increasing LDL and triglyceride levels and decreasing HDL levels. It also raises the blood pressure, which can damage the arterial endothelium. The nicotine in cigarettes induces vasospasm and increases blood viscosity and clotting

factor concentrations, which helps diminish arterial circulation.

If peripheral vascular disease is untreated, your patient may develop infections or even gangrene in her legs, which may lead to amputation. More than half of all nontraumatic amputations of the lower leg are caused by peripheral vascular disease in patients with diabetes.

Signs and symptoms

Intermittent claudication—cramping or aching pain in the calf, thigh, or buttock while walking that's relieved by rest—is commonly the chief symptom of peripheral vascular disease. Total or partial arterial occlusion, which causes the pain, prevents sufficient blood from reaching the muscle that's being used. The patient may also experience leg pain at night that's relieved by standing.

Other signs and symptoms include:
- diminished or absent pulses distal to the occlusion
- shiny, scaly skin
- loss of subcutaneous fat and tissue
- hair loss of the leg or foot
- thickened toenails from fungal infections
- slow capillary refill
- skin blanching of the foot when it's elevated
- gangrene
- wounds that don't respond to treatment
- ulcerations over bony prominences and pressure points of the feet and toes
- cold or numb feet.

Keep in mind that patients with neuropathy may not experience the typical signs and symptoms—especially pain—because of nerve damage associated with peripheral or autonomic neuropathy.

Diagnostic tests

To diagnose peripheral vascular disease, the physician may use Doppler ultrasonography, plethysmography, or arteriography.

Doppler ultrasonography, a noninvasive test, evaluates how fast blood flows through an artery and confirms arterial occlusion. This test uses a transducer to direct high-frequency sound waves toward the artery that's being evaluated. When the sound waves strike red blood cells (RBCs)

Understanding impaired collateral circulation

Collateral circulation develops in response to an arterial occlusion, as shown in the first three illustrations. In the first illustration, arterial blood flow is normal. In the second, collateral circulation develops to bypass a partial arterial occlusion. In the third, collateral circulation bypasses a total arterial occlusion, providing blood, oxygen, and nutrients to the area beyond the occlusion and preventing tissue ischemia and infarction.

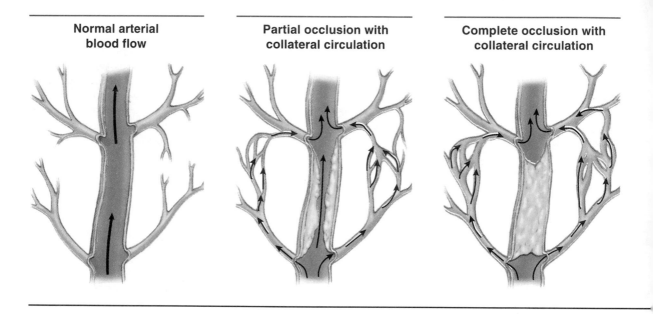

| Normal arterial blood flow | Partial occlusion with collateral circulation | Complete occlusion with collateral circulation |

moving through the artery, they're reflected to the transducer. The frequency with which the sound waves are reflected indicates the speed and strength of the blood flow. The sound waves are amplified and then recorded.

To localize an occlusion, blood pressure readings are taken at the thigh, calf, and ankle of the affected leg during Doppler ultrasonography. If the systolic blood pressure at one of these sites is more than 20 mm Hg lower than the brachial systolic blood pressure, arterial occlusion probably exists at or near the site.

Plethysmography detects blood volume and pressure in a limb using a plethysmograph (a pulse volume recorder). It's especially useful when blood vessels are calcified. During plethysmography, blood pressure is measured at the thigh, calf, and ankle. If the systolic blood pressure at one of these sites is more than 20 mm Hg lower than the brachial systolic blood pressure, arterial occlusion probably exists at or near the site. While

blood pressure is measured, the plethysmograph displays the blood flow as sound waves on a strip, similar to an ECG tracing. Decreased amplitude in the sound waves indicates arterial occlusion.

If the physician suspects serious ischemia, he may order arteriography of your patient's legs. This invasive test can determine the severity and location of an arterial occlusion as well as the quality of the patient's collateral circulation. Because arteriography uses radiographic dye, it carries the risk of causing renal insufficiency and acute renal failure. To reduce the risk, the physician may prescribe mannitol before the procedure, use minimal dye during the procedure, and order fluids afterward.

Treatment

As with other chronic complications of diabetes, encourage your patient to modify risk factors as-

Unfortunately, many diabetic patients who have peripheral vascular disease can't develop good collateral circulation when an artery becomes occluded. This puts them at risk for tissue ischemia and infarction, which may lead to gangrene and amputation.

Poor collateral circulation

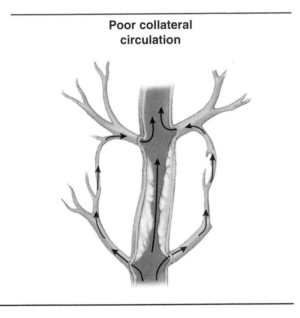

sociated with atherosclerosis, such as cigarette smoking and hypertension. And make sure that her plan of care includes exercise, diet, and, if necessary, drugs to control cholesterol levels.

Management of foot problems

Foot ulcers can lead to serious complications. If your patient has poor circulation, which impedes healing, she may develop ischemia or gangrene and may require amputation of her toes or foot. Meticulous foot care, along with tight blood glucose control and other measures, can help prevent these complications. In fact, up to 50% of amputations performed on patients with diabetes could be avoided with aggressive foot care.

If your patient has a foot ulcer and you suspect an infection, obtain a wound culture to check for bacteria. If she has an infection, the physician will prescribe an antibiotic. An infected wound may require incision, drainage, or debridement. If the physician suspects osteomy-

elitis, the patient will undergo tests, such as a nuclear bone scan.

Keep in mind that blood glucose levels usually climb in response to infection, increasing the patient's insulin requirements. To promote wound healing, your patient should control her blood glucose levels to avoid hyperglycemia. If levels reach 200 mg/dl, macrophages and other white blood cells (WBCs) can't fight the infection effectively. If your patient has an infected wound, be sure to monitor her for complications of severe hyperglycemia, such as DKA.

Drug therapy

The physician may prescribe pentoxifylline to help ease your patient's symptoms of intermittent claudication. This drug increases RBC flexibility and decreases blood viscosity, plasma fibrinogen, and platelet aggregation. This, in turn, improves blood flow and enhances tissue oxygenation. The physician may also prescribe platelet inhibitors, such as aspirin or ticlopidine, to help slow the progression of atherosclerosis.

Surgery

Several surgical options are available for treating peripheral vascular disease, including aortobifemoral bypass, axillofemoral or axillobifemoral bypass, and femoropopliteal bypass (see *Bypass surgery for peripheral vascular occlusion,* pages 94 and 95).

The procedure of choice depends on the location and severity of the patient's arterial occlusion and on her overall medical condition. Before reconstructive surgery is performed, the physician will treat other medical problems that may interfere with healing, such as infection.

Bypass grafting is done with grafts made of Dacron, polytetrafluoroethylene, or other synthetic materials. Sometimes, one of the patient's veins is used for the bypass. However, the vein that's used must be free from disease. By restoring circulation to the affected limb through a bypass, the physician may be able to avoid or minimize amputation.

Bypass surgery is indicated for intermittent claudication only if the patient has unresponsive foot ulcers, infections, or gangrene or if the pain interferes with her occupation. If the occlusion is isolated, percutaneous transluminal angioplasty of the femoral, iliac, or popliteal artery may be performed. It may be used with laser angioplasty to open the artery and enhance blood flow.

Bypass surgery for peripheral vascular occlusion

These illustrations show three common surgical procedures used to bypass peripheral arterial occlusions.

Aortobifemoral bypass graft

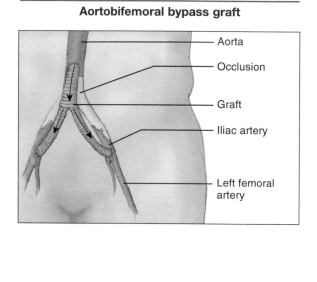

- Aorta
- Occlusion
- Graft
- Iliac artery
- Left femoral artery

Axillobifemoral bypass graft

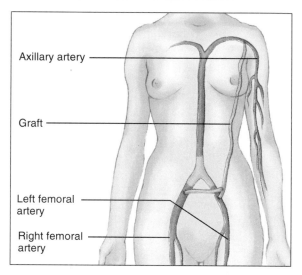

- Axillary artery
- Graft
- Left femoral artery
- Right femoral artery

Nursing considerations

Your nursing interventions should focus on providing foot care, monitoring your patient's response to the prescribed drugs, and promoting circulation after surgery.

Foot care

The primary goal of nursing care in patients with diabetes and peripheral vascular disease is to help reduce the risk of foot and leg amputations. Therefore, protect the patient's legs and feet from even minor traumas, which can lead to infection, ulcers, and ultimately loss of function.

Thoroughly assess your patient's legs and feet for signs of impaired skin integrity, such as pressure areas or skin tears. If your patient has peripheral or autonomic neuropathy, she may have decreased sensations of touch, pain, or temperature, so examine her legs and feet routinely for signs of breakdown. Check her pedal pulses, foot temperature, capillary refill, and skin color. Also, assess her for changes in feeling, such as numbness or tingling.

Provide your patient with meticulous foot care. To prevent pressure on her legs and feet, make sure she changes position every 2 hours and performs range-of-motion exercises, if possible. Wash her feet with warm water and mild soap, and dry them well, particularly between the toes. Inspect her feet and apply moisturizing cream every day but not between her toes. Use protective padding, foot cradles, or an alternating-pressure mattress to reduce the risk of pressure injuries. To prevent constriction and impaired circulation, don't use elastic antiembolism stockings.

Although your patient's activity may be restricted, make sure she wears appropriate footwear, even for short distances. Shoes or slippers that don't fit properly can cause further injury and lengthen her hospital stay.

Monitor your patient for signs and symptoms of wound infection, including redness, swelling, or foul-smelling, purulent drainage. Obtain a transferase and aspartate aminotransferase levels, which indicate liver dysfunction.

Postoperative circulation

If your patient has a bypass graft, your primary goal after surgery is to promote and maintain circulation through the new grafts. So monitor the neurovascular status of her feet and legs. Immediately report signs or symptoms of graft occlusion, such as severe pain, loss of pulses, cold hands or feet, or new complaints of numbness or tingling.

Position your patient so that her knees aren't flexed, which might impair her circulation and compromise the patency of the graft. Also, make sure she doesn't sit in one position for a long period. Elevate the affected leg to reduce edema. Instruct her not to cross her legs and to avoid keeping the affected leg in a dependent position for a prolonged period.

Patient teaching

Your two most important responsibilities in educating your patient and her family are teaching them about risk factor reduction and giving them foot care guidelines.

Help your patient assess her risk factors for peripheral vascular disease, such as smoking or hypertension, and develop a plan to reduce these risks. If she smokes, emphasize the importance of stopping.

When you begin teaching your patient about foot care, find out if she can see and examine her feet. Teach her how to care for her feet by examining them every day, keeping them clean and dry, and wearing properly fitting shoes (see *Peripheral vascular disease: Selecting the right shoes,* page 96). Explain that increasing her mobility will promote blood circulation to her legs and feet. Low-impact exercises, such as swimming and walking, will also improve circulation. Tell her to avoid crossing her legs or standing for long periods because these actions may impede blood circulation. Refer her to a podiatrist who will trim thickened, fungal toenails and evaluate and treat pressure points.

If your patient had surgery to bypass an arterial occlusion, advise her to contact the physician immediately if she develops signs and symptoms of graft occlusion, such as pain, numbness, or coldness in the leg or foot.

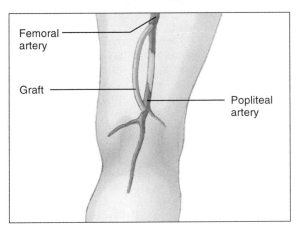

Femoropopliteal bypass graft

Femoral artery

Graft

Popliteal artery

culture of any open or draining lesion, and begin antibiotic therapy as prescribed. If your patient is taking antibiotics, make sure she drinks at least eight 8-ounce glasses of fluid every day, and assess her renal function daily. Dress an infected wound with a wet-to-dry dressing and change it several times a day to achieve mechanical debridement. (Remember that the dressing helps lift off dead surface skin, which promotes new tissue growth.) If the wound isn't infected, dress it with an occlusive dressing that retains moisture and enhances cell migration and healing.

Drug response

If your patient is taking pentoxifylline, check for headaches, dizziness, nausea, or vomiting. Monitor her WBC count for signs of neutropenia. If she's taking ticlopidine, closely monitor her complete blood cell count and WBC differential for adverse effects, such as neutropenia. Also, evaluate her liver function tests for elevated alanine amino-

HEALTH PROMOTION

Peripheral vascular disease: Selecting the right shoes

Advise your patient to purchase shoes that are made of natural material, such as leather. Explain that synthetics don't allow enough air circulation. If she has decreased sensation in her feet, suggest that she take a family member along when she buys new shoes. She can ask the family member to feel her foot through the shoe to make sure it isn't too tight. If necessary, tell her how to order adaptive footwear, such as extra-depth or specially constructed shoes.

If your patient has an orthotic insert and she's buying regular shoes, tell her to make sure she has enough room between the sole and upper part of the shoe for the insert. Explain that orthotics help avoid pressure sores by dispersing pressure evenly across her foot. If she has foot deformities, such as claw toes, tell her to make sure that her toes don't rub against her shoe.

Tell your patient that good running shoes made of soft fabric may be an acceptable alternative to custom-made shoes. Advise her to se-

lect running shoes that have a wide toe area and a thick sole and that lace up the front, not the side. Explain that by wearing comfortable running shoes, she'll have better balance and walk more comfortably.

Encourage her to avoid high heels because they increase pressure on the ball of the foot and may decrease sensation. Instead, she should buy low heels or flats.

Wearing new shoes
Advise your patient to wear new shoes for about 2 hours and then examine her feet for pressure areas—red spots that may turn into blisters. If she finds no pressure areas, she can continue to wear the shoes for a few more hours and then examine her feet again. If she still finds no pressure areas, she should increase the wearing time slowly over a few days. If she does notice pressure areas, she should avoid wearing the shoes because a foot ulcer may develop.

If your patient has a home care nurse, she can assess the home for safety, noting potential hazards—such as scatter rugs, electrical cords, and poorly lit staircases—which can cause accidents that result in traumatic lesions. The home care nurse will work with the patient and her family to make the home safer.

Peripheral neuropathy

Peripheral neuropathy, the most common form of neuropathy, usually affects the legs and feet. The sensory nerves are affected by atrophy and loss of the longer peripheral nerve axons. Symptoms begin in the toes and move up. Typically, the disease affects both legs.

Signs and symptoms

The signs and symptoms of peripheral neuropathy depend on the type and amount of nerve fiber damage. Small peripheral nerve damage

can produce many painful or uncomfortable symptoms, including numbness, paresthesia (spontaneous uncomfortable sensations, such as tingling), dysesthesia (contact paresthesia, such as pain from clothing or bedsheets), severe hyperesthesia (extreme sensitivity of the skin's touch and pain receptors), and frank pain that the patient may describe as pins and needles, burning, shooting or stabbing, or bone deep and aching or tearing. Large fiber damage is commonly associated with foot deformities and may not cause pain or paresthesia. Instead, it may produce impaired balance, diminished proprioception, decreased sense of joint position, absent or reduced vibration sensation, impaired sensation of touch or pressure, depressed or absent ankle reflexes, and sensory ataxia. Most patients experience small and large nerve fiber damage at the same time.

In acute painful peripheral neuropathy, pain usually develops and then subsides in less than 6 months. It's commonly accompanied by an abrupt weight loss. In chronic painful peripheral neuropathy, symptoms appear and stabilize, or they may disappear and be replaced by sensory deficits, such as numb or cold hands or feet.

If your patient with peripheral neuropathy has impaired sensation but no loss of motor function, she may develop neuropathic arthropathy (Charcot's joint). This complication commonly affects the small joints of the foot, such as the tarsals and metatarsals. In the early stages, your patient's foot may be swollen, red, and painless. As the condition progresses, your patient may experience fractures, fragmentations, and disarticulations. If she continues to walk on the foot, she's likely to develop foot deformities, such as a flattened arch. Rarely does surgery, such as closed reduction and internal fixation, correct this degenerative deformity. Over time, the affected joint deteriorates further and ulcers and ischemia occur, leaving the patient unable to bear weight. Ultimately, she may require amputation of the affected part of her foot or leg.

If your patient experiences motor dysfunction, she may develop muscle weakness, foot muscle atrophy, edema, and footdrop. If large fiber damage occurs, she may also develop calluses, ulcers, or structural deformities of the foot. Foot deformities result from tendon shortening (contracture), which leads to decreased toe mobility, difficulty with weight bearing, and the following abnormalities:

- claw toes (toe dorsiflexion at the metatarsophalangeal joint and flexion at the interphalangeal joint)
- hammer toes (toe extension at the metatarsophalangeal joint with flexion of the proximal interphalangeal joint)
- cock-up deformities (flexion of the interphalangeal joint with extension of the metatarsophalangeal joint of the great toe)
- toe crowding
- loss of plantar arches
- metatarsal head prominence with loss of fat pad and callus formation as a result of weight-bearing pressures.

Foot ulcers commonly occur around these abnormalities and, because of the patient's diminished sensation, may go unnoticed until an infection develops.

Diagnostic tests

The physician usually diagnoses peripheral neuropathy by excluding other causes of your patient's signs and symptoms. Typically, the physi-

cian will assess her neurologic function, evaluating her deep tendon reflexes and muscle strength and testing how well she senses temperature, light touch, sharp and dull sensations, vibration in her feet, and changes in the position of her toes.

Temperature sensation in the feet and legs can be assessed by touching a cool metal object, such as a tuning fork, to the skin and asking your patient to describe the temperature. Light touch can be assessed by touching the skin with a wisp of cotton or a monofilament device and asking her to describe the location of the sensation. Sharp and dull sensation can be assessed by asking your patient to close her eyes and then alternately touching her feet with the dull and sharp ends of an object, such as a paper clip, and asking her to describe the sensation. Vibration sensation is assessed by placing a vibrating tuning fork on the distal first metatarsal head or the malleolus of your patient's ankles and asking her to tell you when the vibration stops. To assess your patient's position sense, ask her to close her eyes; then flex and extend her great toe and have her describe its position.

Treatment

If your patient maintains better blood glucose control, her pain and other symptoms may decrease. As nerve cells regenerate with improved blood glucose levels, your patient's pain may worsen initially, but it will decrease over time.

To prevent foot complications, your patient may need to use lamb's wool padding to protect her feet from trauma. The physician may also refer her to a podiatrist, who will assess her feet regularly and gently file any callused areas, if necessary. Your patient may also need a referral to an orthotic or other foot care specialist to fit her for custom-made shoes, molded insoles, or other orthotic devices to protect her feet. In some cases, your patient may require bed rest or crutches. Some patients with foot ulcers have casts applied so that they can walk while the ulcers heal. The cast redistributes foot pressure so that the ulcerated area bears much less weight than it would normally.

For pain associated with peripheral neuropathy, the physician may prescribe:

- a nonnarcotic analgesic, such as ibuprofen or sulindac
- tramadol hydrochloride
- phenytoin or carbamazepine

- a tricyclic antidepressant, such as amitriptyline, alone or with a phenothiazine derivative
- mexiletine
- topical capsaicin 0.075%.

Narcotic analgesics usually aren't prescribed because peripheral neuropathy is a chronic condition, and the patient would risk developing an addiction. However, other therapeutic options may include transcutaneous electrical nerve stimulation (TENS) therapy or referral to a pain control clinic.

Nursing considerations

When caring for a patient with peripheral neuropathy, one of your greatest challenges is to help reduce or relieve her symptoms, especially severe pain. To help alleviate discomfort from paresthesia, encourage your patient to walk. In many cases, this helps reduce the tingling sensations. To help block painful sensations, you can gently massage her affected foot or leg.

For the pain of dysesthesia, use the TENS unit, as prescribed. Also, give your patient information about alternative approaches to pain control, including guided imagery, meditation, and progressive relaxation therapy. These methods may be helpful alone or with drug therapy (see *Easing pain with alternative techniques*).

The pain of hyperesthesia is more difficult to control. Body stockings or pantyhose can be used to keep clothes away from your patient's hypersensitive skin, but for some patients this may actually increase the pain. During periods of hyperesthesia, your patient may experience extreme pain from the simplest tasks, such as pulling up a zipper or putting on her shoes. To help, focus on the things that cause your patient particular pain. For instance, have her wear loose-fitting clothing if zipper pulling is painful, or use a bed cradle if covers cause her pain.

Thoroughly assess your patient's legs and feet for impaired skin integrity, such as pressure areas, skin tears, fissures, or small cracks. Remember, you can't rely on your patient's reports of pain or discomfort before taking action because she may have diminished sensation in her legs or feet. Check her pedal pulses, foot temperature, capillary refill, and skin color. Assess her legs and feet for any changes in feeling, such as numbness or tingling. Also, assess her ability to feel touch, using a monofilament device.

Provide meticulous foot care for your patient. Wash and inspect her feet daily and apply a moisturizing cream except between her toes. To prevent pressure on her legs and feet, make sure she changes position at least every 2 hours, and performs range-of-motion exercises as tolerated. Use protective padding, foot cradles, or an alternating-pressure mattress to reduce the risk of pressure injuries.

Although your patient's activity may be restricted, make sure she has appropriate footwear, even for short distances. Advise her to purchase footwear that's made of natural material, such as leather, and to avoid synthetic material because it doesn't allow enough air circulation for her feet. If needed, adaptive footwear, such as extra-depth or custom-made shoes, should be ordered before the patient is discharged.

Monitor your patient's response to her prescribed drug. If it doesn't reduce her symptoms, discuss other drug options or complementary treatments with the physician.

Assess your patient for signs and symptoms of hyperglycemia, and monitor her blood glucose levels frequently. Although the pain of peripheral neuropathy may worsen temporarily when blood glucose levels are brought under control, most researchers believe this means the nerves are being repaired.

Patient teaching

If your patient experiences painful paresthesia, especially at night, tell her to stretch gently or to get up and walk around. Also, teach her how to safely massage her feet and legs, and explain that this sometimes helps to block pain sensations. If appropriate, teach your patient how to safely use the TENS unit. Teach her about guided imagery, meditation, progressive relaxation techniques, exercise, and therapeutic massage.

Teach your patient the importance of foot care, and review safety measures she can take to prevent trauma. For instance, advise her to avoid prolonged standing and strenuous weight-bearing exercises. Tell her to wear well-cushioned, properly fitting shoes and to walk in well-lit areas where the ground is smooth.

If your patient has decreased temperature sensation, advise her to prevent severe burns by checking the water temperature with a part of her body that's sensitive to temperature, such as

HEALTH PROMOTION

Easing pain with alternative techniques

Patients with diabetic neuropathy may experience a wide range of pain and discomfort, from a mild annoyance that lasts only seconds or minutes to extreme pain that lasts for hours or days. Sometimes, mild analgesics can help relieve the pain—but not always. That's when your patient can benefit from nonpharmacologic techniques, such as guided imagery, meditation, and progressive relaxation therapy. To teach your patient these cognitive and behavioral techniques, you'll need her full cooperation.

Guided imagery
Guided imagery, a form of hypnosis, requires your patient to use her imagination in a structured manner to achieve a desired effect. No one knows for sure how guided imagery works. It may simply distract patients from their pain, or it may trigger the release of endorphins by the anterior pituitary gland and hypothalamus, resulting in pain relief. The overall effect is that your patient becomes more relaxed, and her anxiety and blood pressure are reduced.

To perform guided imagery, your patient must concentrate on a pleasant mental image, such as a warm, sunny beach; a desirable feeling, such as comfort; or a pleasant event, such as winning the lottery. At first, you may need to help her by making suggestions. For example, you can ask her to imagine that she's lying on a warm, sunny beach and then describe some of the sights, sounds, and smells. Over time, your patient will learn to make her own mental connection with pleasant scenes and events. For guided imagery to work, your patient must be able to concentrate for at least 5 minutes without distraction.

Meditation
When using guided imagery, you and your patient can participate together, but meditation is a solitary act. To meditate effectively, your patient must become self-focused and block out all distractions. This may be difficult to achieve in a noisy hospital environment. Meditation calls on a patient's ability to maintain inner control, effectively self-regulating her bodily functions. Some patients find music and chanting helpful; others rely on objects that provide a visual focus. Whatever the technique, many patients who use meditation achieve a level of relaxation and pain relief similar to that achieved with drugs.

Progressive relaxation therapy
Progressive relaxation therapy, a form of relaxation exercise, involves the sequential tightening and relaxing of various muscle groups. As with guided imagery, you can help your patient relax and relieve pain by guiding her through the exercise. Furthermore, you can teach your patient's caregiver how to perform this technique.

For best results, the room should be quiet, free from distractions, and dimly lit. You must first help your patient become quiet and relaxed so that she's receptive to your instructions. Using a soothing voice and playing soft music may help. Then, ask your patient to focus on one muscle group, for example the muscles in her left thigh. Ask her to tighten these muscles with all of her strength and then after several seconds to release and completely relax them. Repeat this procedure with all muscle groups. As this therapy progresses, the patient not only becomes distracted from her pain but also achieves muscular relaxation and in many cases goes to sleep.

---

her forearm. If she experiences abnormal cold sensations, advise her to wear thin gloves in the spring or fall. When temperatures drop, she should wear heavier, insulated gloves. Tell her that mittens may be warmer than gloves. If cold feet are a problem, tell her to wear comfortable insulated socks with her shoes.

Review with your patient the name, dosage, action, and adverse effects of all her prescribed drugs. If she's using topical capsaicin, tell her to wear gloves when she applies it, avoid contact with her eyes, and wash her hands immediately after application. Also, warn her that she may experience transient burning of the affected area after applying capsaicin.

Encourage your patient to avoid drinking alcohol. Explain that alcohol abuse may contribute to the progression of peripheral neuropathy. If appropriate, refer your patient to a counselor or to Alcoholics Anonymous. If she smokes, encourage her to stop. Explain that cigarette smoking can worsen her condition and that stopping may slow its progress.

Explain that your patient should have her feet inspected at least four times a year and that a physician should perform a thorough physical examination and neurologic assessment at least once a year.

Autonomic neuropathy

Autonomic neuropathy affects the autonomic nervous system. For this reason, it can produce symptoms in virtually every body organ, can cause wide-ranging dysfunction, and typically coexists with peripheral neuropathy. Autonomic neuropathy increases your patient's risk of developing other acute and chronic debilitating complications, which require early detection and education to prevent further problems.

Signs and symptoms

The signs and symptoms of autonomic neuropathy depend on the body organ affected. However, because nearly all of the gastrointestinal (GI) system has autonomic innervation, gastroparesis and other GI problems are common. Autonomic neuropathy also may cause cardiovascular, genitourinary, vision, and endocrine problems.

Gastrointestinal problems
When autonomic neuropathy affects the nerves of the stomach, gastric emptying of liquids and solids may be delayed. The upper and lower GI tract may be affected.

Damage to the efferent autonomic nerves, which transmit impulses from the brain to the intestine, causes impaired motility, usually in the colon, and poor contraction of the smooth muscles of the stomach. When this happens, a patient may experience episodes of constipation alternating with diarrhea. Diarrhea can also result when decreased motility of the small intestine leads to overgrowth of normal intestinal bacteria. Or diarrhea may result when autonomic neuropathy causes increased motility.

Constipation is more common than diarrhea; however, diarrhea can be devastating. It can alter your patient's social life and leave her depressed. Diarrhea, which may be preceded by abdominal cramping and pain, usually occurs after meals or at night. It may be associated with steatorrhea or fecal incontinence.

Cardiovascular problems
Orthostatic hypotension, a drop in systolic blood pressure of more than 30 mm Hg or a drop in diastolic blood pressure of more than 10 mm Hg within 2 minutes of rising from a lying position, occurs in late stages of autonomic neuropathy. Orthostatic hypotension can occur without symptoms, but it is commonly accompanied by dizziness, light-headedness, weakness, visual impairment, and syncope.

Your patient is also at risk for cardiovascular abnormalities, such as cardiac denervation syndrome. In this syndrome, your patient maintains a fixed heart rate during stress, exercise, altered breathing patterns, or sleep. This can lead to arrhythmias and possibly cardiac arrest. Patients with this syndrome are at risk for developing myocardial ischemia or an MI without pain. Because of the lack of pain, they may not seek treatment.

Genitourinary problems
Genitourinary autonomic neuropathy can affect your patient's bladder and sexual function. Afferent nerve fibers transmit sensations of bladder fullness to the brain. Efferent nerve fibers then promote bladder contraction during urination, and efferent sympathetic nerves maintain sphincter tone. In autonomic neuropathy, damage can occur to all of these nerves, leading to neurogenic bladder.

The signs and symptoms of neurogenic bladder usually develop slowly. In the early stages, the sensation of the need to void may be blunted. Later, the urine stream may become weak and prolonged, leading to difficulty in emptying the bladder and overflow incontinence.

Untreated neurogenic bladder commonly leads to UTIs as a result of urinary stasis. Your patient may develop pyelonephritis or incontinence. Frequent UTIs may speed the deterioration of your patient's renal function. If your patient has had more than two UTIs in a year or has a palpable bladder or incontinence, her bladder function should be further evaluated.

Up to 75% of men and 35% of women with diabetes experience sexual problems caused by dia-

Diabetic neuropathy and sexual dysfunction

Sexual dysfunction commonly develops in people who have diabetic autonomic neuropathy. That's because diabetic neuropathy affects the parasympathetic fibers that regulate erections in men and vaginal lubrication in women. It also affects the sympathetic nervous system, which mediates orgasm and ejaculation.

Sexual dysfunction in men

Men with autonomic neuropathy may experience retrograde ejaculation (semen ejaculation into the urinary bladder) or impotence. Retrograde ejaculation results from damage to the efferent sympathetic nerves. These nerves normally coordinate the simultaneous closure of the internal vesicle sphincter and relaxation of the external vesicle sphincter during ejaculation. Signs and symptoms of retrograde ejaculation include cloudy urine after intercourse, infertility, and a decreased volume of ejaculate.

If your patient has incomplete retrograde ejaculation or the problem has recently been diagnosed, the physician may advise him to have intercourse when his bladder is distended. Other therapeutic options include taking an antihistamine or desipramine to restore ejaculation.

A patient who's impotent can't attain or maintain an erection despite having a normal sex drive. When evaluating whether impotence results from autonomic neuropathy, the physician will consider other possible causes, such as drugs, alcohol use, hormonal deficiencies, and psychological problems. The physician may evaluate the patient's serum hormone levels and penile blood flow and pressure measurements to help make the diagnosis, or the physician may refer the patient to a urologist for further evaluation.

Because a patient with impotence may be hesitant to discuss his sexual concerns, you may have to bring up the subject yourself. For instance, you can say, "Many of my patients who have diabetes complain of impotence. Has this been a problem for you?" If he acknowledges the problem, explore it with him. Ask if anything seems to make the problem better. If he's uncomfortable talking with you, give him an educational pamphlet or suggest that he discuss it with the physician.

Explain to your patient that effective and acceptable treatments are available. For example, vacuum devices can be used to draw blood into the penis to produce an erection. Or a rigid or semirigid penile prosthesis can be surgically implanted. The physician may also prescribe alprostadil, which the patient administers intracavernously shortly before sexual intercourse, or silenafil, which he takes orally ½ to 4 hours before sexual intercourse.

Sexual dysfunction in women

Women with diabetic autonomic neuropathy may experience difficulties with arousal, diminished vaginal lubrication, and anorgasmy despite a normal sex drive. Symptoms include dyspareunia (painful intercourse) and a delayed orgasm or none at all. If your patient is experiencing these symptoms, advise her to use a vaginal lubricant and to ask the physician for a referral to a gynecologist for further evaluation. Her gynecologist may prescribe an estrogen cream.

---

betic neuropathy (*see Diabetic neuropathy and sexual dysfunction*).

Vision problems

The iris is innervated by parasympathetic and sympathetic nerve fibers. The sympathetic nerve fibers that cause the pupils to dilate are generally more severely affected by autonomic neuropathy. If this is the case, your patient may report difficulty adapting to changes in lighting.

Endocrine problems

Normally, during hypoglycemic episodes, the body responds by increasing the secretion of glucagon, epinephrine, growth hormone, and cortisol. In autonomic neuropathy, the secretion of glucagon and epinephrine are greatly diminished. Therefore, your patient may not be able to recover from a hypoglycemic episode, and severe hypoglycemia can develop.

Patients with long-term diabetes may not experience the typical, early warning signs and symptoms of hypoglycemia, such as anxiety, nervousness, sweating, and palpitations. Instead of developing those adrenergic effects, they may display signs and symptoms of neuroglycopenia, such as lethargy, irritability, confusion, loss of consciousness, or seizures.

Diagnostic tests

Diagnosis of autonomic neuropathy depends on your patient's signs and symptoms. If she has a GI symptom, such as constipation, perform a thorough health history to rule out other possible causes, such as inadequate fluid or fiber intake, drugs, inactivity, or other illnesses. A diagnosis of gastroparesis is based on health history, physical examination, and certain diagnostic tests. A physician may order an esophagogastroduodenoscopy and an upper GI series to rule out intestinal obstruction or a gastric emptying nuclear scan to diagnose delayed gastric emptying.

Orthostatic hypotension is diagnosed by measuring your patient's blood pressure while she lies down and then stands up. Orthostatic hypotension is present if her systolic blood pressure drops more than 30 mm Hg or her diastolic blood pressure drops more than 10 mm Hg within 2 minutes of standing up.

The physician may be able to detect cardiac denervation by measuring your patient's pulse or heart rate as she takes about six deep breaths per minute, performs the Valsalva maneuver or exercises, and then takes another six deep breaths per minute. If her heart rate doesn't vary, she probably has cardiac nerve damage. Cardiac arrhythmias can be detected with a 12-lead ECG or continuous monitoring of the heart rate and rhythm for 24 hours.

If a bladder infection is suspected, obtain a urine sample for culture and sensitivity testing. After your patient voids, if urinary catheterization produces more than 150 ml of urine, she may have neurologic impairment of the bladder. Ultrasound testing of her bladder will probably confirm neurologic impairment.

An ophthalmoscopic examination performed in a dark room can detect a pupillary abnormality. If the patient has such an abnormality, her pupils will dilate slowly.

Treatment

The treatment of autonomic neuropathy depends on the patient's signs and symptoms and the body organ affected. However, blood glucose control is helpful no matter which organ is affected.

Gastroparesis can make it difficult to balance insulin doses with food absorption. Thus, a patient should monitor her blood glucose levels before and after meals and adjust her insulin dosage. Short-acting insulin, such as Lispro, may not be appropriate for a patient with delayed gastric emptying. That's because this type of insulin begins to work in 5 to 15 minutes, when food may not yet be available.

If your patient develops constipation, treatment includes adequate fluid intake; increased physical activity; increased fiber intake; stool softeners, such as psyllium; judicious use of laxatives; and drugs, such as metoclopramide or cisapride, to stimulate gastric motility.

If your patient has diarrhea, her physician may prescribe drugs to slow intestinal motility, including loperamide, codeine, or diphenoxylate hydrochloride with atropine. The physician also may prescribe a high-fiber diet and psyllium to increase stool bulk and consistency. If your patient has diarrhea related to overgrowth of intestinal bacteria, her physician may prescribe a broad-spectrum antibiotic with anaerobic coverage, such as tetracycline or metronidazole. Your patient may benefit from biofeedback, relaxation, and bowel training, so discuss these treatment options with the physician.

A patient with diarrhea may benefit from a liquid, low-fat diet consisting of several small meals a day. This diet is effective when used with drugs taken one-half hour before eating. If your patient has severe diarrhea, the physician may prescribe total parenteral nutrition or jejunostomy tube feedings.

If your patient has orthostatic hypotension, treatment includes increasing her venous pressure by using supportive elastic body stockings applied while she's lying down. Hypovolemia can be corrected by good blood glucose control, adequate salt intake, or fludrocortisone. The physician may prescribe a drug, such as ephedrine, to increase the heart rate and blood pressure through vasoconstriction.

No treatment is available for cardiac denervation. However, if the patient has periods of sustained sinus bradycardia or heart block that produce life-threatening symptoms, such as severe hypotension, she may need a permanent pacemaker. The physician may prescribe theophylline and terbutaline to increase the patient's resting heart rate.

For a patient with bladder dysfunction, treatment focuses on improving bladder function and preventing UTIs. Specific interventions may include treatment with antibiotics for UTIs or a parasympathomimetic drug, such as bethanechol, to improve bladder nerve contraction.

Nursing considerations

Autonomic neuropathy can profoundly affect your patient's life. She'll need current, accurate information and a great deal of emotional support. Because autonomic neuropathy rarely causes an isolated problem, you'll need to address all of the complications your patient experiences.

If your patient has GI symptoms, monitor her bowel status to prevent or treat constipation or diarrhea. If she has diarrhea, and particularly if she's incontinent, be sure to keep her skin clean and dry to prevent breakdown. Assess her for signs and symptoms of gastroparesis, such as loss of appetite, abdominal pain, and bloating. Administer drugs as prescribed and monitor the patient for adverse effects. Be sure to refer her to a dietitian who will monitor her progress.

If your patient has gastroparesis and experiences hypoglycemia, place a simple sugar, such as jelly, glucose gel, or cake icing, under her tongue or against her cheek, where it will be absorbed into the bloodstream. Ensure that your patient receives her meals and snacks as planned to prevent hypoglycemia. Remember that her body may not respond as quickly or effectively to hypoglycemia because of decreased glucagon secretion, so be prepared to administer glucagon or parenteral glucose.

To prevent orthostatic hypotension and symptoms of cardiac denervation, tell your patient to perform simple leg exercises before rising from a seated position. This causes the brain to release stimulating catecholamines that raise her blood pressure, preparing her body to adjust to the position change. If she's reclining, she should sit up slowly, then flex and extend her legs at the side of the bed. If she feels dizzy or light-headed, tell her to remain seated until the symptoms subside. Monitor orthostatic pulse rate and blood pressure measurements. And stand at her side to support her if needed.

If your patient with autonomic neuropathy also has CAD, let her know that she may not experience the typical signs and symptoms of myocardial ischemia or an MI, such as chest pain.

Teach her to be alert for other signs and symptoms, such as fatigue, shortness of breath, and palpitations. Explain the importance of routine physical examinations and electrocardiography.

If your patient has bladder dysfunction, palpate her bladder to detect urine retention. If she has urine retention, plan to:
• routinely palpate her bladder for fullness
• schedule urination every 2 hours while she's awake
• apply manual suprapubic pressure (Credé's method) to ensure that the bladder empties sufficiently.

If retention is severe, intermittently perform urinary catheterization.

Monitor your patient for signs and symptoms of UTI, such as dysuria and foul-smelling urine. If she develops urinary incontinence, keep her skin clean and dry to prevent excoriation and breakdown.

If your patient experiences sexual dysfunction, encourage her to discuss her problems with you or the physician and, if appropriate, obtain a referral to a urologist or counselor.

If you detect pupil abnormalities in your patient, notify the physician. Also, make sure that her environment is safe and that the lighting is adequate to help prevent falls.

Patient teaching

Your teaching topics depend on your patient's specific treatment. For GI dysfunction, teach her about her diet and meal planning. Advise her to check her blood glucose levels frequently, and reinforce the importance of using blood glucose levels to detect hypoglycemia and hyperglycemia. To promote optimal GI function, instruct your patient to consume enough fluid and fiber to prevent constipation. Also, advise her to use laxatives judiciously. Teach her relaxation exercises and biofeedback techniques.

Teach your patient with a dysfunctional bladder to schedule urination every 2 hours to help keep her bladder empty and to reduce the risk of UTI. Review the signs and symptoms of UTI, such as dysuria, fever, and chills, and tell her to contact her physician immediately if she experiences them. Teach her Credé's method to help empty her bladder: She should place a cupped hand directly over her bladder, push in

Recognizing focal neuropathies

Focal neuropathies include cranial neuropathy, mononeuropathy, radiculopathy, and plexopathy.

Cranial neuropathy
Cranial neuropathy, also called ophthalmoplegia, affects the third cranial nerve. Typically, it begins suddenly and causes eye pain, headache, and dysesthesia of the upper lip. These symptoms usually occur several days before the patient develops facial palsy. She may develop pronounced ptosis and an inability to move her eye from side to side or up and down. Cranial neuropathy occurs most commonly in the elderly.

To alleviate accompanying double vision, your patient can use an eye patch. After several weeks, her pain should subside, and the muscular function of her eye should return. After 3 to 5 months, she should recover completely.

Mononeuropathy
Mononeuropathy is an isolated neuropathy of one or several nerves. Carpal tunnel syndrome, which results from compression or entrapment of the median nerve in the wrist, is the most common form of mononeuropathy.

Mononeuropathy of the ulnar nerve at the elbow leads to weakness and loss of sensation on the palm side of the ring and fourth fingers. Wristdrop develops with mononeuropathy of the radial nerve; footdrop develops from mononeuropathy of the lateral cutaneous nerve in the thigh and the peroneal nerve at the head of the fibula.

Treatment options include surgical release of the nerve, physical therapy, and protection from further trauma with wrist splints, elbow pads, or ankle braces.

Radiculopathy
Radiculopathy, also known as intercostal neuropathy, results from damage to the root of a single nerve. Signs and symptoms of radiculopathy include pain in the affected area of the chest or abdominal wall, dysesthesia that worsens at night, and diminished or no skin sensation. The patient may also experience profound weight loss. A nonnarcotic analgesic, such as ibuprofen, may help control the pain, which generally subsides in 6 to 24 months.

Plexopathy
Plexopathy, or femoral neuropathy, commonly affects the sacral plexus and femoral nerves, causing pain that extends from the hip to the anterior and lateral surfaces of the thigh. A patient may experience disabling muscle weakness when she flexes or extends her knee. Pain is usually worse at night and occurs mostly among the elderly.

The patient may use a nonnarcotic analgesic, such as ibuprofen, to relieve her pain. The pain generally goes away spontaneously but may recur periodically.

---

and down, and then massage her bladder to empty it. Also, teach her to palpate her bladder to check for fullness. If your patient must perform self-catheterization, teach her clean technique.

If your patient doesn't have a prescription for glucagon, talk with the physician. Make sure the patient's family and friends know how and when to administer glucagon and when to call for help.

Advise your patient with abnormal pupillary response to use a night-light and keep a flashlight by her bed in case she needs to get up during the night. Also tell her to avoid driving at night. Inform her that her abnormal pupil response and decreased peripheral sensation may cause her to lose her sense of balance easily.

Advise her to keep her environment well lit and free from clutter.

Focal neuropathy

Focal neuropathy, which is less common than peripheral or autonomic neuropathy in patients with diabetes, is dysfunction of a single nerve or group of nerves (see *Recognizing focal neuropathies*). Usually affecting middle-aged and elderly patients, focal neuropathy usually causes acute, localized pain. This form of nerve dysfunction may occur after acute occlusion of a blood vessel produces ischemia. Focal neuropathy has a sudden onset and is self-limiting: The patient's symptoms improve or disappear 2 weeks to 24 months after they appear.

DIABETES MELLITUS

Suggested Readings

Anderson LA, Bruner LA, Satterfield D. Diabetes control programs: new directions. *Diabetes Education.* 1995;21(5):432-438.

Anderson LA, Fogler J, Dedrick RF. Recruiting from the community: lessons learned from the diabetes care for older adults project. *Gerontologist.* 1995;35(3):395-401.

Barnwell M, Raskopf V, Kimball R, Tapler D. *Diabetes: Skidmore-Roth Outline Series.* El Paso, Tex: Skidmore-Roth Publishing, Inc; 1995.

DeFronzo RA. *Current Therapy of Diabetes Mellitus.* St Louis: Mosby, Inc; 1998.

Eberhardt MS, Lackland DT, Wheeler FC, German RR, Teutsch SM. Is race related to glycemic control? an assessment of glycosylated hemoglobin in two South Carolina communities. *J Clin Epidemiol.* 1997;47(10):1181-1189.

Engelgau MM, Thompson TJ, Smith PJ, et al. Screening for diabetes mellitus in adults: the utility of random capillary blood glucose measurements. *Diabetes Care.* 1995;18(4):463-466.

Fujii K, Abe I, Ohya Y, et al. Association between hyperinsulinemia and intima-media thickness of the carotid artery in normotensive men. *J Hypertens.* 1997;15(2):167-172.

Funnell MM, Herman WH. Diabetes care policies and practices in Michigan nursing homes, 1991. *Diabetes Care.* 1995;18(6):862-866.

Goldschmid MG, Barrett-Connor E, Edelstein SL, Wingard DL, Cohn BA, Herman WH. Dyslipidemia and ischemic heart disease mortality among men and women with diabetes. *Circulation.* 1994;89(3):991-997.

Haire-Joshu D. *Management of Diabetes Mellitus: Perspectives of Care across the Life Span.* 2nd ed. St Louis: Mosby, Inc; 1996.

Herman WH. From research to practice. *Diabetes Spectrum.* 1995;8(3):153. Commentary.

Herman WH, Fajans SS, Ortiz FJ, et al. Abnormal insulin secretion, not insulin resistance, is the genetic or primary defect of MODY in the RW pedigree. *Diabetes.* 1994;43(1):40-46.

Herman WH, Smith PJ, Thompson TJ, Engelgau MM, Aubert RE. A new and simple questionnaire to identify people at increased risk for undiagnosed diabetes. *Diabetes Care.* 1995;18(3):382-387.

Hillson R. *Practical Diabetes Care.* New York: Oxford University Press; 1996.

Kannel WB. Cardiovascular risk factors in the elderly. *Coron Artery Dis.* 1997;8(8-9):565-575.

Lewis SM, Collier IC. *Medical-Surgical Nursing: Assessment and Management of Clinical Problems.* 4th ed. St Louis: Mosby, Inc; 1995.

Malarcher AM, Ford ES, Nelson DE, et al. Trends in cigarette smoking and physicians' advice to quit smoking among people with diabetes in the United States. *Diabetes Care.* 1995;18(5):694-697.

McCance KL, Huether SE. *Pathophysiology: The Biological Basis for Disease in Adults and Children.* 3rd ed. St Louis: Mosby, Inc; 1997.

Report of the expert committee on the diagnosis and classification of diabetes mellitus. *Diabetes Care.* 1997;20(7):1183-1197.

Shorr RI, Ray WA, Daugherty JR, Griffin MR. Antihypertensives and the risk of serious hypoglycemia in older persons using insulin or sulfonylureas. *JAMA.* 1997;278(1):40-43.

Suissa S, Garbe E. Risk of hypoglycemia with antihypertensive medication. *JAMA.* 1997;278(19):1570.

Will JC, German RR, Schuman E, Michael S, Kurth DM, Deeb L. Patient adherence to guidelines for diabetes eye care: results from the diabetic eye disease follow-up study. *Am J Public Health.* 1994;84(10):1669-1671. Abstract.

HYPERTENSION

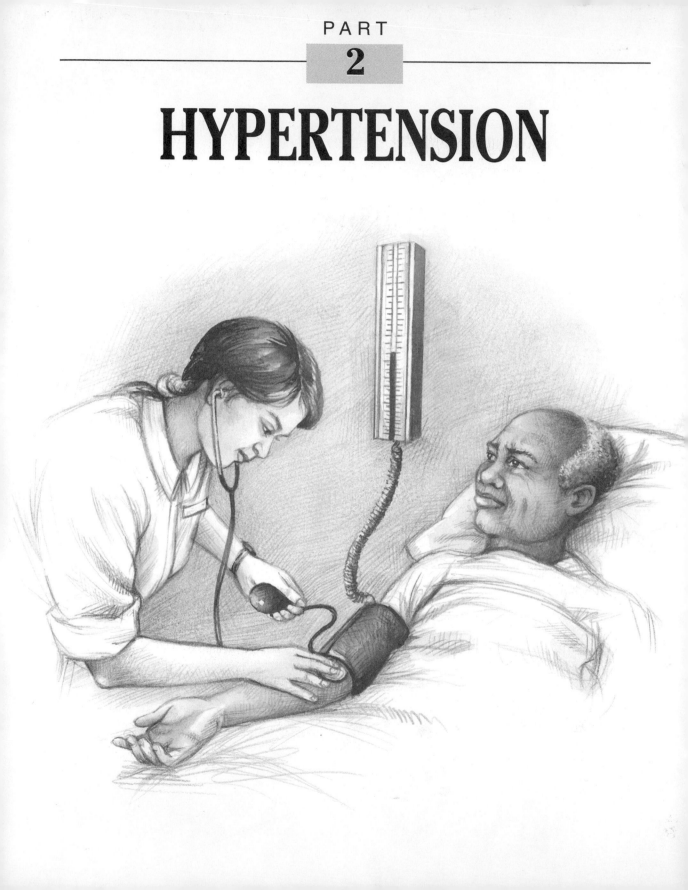

6

HYPERTENSION

Overview

Hypertension affects about 20% of adults and occurs increasingly with age. Typically, the disease is more common:

- among African-Americans than whites
- among less educated people of both races
- in lower socioeconomic groups
- in men from young adulthood to age 55
- in postmenopausal women
- among African-Americans and whites living in the southeastern United States.

About 58 million Americans have hypertension. And although hypertension control has improved considerably over the past 20 years, mostly because of large-scale education programs to increase public awareness, many people with this dangerous disease still don't know they have it.

Typically, hypertension is detected during routine physical examinations or at health fairs. After the condition has been diagnosed, treatment usually consists of lifestyle modifications and antihypertensive drug therapy, depending on the severity of the hypertension.

Blood pressure: Normal and abnormal

The term *blood pressure* refers to the force exerted by the blood against the arterial wall, usually the brachial artery wall. A blood pressure of 120/80 mm Hg is considered normal. The "120 mm Hg" is the systolic pressure—the force exerted against the arterial wall when the heart's ventricles contract. During systole of the cardiac cycle, the elastic walls of the aorta and arteries stretch as more blood enters the ventricles. Ventricular pressure builds, causing the ventricles to contract and the aortic valve to open. The peak pressure of blood being forced through the aorta is the systolic pressure.

The "80 mm Hg" of a normal blood pressure is the diastolic pressure—the force exerted against the arterial walls when the ventricles are relaxed. During diastole of the cardiac cycle, the aortic valve closes, followed by a passive elastic recoil of the arterial walls, with a minimum amount of pressure being exerted against them. The pressure in the arteries continues to decrease during diastole, which allows the ventricles to fill with blood in preparation for the next ventricular contraction.

Patients with hypertension have either high systolic pressure, high diastolic pressure, or both. High systolic pressure is 140 mm Hg or more; high diastolic pressure is 90 mm Hg or more.

A single elevated blood pressure reading doesn't necessarily indicate hypertension because factors such as stress, anxiety, or pain can temporarily elevate blood pressure. A physician diagnoses hypertension when a patient's blood pressure is elevated at two different examinations. During each, readings should be taken when the patient is seated and resting comfortably. During the initial evaluation, blood pressure readings should be obtained in both arms. On subsequent evaluations, they should be taken from the arm with the higher reading.

Types of hypertension

Hypertension is commonly classified in two ways: according to how severe it is and according to whether or not its cause is known.

Classifying hypertension

The severity of a patient's hypertension is classified based on his systolic and diastolic blood pressure readings. The information in this table is based on the Fifth Report of the Joint National Committee on Detection, Evaluation, and Treatment of High Blood Pressure from the National Institutes of Health.

Category	Systolic pressure (mm Hg)	Diastolic pressure (mm Hg)
Normal blood pressure	< 130	< 85
High normal blood pressure	130–139	85–89
Stage 1 (mild) hypertension	140–159	90–99
Stage 2 (moderate) hypertension	160–179	100–109
Stage 3 (severe) hypertension	180–209	110–119
Stage 4 (very severe) hypertension	≥ 210	≥ 120

Classifying hypertension by severity

The current system for classifying blood pressure in people over age 18 defines normal and high normal blood pressure and four categories of increasingly severe hypertension (see *Classifying hypertension*).

A patient who has a reading of 130/85 mm Hg or less and who doesn't take antihypertensive drugs has normal blood pressure. However, a patient in this category still has some cardiovascular risk unless his blood pressure is less than 120/80 mm Hg. If a patient has unusually low readings, he should be evaluated further.

A patient in the high normal category has a systolic reading between 130 and 139 mm Hg and a diastolic reading between 85 and 89 mm Hg. A patient in this category has an increased risk of developing hypertension and should frequently

have his blood pressure monitored. He should also be counseled on lifestyle changes that can reduce his blood pressure.

The four stages of hypertension indicate a patient's increased risk of developing hypertension-related complications such as a cerebrovascular accident (CVA), cardiovascular disease, and renal disease.

All stages of hypertension require treatment, though the specific treatment will vary. If left untreated, hypertension results in damage to organs such as the brain, heart, and kidneys. When noting the stage of a patient's hypertension, you should also identify any organ disease and additional risk factors. For example, a patient with a blood pressure of 142/94 mm Hg and left ventricular hypertrophy plus diabetes should be classified as having stage 1 hypertension with organ disease (left ventricular hypertrophy) and a major risk factor (diabetes).

If a patient's systolic and diastolic blood pressures fall into two different categories, he should be classified based on the more severe pressure reading. For example, 160/92 mm Hg should be classified as stage 2 hypertension based on the systolic pressure reading. However, a reading of 205/125 mm Hg should be classified as stage 4 hypertension based on the diastolic reading.

Stages 1 and 2 hypertension
Patients with stage 1 (mild) hypertension have systolic blood pressure readings of 140 to 159 mm Hg and diastolic blood pressure readings of 90 to 99 mm Hg. Stage 2 (moderate) hypertensive patients have systolic blood pressure readings between 160 and 179 mm Hg and diastolic readings between 100 and 109 mm Hg. Of the four stages of hypertension, stage 1 is the most common in adults.

The typical treatment of stages 1 and 2 hypertension involves lifestyle modification and, initially, a single antihypertensive drug, such as a diuretic or a beta-blocker. Some physicians may withhold drugs from patients with diastolic pressures in the 90 to 94 mm Hg range. However, such patients should be examined in 3 to 6 months to determine if their blood pressure has risen or if they've experienced cardiac and vascular changes.

Stages 3 and 4 hypertension
A patient with stage 3 (severe) hypertension has a systolic blood pressure reading between 180 and

209 mm Hg and a diastolic blood pressure reading between 110 and 119 mm Hg. And the patient with stage 4 (very severe) hypertension has a systolic blood pressure reading of 210 mm Hg or more and a diastolic reading of 120 mm Hg or more.

Treatment of stages 3 and 4 hypertension also includes lifestyle modification. However, the patient may also need a second or third antihypertensive drug (see *Follow-up care for hypertensive patients*).

Classifying hypertension by cause

Hypertension is also classified based on whether or not the underlying cause is known.

Primary hypertension
More than 90% of hypertensive patients have primary hypertension (also called essential or idiopathic hypertension), with the onset generally occurring between ages 30 and 50. Although the cause of primary hypertension isn't known, certain risk factors may contribute to the disease (see *Risk factors for primary hypertension,* page 110).

Advanced age
A patient's chances of developing hypertension increase as he ages because of structural and functional changes in the peripheral vascular system. These changes include atherosclerosis, the loss of connective tissue elasticity, and a decreased relaxation of vascular smooth muscle, which reduces the ability of the vessels to distend and recoil. With advanced age, a patient's heart becomes stiffer and less efficient. Additional peripheral vascular resistance increases the work required to pump blood throughout his body.

Sex
Hypertension occurs more commonly in men until middle age; after middle age, it occurs more in women. The disease is more likely to cause complications and death in men.

Ethnic group
In the United States, whites are less likely to have hypertension than African-Americans, Cubans, Puerto Ricans, and Mexican-Americans. African-Americans are at greatest risk because they tend to have low plasma renin levels and a decreased

Follow-up care for hypertensive patients

Category	Follow-up action
Normal blood pressure	Recheck blood pressure in 2 years.
High normal blood pressure	Recheck blood pressure in 1 year.
Stage 1 hypertension	Confirm hypertension within 2 months.
Stage 2 hypertension	Evaluate patient or refer for care within 1 month.
Stage 3 hypertension	Evaluate patient or refer for care within 1 week.
Stage 4 hypertension	Evaluate patient or refer for care immediately.

ability to rid the body of excess sodium. African-Americans have twice the risk of developing hypertension, a greater tendency to develop severe hypertension, and a higher death rate from hypertension.

Family history
Genetics seems to be a risk factor for some hypertensive patients. Although the inherited traits leading to high blood pressure haven't been determined, certain families have elevated intracellular sodium levels and lowered potassium-to-sodium ratios. Also, studies show a relationship between blood pressure and environment for genetically similar family members. From these studies, researchers estimate that 25% to 61% of all hypertension cases are linked to genetics.

Obesity
Generally, the greater a person's weight, the higher his blood pressure. Just a 10-pound weight loss can significantly decrease a person's blood pressure and may reduce the dose of antihypertensive drug needed.

Upper-body fat is more dangerous than fat in the hips and thighs. In particular, patients with increased intra-abdominal fat are at risk for devel-

Risk factors for primary hypertension

When assessing patients, use this list of risk factors as a quick reference:
- advanced age
- sex
- ethnic group
- family history
- obesity
- tobacco use
- high-sodium diet
- high-fat diet
- heavy alcohol consumption
- sedentary lifestyle
- stress
- excess renin
- mineral deficiencies
- diabetes.

oping hypertension. Also, women with a waist-to-hip ratio greater than 0.85 and men with a waist-to-hip ratio greater than 0.95 have an increased risk of developing hypertension.

Tobacco use
Although smoking and hypertension haven't been conclusively linked, patients who stop smoking decrease their risk of developing cardiovascular disease. In fact, a hypertensive patient who does not smoke is three to five times less likely to suffer a myocardial infarction (MI) or CVA than a patient with hypertension who does smoke. Also, smoking interferes with the action of some antihypertensive drugs such as propranolol.

High-sodium diet
For patients with primary hypertension, ingesting high-sodium foods or beverages may trigger an excessive release of natriuretic hormone, which indirectly increases blood pressure. Also, sodium intake may stimulate vasopressor mechanisms within the central nervous system (CNS), causing water retention and high blood pressure. Usually, blood pressure decreases when sodium intake is restricted.

Although almost everyone in Western countries consumes a high-sodium diet, only about 20% develop hypertension. Thus, a person must be sensitive to sodium to some degree for high-sodium intake to trigger the development of hypertension.

High-fat diet
Foods with a high fat content have an indirect effect on blood pressure. A high-fat diet contributes to obesity and hyperlipidemia, which increase a patient's risk of cardiovascular complications. Hyperlipidemia, an excess of lipids in the plasma, increases the risk of atherosclerosis. Thus, hypertensive patients should be encouraged to eat a low-fat diet to reduce the risk of cardiovascular complications.

Heavy alcohol consumption
Alcohol consumption increases blood pressure; the greater a patient's daily consumption, the higher his blood pressure. Patients who drink excessive amounts of alcohol may be twice as likely to develop hypertension as patients who drink very little. Between 5% and 11% of all cases of hypertension result from excessive alcohol consumption.

Sedentary lifestyle
A patient's risk of developing hypertension increases by as much as 25% with a sedentary lifestyle. A hypertensive patient should be encouraged to exercise as a way to better his overall cardiovascular health. The activity doesn't need to be strenuous; moderate activity, such as a brisk 30-minute to 45-minute walk three to five times a week, is sufficient. By maintaining regular aerobic activity, a hypertensive patient can decrease his systolic blood pressure by about 10 mm Hg.

Stress
A patient's blood pressure can temporarily increase as part of a normal protective, physiologic response to stressors such as anger, fear, and physical pain. However, if such stressors persist, increased vasoconstriction, an increased heart rate, and stimulation of renin release can cause continued high blood pressure. Thus, patients who are exposed to repeated stress have an increased risk of hypertension.

Excess renin
In some patients with primary hypertension, the kidneys secrete excess quantities of renin, resulting in the conversion of angiotensinogen to an-

giotensin. Angiotensin causes arteriole constriction and an increase in aldosterone levels, followed by electrolyte and water retention and, subsequently, hypertension. Between 10% and 17% of hypertensive patients have elevated plasma renin levels and are classified as having high-renin primary hypertension.

Mineral deficiencies
Patients with potassium, calcium, and magnesium deficiencies may experience increased blood pressure. A person can maintain normal potassium levels by changing his diet. Taking calcium supplements may reduce blood pressure in some patients, but it's not recommended to prevent hypertension. Taking magnesium supplements to control hypertension isn't recommended either.

Diabetes
Diabetic patients commonly develop hypertension, and they do so at an early age. In patients with both diabetes and hypertension, complications are severe.

Secondary hypertension
Only 5% or fewer hypertensive patients have secondary hypertension. If a patient over age 50 suddenly develops hypertension, especially if it's severe, suspect a secondary cause, such as a disease that increases cardiac output (CO) or peripheral vascular resistance. After the cause has been identified and treated, generally with surgery or drug therapy, the patient's blood pressure should return to normal.

To identify the cause of secondary hypertension, a physician will order a basic workup that evaluates a patient's cardiac, renal, endocrine, and neurologic systems. Abnormalities in these systems commonly cause hypertension in young hypertensive patients, severely hypertensive patients, and hypertensive patients who don't respond to standard antihypertensive therapy.

Cardiovascular disorders
Coarctation of the aorta, a localized narrowing or constriction of the lumen of the aorta, is a vascular defect that commonly causes hypertension. Generally, the disorder is diagnosed in children.

Coarctation may occur anywhere along the aorta, but it most commonly occurs just beyond the origin of the left subclavian artery. When the condition is severe, the constriction of the lumen produces absent or markedly diminished femoral pulses as well as bruits heard throughout the posterior thorax.

Coarctation of the aorta can be detected by carefully timing the appearance of the patient's femoral pulse with his radial or brachial pulse to determine if a substantial delay exists between pulses. If so, the patient's blood pressure should be taken in both arms and his legs. The blood pressure of a patient with coarctation of the aorta will be elevated in the arms and reduced in the legs.

Surgical repair is usually required to correct coarctation of the aorta. Following surgical repair, only 5% to 10% of patients still have hypertension.

Subclavian artery stenosis also causes hypertension. If a patient has subclavian artery stenosis, his pulse in one arm will be absent or significantly diminished, and his blood pressure in that arm will be significantly lower than in his other arm.

Renal disorders
Renovascular stenosis is the most common cause of hypertension that can be reversed by surgery or percutaneous transluminal angioplasty. Stenosis of one or both renal arteries can produce severe hypertension and a loss of kidney function. Arterial fibromuscular dysplasia, fibrosis of the muscular layer of the artery wall, is the most common cause of renovascular hypertension in patients under age 40; atherosclerosis is the most common cause of renovascular hypertension in older patients.

Systolic bruits in the upper abdominal quadrants may indicate renovascular stenosis or renal arteriovenous malformation. If the bruit is continuous and extends into diastole, the stenosis is severe.

Hypertension can also result from renal parenchymatous disease, a consequence of acute and chronic glomerulonephritis, chronic pyelonephritis, polycystic kidney disease, collagen vascular disorder, intercapillary glomerulosclerosis, and interstitial nephritis. Many hypertensive patients with renal parenchymatous disease develop chronic renal failure. Generally, the treatment of choice for their condition is a diuretic and a diet limiting them to a daily intake of 2 grams of sodium and 40 to 50 grams of protein. Eventually, these patients may also need dialysis.

Though rare, renin-producing tumors also cause hypertension. These tumors, including

Wilms' tumor found in infants and children, arise from either the cortex or pelvis of the kidney and may be benign or malignant. The malignant form is more common, and the treatment is usually radical nephrectomy and, possibly, radiation therapy.

Endocrine disorders

Pheochromocytoma, an abnormal growth of new tissue on the adrenal medulla, produces excessive catecholamines, causing hypertension. These tumors occur most commonly in patients ages 40 to 60, and about 90% of them are benign.

A patient with pheochromocytoma may experience severe headaches, profuse sweating, palpitations, and pronounced pallor caused by a sudden release of catecholamines resulting in a hypertensive crisis. These attacks can be triggered by physical activity, postural changes, emotional distress, hypoglycemia, and surgical trauma. An attack may also be provoked when the tumor is palpated.

If left untreated, a patient with pheochromocytoma can develop diabetes, cardiomyopathy, and hypertension, any of which can result in death. The usual treatment is surgical removal of the tumor, which relieves hypertension in about 75% of patients. The remaining 25% can usually manage their hypertension with antihypertensive drug therapy.

Caused by excessive aldosterone secretion of the adrenal gland, primary hyperaldosteronism is another endocrine disorder that causes hypertension. This condition is more common in women ages 20 to 50. Suspect it in hypertensive patients who have hypokalemia and don't take diuretics.

The three causes of primary hyperaldosteronism are unilateral adrenocortical adenoma, adenomatous hyperplasia, and adrenocortical carcinoma. Unilateral adrenocortical adenoma alone causes 80% to 85% of the cases of primary hyperaldosteronism.

Physicians typically treat primary hyperaldosteronism by surgically removing the tumor. Unfortunately, surgery generally doesn't cure hypertension resulting from adenomatous hyperplasia.

Cushing's syndrome, another cause of hypertension, results from either prolonged treatment with large doses of glucocorticoids or excess cortisol production by the adrenal cortex, which is most commonly caused by a pituitary tumor. In either case, hypertension results from the mineralocorticoid effects of the hyperfunctioning adrenal tissue. When a pituitary tumor causes Cushing's syndrome, the usual treatment consists of surgical removal.

Hypertension can also be caused by acromegaly—a chronic metabolic condition resulting from excessive production of growth hormone in the anterior pituitary. The condition is characterized by enlargement and elongation of the bones of the face, jaw, and extremities. Although one-third of patients with acromegaly have hypertension, it's usually not severe, and the treatment of acromegaly—surgery, radiation, and drugs—usually alleviates the hypertension.

Neurologic disorders

A patient who has sustained a spinal cord injury above the T7 level is at risk for hypertension because of autonomic hyperreflexia, a potentially life-threatening complication resulting from the sympathetic neurons' loss of control over their sympathetic outflow. Stimulation of nerves below the injury, such as from fecal impaction, urine retention, or tactile stimulation, can cause reflex sympathetic activity along the spinal cord resulting in hypertension, bradycardia, severe headache, sweating, blurred vision, a flushed feeling, and nasal congestion. Any quadriplegic who complains of a headache should have his blood pressure promptly checked to determine if hypertension exists as a possible result of autonomic hyperreflexia.

When a patient with a spinal cord injury develops hypertension, his systolic blood pressure may rise to 300 mm Hg, and if the condition is left untreated, he may have a CVA or die. Treatment of autonomic hyperreflexia consists of immediately removing the source of the nerve stimulation, such as bladder distention. If the patient's hypertension persists, his physician may prescribe antihypertensive drugs.

Patients with brain injuries are also at risk for hypertension. When a patient's brain is injured, his intracranial pressure increases, and the blood volume and flow to his brain becomes passively controlled by the pressure in his systemic circulation. So a patient who sustains a brain injury has an elevated blood pressure because of the autoregulatory and compensatory mechanisms within the brain trying to maintain optimal cerebral perfusion pressure.

Drugs

Many prescription and over-the-counter (OTC) drugs can increase blood pressure or interfere with other drugs used to treat hypertension. Oral contraceptives, for example, cause a small increase in systolic and diastolic blood pressure. Hypertension is two to three times more common in patients who use oral contraceptives for more than 5 years than in patients who haven't used them at all. A patient who uses oral contraceptives has an increased risk of developing hypertension, with increasing age, duration of use, and body weight.

Estrogen, when used as a postmenopausal replacement therapy, increases blood pressure in some women. All women receiving hormone replacement therapy should have their blood pressure routinely monitored.

Cyclosporine, which is used as an immunosuppressant to prevent organ rejection in transplant recipients, causes vasoconstriction and reduces renal blood flow. Cyclosporine also increases the reabsorption of sodium, water, and urea and has a direct toxic effect on the nephrons. Vasoconstriction and sodium retention lead to hypertension in 50% to 70% of organ transplant recipients taking cyclosporine and in about 20% of nontransplant patients taking the drug for other reasons. Similarly, corticosteroids used to produce immunosuppression in organ transplant recipients can cause hypertension.

Monoamine oxidase (MAO) inhibitors, which are used for treating depression, can cause a severe hypertensive crisis. This condition results from an interaction of the MAO inhibitors with foods such as cheese, bananas, beer, wine, yeast, yogurt, and meat extracts containing tyramine, dopa, or serotonin. Patients who use MAO inhibitors should have their blood pressure monitored regularly.

Erythropoietin—a hormone that acts on bone marrow cells to stimulate red blood cell (RBC) production—causes increased blood pressure in one-third of patients with end-stage renal disease. Although the exact mechanism of action is unknown, erythropoietin may increase systemic vascular resistance by increasing blood viscosity and reversing hypoxic vasodilation.

Nonsteroidal anti-inflammatory drugs (NSAIDs) can increase blood pressure by blocking the production of prostaglandins in the kidneys, which leads to sodium and water retention. These drugs also antagonize the effects of some antihypertensive drugs, such as diuretics, by blocking sodium excretion. And NSAIDs cause vasoconstriction by affecting the renin-angiotensin-aldosterone system. African-Americans, diabetic patients, and the elderly are most vulnerable to the effects of NSAIDs. Keep in mind that the elderly commonly use NSAIDs for arthritis.

Cold remedies, nasal decongestants, and appetite suppressants also can cause hypertension. Generally, cold remedies and nasal decongestants are powerful vasoconstrictors that increase systolic and diastolic blood pressures. Appetite suppressants such as amphetamines, however, increase blood pressure by stimulating the CNS. Other types of appetite suppressants, such as dexfenfluramine, can cause primary pulmonary hypertension without affecting systemic blood pressure. Patients with advanced atherosclerosis, cardiovascular disease, or moderate to severe hypertension shouldn't take appetite suppressants.

Alcohol and cocaine

Both alcohol and cocaine cause hypertension. Excessive ingestion of alcohol can cause a patient to exacerbate his preexisting hypertension, or it can induce hypertension. And cocaine produces devastating effects on blood pressure by increasing the release of norepinephrine, a powerful vasopressor produced by the body in response to hypotension and stress. This can result in acute hypertension, tachycardia, tremor, and seizures as well as coronary artery vasoconstriction from a CVA or MI.

Poisons

Many poisons can elevate blood pressure and cause hypertension. Some common poisons include cyanide, phencyclidine, and black widow spider venom. Treatment varies depending on the poison, and it usually relieves the poison-induced hypertension.

Pregnancy

Pregnancy-induced hypertension can threaten the lives of both the mother and infant. It causes elevated blood pressure, proteinuria, and edema and may lead to abnormalities in the mother's coagulation system and liver function. The only treatment for pregnancy-induced hypertension is delivery of the infant.

Stress

For some patients, even mild stress can cause a rise in blood pressure. In response to a stressful event, the patient perceives a stressor, and his body initiates a fight-or-flight reaction. Physical signs and symptoms of stress-induced hypertension include decreased gastrointestinal motility, pupil dilation, and increased perspiration, all of which result from sympathetic nervous system stimulation that causes increased blood pressure and increased heart and respiratory rates.

With the white-coat phenomenon, a patient has elevated blood pressure readings in his physician's office or the hospital but normal readings elsewhere. To determine if a patient has true hypertension, a physician may order repeated measurements over time or ambulatory measurements.

In postoperative patients, stress-related hypertension commonly results from sympathetic stimulation caused by pain, bladder distention, hypothermia, or respiratory compromise.

Sleep apnea

Sleep apnea can contribute to the development of hypertension. During apnea, the tongue and soft palate relax and fall back, obstructing the airway either partially or completely. As a result, the patient can't breathe. His oxygen levels fall, and carbon dioxide levels rise, resulting in acidosis and vasoconstriction of the pulmonary arterioles. Eventually, the patient partially awakens, gasps, and reopens his airway. Episodes of apnea may last from 15 to 90 seconds and occur repeatedly during the night.

Diseases causing vasculitis

Scleroderma, polyarteritis nodosa, lupus erythematosus, rheumatoid arthritis, and nonspecific arthritis may cause vasculitis in some patients. About one-half of these patients subsequently develop hypertension because of the effect the diseases have on the arterioles and major arteries.

Complications of untreated hypertension

Hypertension is sometimes called the "silent killer" because many people don't know they have it. If left untreated, chronic systolic and diastolic hypertension damages the walls of systemic blood vessels and organs such as the heart, brain, kidneys, and retina. Eventually, this organ damage can result in coronary artery disease (CAD), CVA, renal failure, and blindness (see *Complications of hypertension*).

Coronary artery disease

Hypertension is the main risk factor for developing CAD from atherosclerosis. With hypertension, atherosclerotic plaque forms in the inner lining of the artery at an accelerated rate. As the artery narrows, more force is needed to pump blood through it, creating an even further elevation in blood pressure.

Cerebrovascular accident

Hypertension is also a serious risk factor of CVA. In fact, hypertension is a leading cause of transient ischemic attacks and CVAs resulting from cerebral thrombosis, intracerebral hemorrhage, and emboli.

Cerebral arterial hemorrhage can occur when progressive atherosclerotic changes take place and blood pressure increases in the affected vessels. Eventually, smooth blood vessel tissue is replaced with fibrous tissue, causing vessel walls to become thicker and more rigid. But the vessels also weaken because of intense constriction of the cerebral arterioles and arteries, resulting in the development of microaneurysms that tend to rupture easily.

Renal disease

Hypertension also leads to end-stage renal disease. During the early stage of hypertension, the capillary basement membrane of the glomeruli becomes thickened by atherosclerosis. Hypertension then causes a gradual destruction of the glomeruli, tubules, and nephrons. At first, a patient's glomerular filtration rate may remain normal, but scarring eventually occurs, causing renal failure. Although most hypertensive patients have some degree of renal dysfunction, African-American hypertensive patients have the greatest risk of developing end-stage renal disease.

Retinopathy

Hypertension can also cause retinopathy. The resulting retinal changes are categorized in four stages of increasingly severe vessel damage.

Usually, the early stages go undetected because the patient has no significant signs or symptoms to report and no apparent reason to seek medical attention. However, if his hypertension is left untreated and his condition progresses into the later stages of retinopathy, he may develop retinal lesions, which can cause blurred vision, or papilledema and retinal hemorrhaging, which can result in blindness.

Arterial system

Arteries, the vessels through which blood travels away from the heart, all carry oxygenated blood, except for the pulmonary arteries, which carry oxygen-depleted blood from the heart to the lungs. The arterial system is made up of vessels of various sizes:
- large, usually elastic arteries, such as the aorta and the pulmonary trunk
- medium-sized arteries, which make up most of the arterial vasculature
- large and small arterioles.

   Arteries have nerves bundled along their outer walls. Primarily derived from the sympathetic nervous system, these nerves cause the arteries to contract and relax, thus regulating the flow of blood to various parts of the body.

Arterial walls

All arteries have three distinct layers. The outer layer (tunica adventitia or externa) is made of strong connective tissue with abundant elastic fibers. The middle layer (tunica media) consists of more elastic fibers than smooth-muscle fibers. The inner layer (tunica intima) is a transparent and highly elastic structure that has direct contact with the circulating blood.

   The thickness of each of these layers varies depending on the location of the artery. For instance, large arteries like the aorta or pulmonary arteries typically have a thick tunica media with more elastic fiber than smooth muscle, enabling them to stretch as blood is ejected from the heart during systole and to recoil during diastole. However, arteries located farther away from the heart have less elastic tissue and more smooth muscle. These small-sized to medium-sized vessels are muscular arteries. Together, all arteries help to maintain blood pressure throughout the high-pressure, high-resistance, low-volume arterial system.

   Arteries become arterioles when the diameter of the vessel is less than 0.5 mm. The thick,

Complications of hypertension

Body system	Effects of hypertension
Cardiovascular	• coronary artery disease • left ventricular hypertrophy • intermittent claudication
Neurologic	• transient ischemic attack or cerebrovascular accident • cerebral aneurysm
Renal	• decreased creatinine clearance • proteinuria • microalbuminuria
Visual	• retinopathy

smooth-muscle layer of the arterioles enables them to control the flow of blood through the systemic circulatory system by means of vasodilation and vasoconstriction and push the blood through finer arterial structures, the capillaries (see *Reviewing the structures of arteries and capillaries,* page 116).

Capillaries

Capillaries are the smallest and most numerous vessels in the arterial circulatory system. The walls of the capillaries consist of a fine, transparent, endothelial layer of tissue similar to the inner layer of the arteries. Capillaries have no elastic or muscular tissues, so nutrients and metabolic end products can pass through their thin walls.

   Capillaries are interposed between arterioles and venules, creating networks. These networks permeate all tissues, supplying blood and nutrients. The more active the function of an organ or tissue, the greater the network of capillaries within it. These networks are typically large in bones and ligaments, smaller in glands and mucous membranes, and nearly absent in tendons.

   Capillary networks contain specialized channels called metarterioles and rings of smooth muscle called precapillary sphincters. These sphincters contract and relax, regulating the flow of

Reviewing the structures of arteries and capillaries

As you review these structures, note the artery's thick muscular tunica media, which helps to control the flow of blood into the capillaries. Decreased elasticity in this layer is a major cause of hypertension.

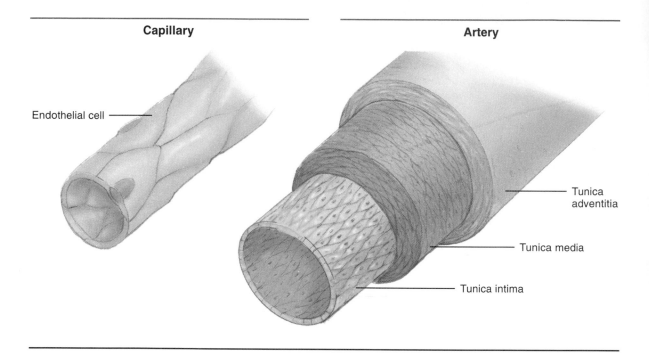

Capillary

Endothelial cell

Artery

Tunica adventitia

Tunica media

Tunica intima

blood through the capillaries. Blood enters the capillary network as arterial blood, and after the exchange of nutrients and metabolic end products takes place, it exits as venous blood returning to the heart through the venous system (see *Inside the capillary network*).

Arterial pressures

To determine if a patient has hypertension, of course, you'll measure his blood pressure. From his blood pressure measurements, you can determine his pulse pressure and mean arterial pressure (MAP). These measurements, in turn, can help you detect related disorders and understand the effects of certain hemodynamic factors on your patient's blood pressure.

Blood pressure

You can measure a patient's blood pressure directly or indirectly. To measure it directly, you'll need an arterial catheter attached to a pressure measuring monitor. To measure it indirectly, you'll need a blood pressure cuff, a stethoscope, and a sphygmomanometer, such as a mercury gravity or aneroid type.

When performed correctly, indirect measurements are within 5 mm Hg of direct measurements. To measure blood pressure indirectly, first place an appropriate-sized blood pressure cuff on the patient's arm. Then, place the bell of the stethoscope over the artery distal to the cuff. Next, inflate the cuff 30 mm Hg beyond the patient's systolic pressure, at which point blood flow in the artery stops. Then, lower the cuff pressure and auscultate for Korotkoff sounds.

Inside the capillary network

Capillary networks—which consist of capillaries, metarterioles, and precapillary sphincters—regulate the flow of blood from the arterioles to the venules. Arrows in this illustration show the flow of blood from an arteriole, through the capillaries and metarterioles, and then into a venule.

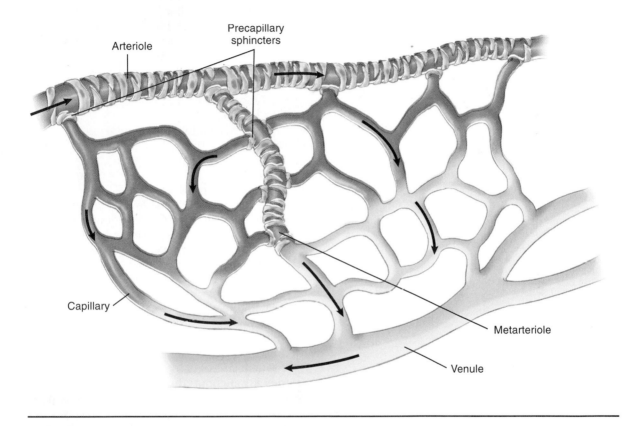

Korotkoff sounds

During auscultation, you'll hear five Korotkoff sounds or phases. Phase 1 is characterized by a faint, clear, rhythmic tapping gradually increasing in intensity. The first sharp thump you hear is the systolic blood pressure, and this sound is produced by blood rushing into the collapsed artery as the pressure in the cuff decreases. The force of the blood determines the intensity of the sound.

Phase 2 begins when murmuring or swishing sounds are produced by blood flowing through the narrowed artery under the pressure cuff and into a wider artery distal to it. The difference in artery widths creates currents that cause the blood and vessel walls to vibrate. These sounds may temporarily disappear, particularly in hypertensive patients, and this silence is called the auscultatory gap. If you don't detect the auscultatory gap, you may underestimate the patient's systolic blood pressure or overestimate his diastolic pressure.

Phase 3 begins when the murmur of phase 2 disappears and the sounds begin to increase in intensity and clarity. In phase 3, the compressed vessel opens during systole but closes during diastole.

Recognizing Korotkoff sounds

To accurately assess your patient's systolic and diastolic blood pressure readings, you need to recognize the variations in the sounds you hear. After you inflate the blood pressure cuff and begin releasing air from it, you'll hear the first of the five Korotkoff sounds described below. In this example, the blood pressure reading is 140/90 mm Hg.

Phase 1 (systolic blood pressure)
A sharp thump, and then tapping.

Phase 2
A murmuring or swishing sound.

Phase 3
The murmuring disappears, and sounds increase in intensity and clarity.

Phase 4 (first diastolic blood pressure)
A softer blowing sound that fades.

Phase 5 (second diastolic blood pressure)
The sounds disappear.

140
130
120
110
100
90
80

Phase 4 occurs when the sounds become muffled and less intense. This phase is referred to as the first diastolic pressure.

Finally, the sounds disappear completely in phase 5, also called the second diastolic pressure. During this phase, the vessel is completely open, and blood flows freely through the artery. At this point, you can palpate a strong radial pulse (see *Recognizing Korotkoff sounds*).

Pulse pressure and mean arterial pressure

You can derive two measurements from a patient's systolic and diastolic blood pressures. These measurements can help in detecting conditions related to a patient's high blood pressure and in understanding the hemodynamic factors that affect blood pressure. One such measurement, pulse pressure, is the difference between the systolic and diastolic pressures. For instance, if a patient's blood pressure is 120/80 mm Hg, his pulse pressure is 40 mm Hg. Normally, a patient's pulse pressure is 30 to 40 mm Hg.

Pulse pressure reflects stroke volume (SV), ejection velocity, systemic vascular resistance, and CO. An increased or widened pulse pressure, such as in a patient with a blood pressure of 160/40 mm Hg, signifies increased SV, which could result from the following conditions:
- high blood pressure
- sinus bradycardia
- complete heart block
- aortic regurgitation
- anxiety
- exercise
- catecholamine production
- arteriosclerosis of the large arteries and aorta.

Increases in pulse pressure reduce a patient's systemic vascular resistance and may appear when a patient has a fever, is in a hot environment, or has been exercising.

A decreased pulse pressure can be caused by factors such as:
- heart failure, which causes reduced ejection velocity
- hypovolemia
- shock.

A patient's MAP is the average pressure in the arteries throughout the cardiac cycle as influenced by CO and vascular resistance. This pressure varies in different parts of the body, from about 100 mm Hg in the aorta and large arteries to about 0 mm Hg at the end of the vena caval system.

To calculate a patient's MAP, use the following formula:

MAP = diastolic pressure + ⅓ pulse pressure

Using this equation, a patient whose blood pressure is 120/80 mm Hg and pulse pressure is 40 mm Hg would have a MAP of 93.2 mm Hg.

Normally, a patient's MAP ranges from 70 to 100 mm Hg. An increased MAP occurs with primary hypertension, arterial disease, and epinephrine release, and a decreased MAP can indicate decreased vascular resistance, cardiac failure, or hypovolemia.

Hemodynamic factors

Various hemodynamic factors, such as SV and CO, affect a patient's blood pressure (see *How hemodynamic factors affect blood pressure*). Fluctuations of these hemodynamic factors can also indicate a related condition.

Stroke volume

A patient's SV, the amount of blood pumped from the left ventricle during systole, is usually about 70 ml per heartbeat. Three factors affect SV: preload, afterload, and contractility.

Preload is the force of blood in the ventricle exerted on the ventricular muscle at the end of diastole. The more the muscle fibers are stretched during diastole, the more forcefully they'll contract during systole.

Afterload is the pressure that causes the ventricular muscle to force the aortic valve open and send blood into the aorta. And contractility is the ability of the myocardium to contract normally.

Decreased SV commonly indicates hypovolemia, increased systemic vascular resistance, or heart failure. Increased SV can result from hypervolemia or decreased systemic vascular resistance.

Cardiac output

A patient's CO, the amount of blood pumped by the ventricles each minute, is usually 5 to 7 liters per minute. You can calculate CO by multiplying a patient's SV by his heart rate for 1 minute.

A decreased CO may indicate that a patient has one of these conditions:
* heart failure
* decreased blood volume
* arterial or venous obstruction
* anaphylactic shock
* septic shock.

An increased CO may indicate that a patient has one of these conditions:
* decreased systemic vascular resistance
* sepsis
* an intrauterine pregnancy.

Systemic vascular resistance

Systemic vascular resistance, the amount of resistance in peripheral blood vessels, also plays a major role in regulating blood pressure. The vasomotor tone of the vessels primarily determines systemic vascular resistance. When vas-

How hemodynamic factors affect blood pressure

Hemodynamic factor	Effect on blood pressure
Stroke volume • increases with fluid overload • decreases with hemorrhaging	• increase • decrease
Cardiac output • increases with metabolic demand (from sepsis, thyroid disease, or pregnancy) • decreases with heart failure	• increase • decrease
Systemic vascular resistance • increases with vasoconstriction • decreases with vasodilation	• increase • decrease
Blood viscosity • increases with polycythemia	• increase
Elasticity of the arterial walls • reduced by arteriosclerosis	• increase

cular resistance is high, a patient's blood pressure rises.

The amount of a patient's circulating blood volume influences his systemic vascular resistance. If blood flow decreases, the body compensates by increasing systemic vascular resistance, making the arteries and arterioles adjust their internal diameter. A small change in the diameter of an artery or arteriole creates a major change in systemic vascular resistance: As the vessel lumen decreases, the resistance increases. This system increases arterial pressure to maintain blood pressure as near normal as possible. In contrast, when systemic vessels dilate and systemic vascular resistance falls, blood pressure decreases.

Blood viscosity and arterial elasticity

Two other hemodynamic factors affecting blood pressure are blood viscosity and elasticity of the arterial walls. Increased blood viscosity, which causes increased blood pressure, results from polycythemia, an abnormal increase of RBC mass in relation to blood plasma.

Decreased elasticity of the arterial walls can also cause increased blood pressure. In many cases, decreased elasticity results from arteriosclerosis.

Blood pressure regulation

The regulation of normal systemic arterial pressure is a complex process involving the nervous, renal, and endocrine systems. In some hypertensive patients, elevated blood pressure may result from abnormal functioning in one or more of these systems.

Nervous system

Comprised of the sympathetic nervous system and the parasympathetic nervous system, the autonomic nervous system coordinates and maintains a steady state among the internal organs and glands of the body.

The vasomotor center of the sympathetic nervous system, located in the medulla, generates energy in times of need, such as during the fight-or-flight response. And the motor area of the sympathetic nervous system, located in the cerebral cortex, is activated during exercise, in turn stimulating the vasomotor center. Postural changes, such as moving from a lying to a standing position, also activate the vasomotor center to maintain blood pressure.

Located throughout the body, sympathetic nervous system adrenergic receptors are categorized as $alpha_1$, $alpha_2$, $beta_1$, and $beta_2$, depending on their location and function. The smooth muscle of the peripheral vasculature contains both alpha and beta receptors. When stimulated, these receptors cause vasoconstriction, resulting in increased systemic vascular resistance.

Through $beta_1$ receptors, a patient's nervous system quickly reacts to a decrease in CO or blood pressure. Secretions of epinephrine and norepinephrine from sympathetic nerve endings and the adrenal medulla increase heart rate and strengthen myocardial contractions. In this way, the body attempts to increase CO and sustain perfusion to vital organs such as the brain and heart.

Two other parts of the sympathetic nervous system, chemoreceptors and baroreceptors, help regulate blood pressure. Located within the aortic arch and carotid arteries, chemoreceptors initiate changes in heart rate and arterial pressure in response to chemical stimulation. When partial pressure of arterial oxygen or pH decreases, chemoreceptors cause blood pressure to increase. When partial pressure of arterial carbon dioxide increases, they cause blood pressure to decrease.

Baroreceptors, specialized nerve receptors located in the aortic arch and carotid arteries, control only temporary changes in the blood pressure. For instance, when a patient's blood pressure increases, the baroreceptors are stimulated and send inhibitory impulses to the sympathetic vasomotor center in the brain, stimulating the vagus nerve. The vagus nerve, under the control of the parasympathetic nervous system, causes dilation of the peripheral arterioles, a reduced heart rate, and decreased cardiac contractility. Subsequently, blood pressure decreases.

When blood pressure decreases, baroreceptors can stimulate the sympathetic nervous system, resulting in constriction of the peripheral arterioles and an increased heart rate. In the hypertensive patient, these baroreceptors become adjusted to an elevated blood pressure level, and they begin to recognize it as normal.

The parasympathetic nervous system conserves and restores energy. However, it plays only a minor role in blood pressure regulation because most blood vessels are innervated by sympathetic nerves. Sympathetic activity increases peripheral vascular resistance; parasympathetic activity does little to alter it. However, changes in blood pressure do occur when the parasympathetic nervous system is stimulated through the vagus nerve, leading to a reduction in heart rate and CO.

Renal system

The kidneys help regulate blood pressure by controlling sodium and extracellular fluid volume. When sodium is retained, water retention increases, leading to increased extracellular fluid volume. Higher extracellular fluid volume increases venous return to the heart, elevates SV, and ultimately elevates blood pressure.

The renal system also has another mechanism for regulating blood pressure—the renin-angiotensin-aldosterone system. Once activated, this system responds to sympathetic stimulation or decreased blood flow through the kidneys. First, renin is secreted from the juxtaglomerular apparatus in the afferent arterioles of the kidney. Renin then converts angiotensinogen to angiotensin I, which is subsequently converted into angiotensin II in the lungs.

Angiotensin II increases blood pressure by way of two different mechanisms. When released, angiotensin II, a potent vasoconstrictor, increases vascular resistance, leading to an immediate increase in blood pressure. Angiotensin II also increases blood pressure by stimulating the adrenal cortex to secrete aldosterone. This secretion causes sodium retention by the kidneys, and elevated sodium levels lead to increased blood volume and increased CO.

The renal medulla secretes prostaglandins, which have a vasodilatory effect on systemic circulation. Prostaglandin secretion decreases vascular resistance and lowers blood pressure by counteracting the vasoconstrictive effects of angiotensin and norepinephrine. In patients with renal failure, prostaglandin production and functioning parenchyma are lost, and without the opposing action of prostaglandin, hypertension can develop.

Endocrine system

When stimulated by the sympathetic nervous system, the adrenal medulla releases epinephrine and norepinephrine. They, in turn, cause vasoconstriction, an increased heart rate, and increased contractility, all of which increase CO and systemic vascular resistance, thereby raising blood pressure.

As discussed, aldosterone causes the kidneys to retain sodium and water, elevating blood pressure by increasing CO. This sodium increase also causes the release of antidiuretic hormone by the posterior pituitary gland. When the kidneys are stimulated to retain water, extracellular fluid volume increases, elevating blood pressure.

Pathophysiology of hypertension

To understand the pathophysiology of primary hypertension, remember that arterial blood pressure is a product of CO and systemic vascular resistance and that CO is a product of heart rate and SV. Thus, any change in heart rate, CO, SV, or systemic vascular resistance affects blood pressure.

Several theories attempt to explain the onset of primary hypertension in at-risk patients. These theories suggest that primary hypertension develops through a combination of mechanisms, such as:

- increased blood volume
- inappropriate autoregulation of blood pressure
- overstimulation of sympathetic nervous fibers in the heart and blood vessels
- water and sodium retention by the kidneys
- hormonal malfunction affecting the kidneys and blood vessels.

In the theory of hypertension induced by increased blood volume, CO increases to keep up with the high volume of blood passing through the heart. The autoregulatory mechanism of the arterial system produces vasoconstriction in an attempt to keep tissue perfusion relatively constant. When the blood volume remains elevated, vasoconstriction causes systemic vascular resistance, leading to hypertension.

Inappropriate autoregulation of the cardiovascular system is another possible cause of primary hypertension. Beginning with elevated CO, hypertension develops through a failure of the autoregulatory mechanism. After CO and blood volume decrease, vascular tone doesn't return to normal. The hypertensive state becomes the new baseline for the cardiovascular system, and autoregulation maintains this elevated blood pressure.

Another theory maintains that the sympathetic nervous system's normal physiologic response to stress may become pathologic, resulting in overstimulation of the sympathetic nervous system and increased vasoconstriction. This overstimulation increases CO and systemic vascular resistance.

Baroreceptors monitor arterial blood pressure. When arterial pressure rises, the baroreceptors stimulate a vagal response, decreasing the heart rate and causing vasodilation. Likewise, when arterial pressure falls, this reflex system causes arterial pressure to rise. The reason this system doesn't function properly in hypertensive patients isn't known, but one theory suggests that baroreceptor sensitivity is reset at a higher level as the body becomes accustomed to the increased blood pressure.

Excessive sodium intake may cause primary hypertension in people with an inherited defect in sodium excretion. In response to elevated blood pressure, diuresis decreases in normally functioning kidneys. Pathologic changes can alter the threshold at which the kidneys excrete water

RESEARCH UPDATE

Systolic hypertension in the elderly

Increased systolic blood pressure used to be considered a normal part of aging. An old rule stated that *100 mm Hg plus the patient's age* was tolerable. Isolated systolic hypertension wasn't a treated condition. However, the results of the Systolic Hypertension in the Elderly Program (SHEP) study changed this way of thinking.

The SHEP study, a double-blind clinical trial, used low doses of chlorthalidone and atenolol to treat systolic hypertension. The participants' blood pressures were then monitored for 4 to 5 years, after which the researchers found a 36% decrease in cerebrovascular accidents, a 25% decrease in coronary artery disease, and a 54% decrease in left ventricular heart failure in the patients who received the chlorthalidone and atenolol. Similar studies in Sweden and the United Kingdom later confirmed these findings.

Currently, the Fifth Report of the Joint National Committee on Detection, Evaluation, and Treatment of High Blood Pressure stresses the importance of systolic blood pressure in evaluating hypertension. Particularly for middle-aged and older patients, systolic hypertension increases the risk of cardiovascular disease, even when diastolic blood pressure is normal.

and sodium, thereby altering the arterial blood pressure.

The onset of primary hypertension in some patients may result from interference with the sodium-potassium pump that controls the movement of sodium and potassium across the cell membrane. Also, hypertension may result from excess renin production, which stimulates the release of aldosterone, causing sodium and water retention and increased arterial blood pressure.

Primary hypertension may also be caused by a hormone preventing sodium and calcium excretion. Intracellular calcium, which promotes smooth-muscle contraction, causes vasoconstriction, resulting in increased peripheral resistance and elevated blood pressure.

Hypertension in the elderly

Systolic hypertension is more common in elderly patients (see *Systolic hypertension in the elderly*). Elevated systolic blood pressure readings are usually caused by increased CO, systemic vascular resistance, or both. The main vascular cause of systolic hypertension is rigidity of the aorta, which develops from arteriosclerosis and increases total peripheral vascular resistance. Normally, the elastic aorta stretches as blood is pumped from the heart, but with decreased elasticity and compliance, systolic pressure increases significantly.

Aging also causes hyaline degeneration of the tunica media of arterioles, reducing lumen size. Further, decreased baroreceptor sensitivity may contribute to increased sympathetic nervous system activity and elevated levels of norepinephrine.

About 45% of the elderly in the United States have systolic blood pressures of 160 mm Hg or higher and diastolic pressures of less than 90 mm Hg—a condition known as isolated systolic hypertension. Generally, this condition reflects a disease process resulting in lost elasticity of the aorta and its large branches. Other than advanced age, this condition is the greatest risk factor of cardiovascular disease in elderly patients.

7

HYPERTENSION

Assessment

At first, many patients with hypertension have no symptoms. As the disease progresses, some patients actually become accustomed to its symptoms—headaches, dizziness, and blurred vision—and view them as insignificant. Thus, diagnosing and treating hypertension may require a thorough patient assessment. This usually includes obtaining and interpreting a patient's health history, performing a physical examination, taking blood pressure readings, and monitoring the results of diagnostic tests.

You also may use your assessment skills to help identify someone who may develop hypertension. And you may use them to evaluate a patient who has just been diagnosed with hypertension, to monitor a hypertensive patient's treatment, and to detect complications resulting from hypertension.

Health history

By guiding a hypertensive patient through the initial phases of detection and education about his condition, you play a leading role in his plan of care. For the first step in this process, obtain the patient's health history, which should include risk factors, medical history, and any social characteristics that might influence his response to the disease or its treatment.

Family history

Hypertension seems to be hereditary. If a patient's parents have hypertension, he has twice the risk of developing it as someone whose parents don't have it. When obtaining a hypertensive patient's family history, ask about his parents, grandparents, siblings, and children. Record their ages and general states of health. If one of these family members is dead, find out the cause of death and the age at the time of death.

Note episodes of hypertension and coronary artery, cerebral, peripheral, or renal vascular disease among family members. If a family member has any of these diseases, the rest of the family has an increased risk of developing them.

Also, ask him if he knows of any complications that occurred during his fetal development (see *How congenital abnormalities lead to hypertension*, page 124).

Risk factors

When assessing a patient's risk of developing hypertension, consider his race, sex, and age. African-Americans have a greater risk of hypertension than whites. Men have a greater risk of hypertension from early to middle adulthood, but women have greater risk after middle age. Also, the risk of hypertension increases with age. Older African-American women have the greatest risk of developing the condition.

A patient's educational level and socioeconomic status and the part of the country where he lives or used to live are also risk factors for hypertension. Less educated people, people from lower socioeconomic groups, and people from the southeastern United States have an increased risk of developing it.

How congenital abnormalities lead to hypertension

Sometimes, the underlying cause of hypertension begins at birth—or earlier. If problems such as maternal anemia and undernutrition caused a low birth weight, your patient may have been born with a smaller number of nephrons, making him less able to maintain adequate renal function. Because the kidneys play such a pivotal role in regulating blood pressure, any damage to them during fetal development can significantly affect blood pressure control later in life.

In utero complications during the first weeks of life may lead to unilateral or bilateral renal agenesis—congenital absence of the kidney. Growth disturbances during the second or third month can result in a congenital malformation such as renal hypoplasia—an incomplete or underdeveloped kidney. And a complication after the fourth month will most likely affect the renal parenchyma, possibly causing polycystic kidney disease.

Of course, some patients won't know if they suffered in utero complications. If the mother's medical records are available, review them for any mention of complications during her pregnancy. If they aren't available and she's still living, have your patient ask her about the course of her pregnancy.

Obesity, a modifiable risk factor for hypertension, doubles a patient's risk of developing the disease. As you interview the patient, note whether he's obese.

Stress also increases a patient's risk. As you know, stress elevates a person's circulating catecholamine level. And catecholamines work directly on the sympathetic nervous system to increase heart rate and blood pressure. Therefore, be sure to note the patient's responses to daily stress. Ask him what type of job he has and whether or not he finds it stressful. Also, ask him whether he uses moderate exercise to reduce tension.

Ask your patient if he drinks alcohol. If he does, ask how much he drinks in an average day. Alcohol abuse can increase his risk of hypertension. Alcohol also interferes with the action of many antihypertensive drugs.

Ask your patient if he smokes. Tobacco has vasoconstrictive effects, thereby increasing a smoker's blood pressure. Smoking also adds greatly to his risk of developing cardiovascular disease.

Allergies

Thoroughly document your patient's allergies; don't simply list the allergies he claims to have. Many patients believe they've had allergic reactions—for example, gastrointestinal (GI) upset from a particular drug—when what they actually experienced was an adverse effect. Thus, for each drug or food that your patient claims an allergy, find out which symptoms he experienced. A true allergic reaction consists of anaphylaxis or threatened anaphylaxis, including hives, itching, edema of the mucous membranes, and life-threatening laryngospasm.

A patient's allergy history helps in determining the treatment of hypertension. For example, thiazide diuretics are among the most commonly used hypertensive drugs. However, an allergy to sulfonamide-derived drugs contraindicates their use.

Diet history

Although no studies have proven the link between sodium and hypertension, increased salt intake can elevate blood pressure by 10%, especially in patients with a sensitivity to salt. Assessing the sodium content of a patient's diet may require some detective work. A patient may not have a good grasp of the sodium sources in his diet, so ask specific questions about the types of foods he eats. For example, if your patient says he has soup for lunch, ask whether it's homemade or canned. Canned soup can have up to 1,000 mg of sodium per serving, and prepackaged soup mixes can also be high in sodium. If the soup is homemade, ask how much salt, garlic salt, artificial flavoring, or other sodium sources are added during cooking.

To further assess his sodium intake, tell your hypertensive patient to keep a dietary log of all the food and drink he consumes over several days. If appropriate, also discuss with the patient's physician the need for a dietary consultation.

The patient's diet history helps you assess his potassium intake. A potassium deficiency may increase blood pressure and the risk of ventricular

Reviewing causes of secondary hypertension

If your patient has a specific disorder or takes certain drugs, he may be at risk for developing secondary hypertension. Renal disorders are the most common cause, but secondary hypertension may result from any of the following:

Renal disorders
- primary sodium retention
- renal parenchymatous disease (chronic nephritis, acute glomerular nephritis, polycystic kidney disease, diabetic nephropathy, hydronephrosis)
- renin-producing tumors
- renovascular disease

Endocrine disorders
- acromegaly
- adrenal cortical disease (Cushing's syndrome, primary aldosteronism)
- hyperparathyroidism
- hyperthyroidism
- hypothyroidism
- pheochromocytoma

Neurologic disorders
- familial dysautonomia
- Guillain-Barré syndrome
- increased intracranial pressure from brain tumor, encephalitis, or respiratory acidosis

- lead poisoning
- quadriplegia
- sleep apnea

Drugs
- estrogen
- glucocorticoids
- mineralocorticoids
- monoamine oxidase inhibitors taken with foods containing tyramine
- sympathomimetics

Acute stress
- alcohol withdrawal
- burns
- hypoglycemia
- pancreatitis
- postoperative stress
- postresuscitation stress
- sickle cell crisis

Other causes
- alcohol
- coarctation of the aorta
- illicit drugs
- increased intravascular volume
- pregnancy
- psychological disturbances

arrhythmias. But a high-potassium intake, preferably from foods such as oranges, bananas, raisins, and dried apricots, can sometimes lower blood pressure. If your patient is taking a diuretic for hypertension, he may need potassium supplements.

The diet history also helps you assess your patient's calcium intake. Calcium deficiency increases a patient's risk of hypertension. And the recommended daily allowance of calcium is 800 to 1,200 mg.

History of present illness

Most patients with hypertension don't have specific symptoms. Though widely considered a symptom of hypertension, headache usually only occurs with severe hypertension. Generally, a patient has pain in the occipital area when he wakes up in the morning, and it subsides spontaneously after a few hours. He may experience related symptoms, including dizziness, palpitations, fatigue, or impotence. If he has hypertensive vascular disease, symptoms may include dizziness from transient cerebral ischemia, visual disturbances from retinal changes, and angina from coronary artery occlusion.

If a patient has secondary hypertension, his signs and symptoms will be specific to the underlying disorder (see *Reviewing causes of secondary hypertension*). Carefully reviewing his signs and symptoms and medical history should help you detect the underlying cause. For example, ask the patient if he has been experiencing headaches, palpitations, or excessive perspiration, which may indicate pheochromocytoma. Weakness and polyuria may be signs of hyperaldosteronism or an adrenal cortical disorder. Claudication of the legs may indicate coarctation of the aorta or peripheral vascular disease. And weight gain and mood swings may indicate Cushing's syndrome.

Ask the patient to describe his symptoms, including their location, intensity, and frequency. Find out what measures he has taken to relieve his symptoms and whether they've been effective. Also, ask him or find out from his medical record when he learned that he has hypertension and when he was last told he had a normal blood pressure reading.

Drug history

Several types of drugs can significantly affect blood pressure, so to rule out secondary hypertension, explore the patient's drug history. Ask if he's using a nasal decongestant for cold or allergy symptoms; the active ingredient in nasal decongestants—usually phenylpropanolamine or phenylephrine—can cause vasoconstriction. Phenylpropanolamine is also the active ingredient in many over-the-counter diet pills, and phenylephrine is the active ingredient in eyedrops used for pupillary dilation. Despite being administered in the eye, these drops also elevate blood pressure.

A patient may be taking corticosteroids for allergies or for inflammatory, respiratory, nervous system, endocrine, hematologic, eye, or skin diseases. Corticosteroid use results in salt and fluid retention, which increases intravascular volume and elevates blood pressure. Corticosteroids also reduce the dilation and permeability of capillaries, resulting in increased blood pressure.

If your patient is a woman, ask if she uses oral contraceptives. Oral contraceptives cause hypertension in 4% to 5% of women and aggravate it in 9% to 16%.

In patients being treated with monoamine oxidase (MAO) inhibitors, hypertensive crisis can result from eating foods containing tyramine—high-protein foods that have undergone protein breakdown by pickling, aging, fermenting, smoking, or bacterial contamination, including aged cheeses, wine, beer, salami, pickled herring, chicken livers, yeast extract, and yogurt. These MAO inhibitors also have many drug interactions—such as levodopa, methylphenidate, and systemic sympathomimetic drugs—that can lead to hypertension.

Cyclosporine and erythropoietin can also raise blood pressure. Used in transplant patients to decrease the chances of organ rejection, cyclosporine causes vasoconstriction and salt retention, which can result in hypertension. Used to stimulate red blood cell (RBC) production by the bone marrow, erythropoietin increases blood pressure in about one-third of patients with end-stage renal disease.

Complications

Patients with long-standing, uncontrolled hypertension have a greater risk of experiencing complications. If a patient has been diagnosed with related complications, ask about the prescribed therapy, his compliance with it, and his response to it.

Ask the patient about any problems with his vision because the eyes are especially sensitive to elevated blood pressure. If a patient complains of visual disturbances, hypertension may have caused injury to his retina.

Hypertension may cause nephrosclerosis, which may lead to renal insufficiency and uremia. Particularly in African-Americans, hypertension commonly results in end-stage renal failure. Ask patients about overly frequent urination, any changes in the amount of urine, recent unexplained weight gain, and dependent edema.

Hypertension may also affect the central nervous system. Cerebral atherosclerosis can lead to transient ischemic attacks (TIAs) or cerebrovascular accidents (CVAs). Therefore, when taking a patient's history, thoroughly explore any neurologic complaints such as transient hemiparesis, aphasia, or loss of consciousness.

Surgical history

A patient's surgical history should include all operations he has had and the type of anesthesia used. The kidneys play a major role in blood pressure regulation, so ask whether he has had surgery involving his kidneys or adrenal glands. Also, any surgery with general anesthesia can affect kidney function and blood pressure. General anesthesia is especially risky for patients with renal failure because it stresses an already fragile organ.

Psychological and social history

A patient's lifestyle can affect his compliance with his prescribed plan of care. To help achieve effective therapy, use the initial interview to identify any lifestyle factors that may interfere with compliance. For example, ask if the patient travels frequently on business. If so, he may find himself in situations that interfere with treatment, such as frequently eating out and drinking with clients. Advise such a patient to select restaurants that offer healthy meals and to limit his alcohol intake.

Also, find out about the patient's work schedule. Some patients work night shifts and have erratic sleep and eating habits. If a patient needs an antihypertensive drug, he'll need help adjusting the dosage schedule to fit his lifestyle.

A patient's support system and culture also can influence his compliance with the treatment plan. If his family, culture, or religion doesn't allow the use of Western drugs, he may disregard the treatment regimen. So assess your patient's personal and cultural beliefs and try to create a plan that he'll follow. For example, your treatment plan may include having the patient lose weight, follow a low-sodium diet, and participate in a planned exercise program.

Determine whether a patient has financial limitations that may affect his compliance. If he has little money, he may buy food instead of filling a prescription. Refer such patients to a social worker or other appropriate person in your facility who can explore financial options to assist with his treatment. If a patient has a prescription plan that requires co-payment, recommend the less expensive alternatives to the physician.

A patient's educational level can affect his understanding of the disease. He may be willing to follow a treatment plan but unable to understand what he's supposed to do. Assess a patient's ability to learn and retain information and then tailor your teaching plan accordingly. For instance, if you suspect that the patient cannot read and needs to know which foods he should avoid, he may learn best with pictures illustrating various foods.

Adverse effects from drug therapy can also interfere with a patient's compliance. Some drugs can alter the taste of food; others can cause impotence. Before drug therapy begins, explain the possible adverse effects and any measures your patient can take to control them. Then during the course of drug therapy, ask him about adverse effects to drugs he's currently taking. Prompt him to discuss sexual difficulties by asking him if he has experienced sexual problems since he started drug therapy. Be sure to assess whether or not he had these problems before he started therapy.

Physical examination

After obtaining a complete health history, examine the patient for the physical findings resulting from hypertension. In particular, if he has reported symptoms related to hypertension or complications caused by hypertension, look for the corresponding signs during the physical examination.

General appearance

Your physical examination should start with an evaluation of the patient's overall appearance. Ask yourself these questions:
- Does he appear well nourished, undernourished, or overnourished?
- Is his face round? Does he have abdominal obesity, which can occur with Cushing's syndrome?
- How is his grooming? This may indicate whether he can perform self-care and how well he'll adhere to his treatment plan.
- Does he appear to be in pain? Assessing his comfort level may help you explore his chief complaint and focus the examination.
- Is he alert? If he has difficulty remaining alert, he may be suffering neurologic changes from hypertension or adverse effects from his antihypertensive drugs.

Height and weight

Measuring a patient's height and weight determines whether he's obese or at his ideal body weight. Obese patients have an increased risk of hypertension, and patients with abdominal obesity have a greater risk than those with excess fat in their hips and thighs.

If a patient's weight is 20% or more than the desirable range for his age, sex, height, and body build, find out whether he has taken any measures to reduce his weight. Ask him what methods have and haven't worked and why he thinks this is so. In coordination with his physician and dietitian, develop a weight-loss diet that's appropriate for him.

With even moderate weight loss, some obese patients experience significantly reduced blood pressure. As a patient decreases his caloric intake, he'll probably also decrease his sodium and saturated fat intake, which will prevent or slow the progression of atherosclerosis.

Vital signs

Take vital signs when assessing a patient's hypertensive status, following the progression of the disease, and determining his response to treatment. If you detect abnormalities in the pulse rate or rhythm or in the quality of respirations, he may have complications from hypertension or an underlying disorder. For instance, if the patient has an irregular pulse or rapid, shallow respirations, he may have developed an arrhythmia resulting from heart failure due to left ventricular hypertrophy.

Neurologic status

Determine the patient's level of consciousness and mental status as he answers your questions during the interview. If you suspect a CVA or TIA, perform a complete neurologic examination to pinpoint any neurologic damage:

- Note the quality, clarity, and content of the patient's speech.
- Test his cerebellar function by observing his gait and his ability to walk heel-to-toe, walk on his heels, walk on his toes, hop in place, and do shallow knee bends.
- Perform Romberg's test and assess the patient's ability to perform rapid alternating movements.
- Check his motor system by assessing muscle tone, muscle strength, and point discrimination.
- Assess his sensory system by checking for pain, temperature, light touch, position, vibration, and discrimination sensations. Compare right and left sides and proximal and distal areas on the limbs.

Abnormal findings may indicate that the patient is experiencing a complication of his hypertension, such as hemiparesis from a CVA.

Head and neck

When examining a patient's head and neck, keep in mind the causes and effects of secondary hypertension. If necessary, perform a funduscopic eye examination. The retinal arteries, the only arteries in the body that can be examined directly, may provide important clues about the severity of a patient's hypertension. Check for papilledema—an elevated and swollen optic disc—and for arteriovenous (AV) nicking, which indicates narrowing and damage to the retinal arteries. As hypertension progresses, you may see further evidence of injury to the retina, such as retinal hemorrhages and exudates.

Examine the neck for jugular vein distention, a sign of heart failure. Auscultate the carotid arteries for bruits and check the patient for other evidence of arteriosclerosis. Palpate the thyroid gland for abnormalities because thyroid dysfunction can also cause secondary hypertension.

Heart and lungs

Perform a cardiac examination to detect any effects of hypertension. Palpate the precordium to detect precordial lifts or heaves and to locate the point of maximal impulse. The presence of a lift or heave or a laterally displaced point of maximal impulse may indicate left ventricular hypertrophy (see *Palpation tips for cardiac assessment*). An increased heart rate and an S_3 or S_4 heart sound may signify that your patient is developing heart failure. You may hear murmurs because of turbulent blood flow through a damaged heart valve. Finally, listen for arrhythmias that may result from myocardial ischemia or a myocardial infarction (MI).

Be sure to auscultate all lung fields, anterior and posterior. If you note crackles and the patient complains of shortness of breath on exertion, your patient may have heart failure or pulmonary edema.

Abdomen

Inspect the patient's abdomen for the truncal obesity and purple striae that result from hypertensive Cushing's syndrome. While auscultating the abdomen, listen carefully for any bruits in the aorta and the renal and iliac arteries. Such bruits may indicate an abdominal aortic aneurysm or renal or iliac artery stenosis.

Palpate the abdomen for masses, such as pheochromocytoma and renin-producing tumors. Also, palpate the patient's kidneys for size, shape, and smoothness. Feel for enlarged or polycystic kidneys to rule out a renal cause of hypertension. Assess his liver and spleen for en-

Palpation tips for cardiac assessment

When palpating the precordium, use the heel of your hand while keeping your fingers slightly elevated to best feel the right ventricle.

To detect the point of maximal impulse, position your fingers as shown. Normally felt as a gentle tap, the point of maximal impulse is located 5 to 7 cm from the left sternal border along the fifth intercostal space. If you don't detect it in the normal position, check for a laterally displaced point of maximal impulse.

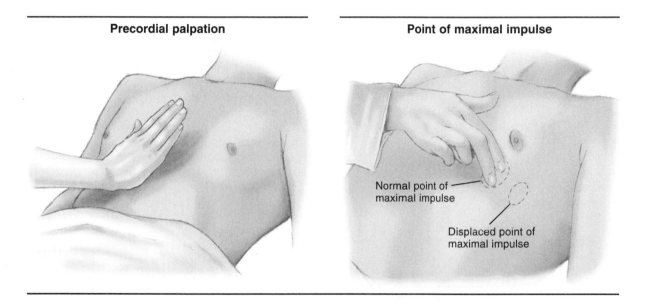

Precordial palpation

Point of maximal impulse

Normal point of maximal impulse

Displaced point of maximal impulse

largement, which may indicate heart failure. And carefully palpate for any abnormalities in the abdominal aorta. Because hypertension can cause abdominal aortic aneurysms and dissecting aneurysms, be alert for any enlargement of the aorta or a pulsatile mass. If a pulsatile mass is visible, don't palpate it because it can rupture.

Arms and legs

Palpate the pulses in the patient's limbs. Bruits in the femoral artery or diminished peripheral pulses could indicate peripheral vascular disease. They may also indicate coarctation of the aorta, a cause of hypertension. Another sign of coarctation of the aorta is higher blood pressure in the arms than in the legs, which can be determined during blood pressure testing. Also, check for pedal edema, a characteristic sign of heart failure.

Diagnostic tests

Diagnosing and treating hypertension requires accurate blood pressure testing. Also, several other tests—blood and urine tests and tests that evaluate the structure and function of the heart and blood vessels—are used to diagnose secondary hypertension, to monitor a patient's response to treatment, and to detect and follow the progress of complications.

Blood pressure

Normally, hypertensive patients have a systolic blood pressure of 140 mm Hg or higher or a diastolic pressure of 90 mm Hg or higher on at least two separate occasions. However, even in healthy people, blood pressure fluctuates depending on the time of day and the activities they've been

Ensuring accurate blood pressure measurement

Before you take a patient's blood pressure, consider these factors, which can distort your reading. Then, as appropriate, take steps to ensure an accurate reading. For instance, if your patient smokes and drinks caffeinated beverages, make sure he hasn't done so for at least 30 minutes before you take his blood pressure.

Patient
- anxiety
- arrhythmias
- bladder distention
- conversation
- medications
- pain
- posture
- recent consumption of large meal or caffeine
- recent physical activity
- recent tobacco use
- time of day

Examiner
- hearing impairment
- knowledge of previous readings
- knowledge of treatment
- procedural error such as diastolic blood pressure recorded at muffling instead of disappearance of sounds
- vision impairment

Environment
- cold or excessively warm room
- loud or repetitive noises

Equipment
- inaccurate mercury level
- incorrect cuff size
- pressure leak in the inflation system
- stethoscope with long or cracked tubing
- stethoscope with no bell or cracked bell
- uncalibrated aneroid manometer
- worn Velcro or ripped cuff fabric

mal, but if the difference is more than 10 mm Hg, the patient may have arterial compression or obstruction on the side with the lower pressure.

If a hypertensive patient's diastolic pressure increases when he stands up from a supine position, he may have primary hypertension. However, if his diastolic pressure decreases when he stands (and he's not taking an antihypertensive drug), he may have secondary hypertension.

Take at least two measurements separated by at least 2 minutes. If the readings from the same arm vary by more than 5 mm Hg, recheck your technique and take additional readings until you obtain two that are similar. In particular, confirm a high reading with at least two subsequent readings. This helps to rule out white-coat syndrome—elevated blood pressure in response to the stress of having a health care professional take the reading. White-coat syndrome occurs about 20% of the time. Several other factors also can influence the accuracy of blood pressure readings (see *Ensuring accurate blood pressure measurement*).

Placing the cuff improperly or using a wrong-sized cuff may result in inaccurate readings. For example, using a regular adult cuff on an obese patient may give an incorrectly high reading (see *Determining blood pressure cuff size*).

You can use either a mercury or aneroid manometer. But remember that aneroid manometers require monthly calibration to ensure their accuracy.

Patient preparation
To prepare the patient for blood pressure measurement, make sure you have him remain seated quietly, in a comfortable environment, for at least 5 minutes. Free his arm from clothing by either rolling up the sleeve or having him remove his long-sleeved shirt and offering him a patient gown, if necessary. Then place the arm in a comfortable position. Make sure his arm doesn't have an AV fistula for dialysis, scarring from brachial artery cutdowns, or lymphedema, which may follow axillary node dissection and radiation therapy.

Palpate for the brachial pulse to make sure it's present. Before applying the cuff, make sure the brachial artery, located at the crease of the antecubital fossa, is positioned at heart level. If the patient is sitting, a table that reaches just above his waist is usually sufficient. If the patient is standing, support his arm at midchest level. The reading can be falsely elevated if he expends effort keeping his arm up.

performing, so assessing hypertension requires several blood pressure measurements.

Obtain at least one reading in both arms with the patient sitting, lying, and standing. A difference of 5 to 10 mm Hg between the arms is nor-

Nursing considerations

If using a mercury manometer, position the gauge vertically with the meniscus at eye level. If using a calibrated aneroid manometer, turn the gauge so that it faces you. Place the cuff on the patient's arm by centering the inflatable bladder over the brachial artery. Securely fasten the lower border of the cuff about 2.5 cm above the antecubital crease.

Falsely low blood pressure readings commonly occur when the cuff isn't inflated high enough. To prevent this, first estimate the patient's systolic blood pressure. Then add 30 mm Hg to this estimated pressure. This number will be the target for subsequent inflations; using it should prevent errors caused by an auscultatory gap. After obtaining the target number, deflate the cuff completely and wait a few minutes before taking an actual measurement (see *Estimating systolic blood pressure,* page 132).

To obtain the patient's blood pressure measurement, place the bell of the stethoscope lightly over his brachial artery. The full rim should be in contact with his arm to create an air seal. Remember, the bell of the stethoscope will allow you to hear low-pitched Korotkoff sounds better than the diaphragm will.

Inflate the bladder quickly to the target level. Then deflate it at a rate of 3 mm Hg per second. As the pressure decreases, note the patient's systolic pressure as the level at which you hear the sounds of at least two consecutive beats.

While continuing to release the pressure in the bladder, listen for the Korotkoff sounds to become muffled and then disappear. Note this level as the patient's diastolic pressure. Usually, the points where the sounds are muffled and where the sounds disappear differ by only a few mm Hg. However, if the difference is more than 10 mm Hg, record both numbers along with the systolic pressure—for example, you might record a patient's blood pressure as 160/90/72.

After the sounds have disappeared, continue listening while the pressure decreases another 10 to 20 mm Hg. Then rapidly deflate the cuff to zero.

If the sounds are difficult to hear, have your patient raise his arm and then open and close his hand five to ten times. Quickly inflate the cuff with his arm raised, then lower it and take a reading. This maneuver should help intensify the Korotkoff sounds.

You may also measure blood pressure in a patient's leg, particularly if you're trying to detect

Determining blood pressure cuff size

To choose the correct blood pressure cuff for your patient, measure the circumference of his upper arm just above the antecubital area. The inflatable bladder of the cuff should have a width of about 40% of your patient's arm circumference, which is 12 to 14 cm for an average adult. The bladder should also be long enough to almost completely encircle his arm.

Arm circumference (cm)	Cuff width required (cm)	Appropriate cuff type
26–33	12	regular adult
33–42	15	large adult
> 42	18	thigh

coarctation of the aorta. Wrap a thigh cuff around his thigh and place the stethoscope bell in the popliteal space. Then obtain the blood pressure measurement just as you would in the arm. If the systolic pressure in the leg is more than 20 mm Hg lower than the brachial systolic pressure, the patient probably has an arterial occlusion.

Another simple technique—the cold pressor test—can be used to enhance blood pressure measurement and help identify the severity of hypertension (see *What the cold pressor test can tell you,* page 133).

Blood tests

Although blood tests aren't used to detect hypertension, they are useful for identifying the effects of hypertension and the causes of secondary hypertension. They can also help in monitoring a patient's response to hypertensive treatment.

Electrolyte levels

Serum electrolyte testing is used to determine the body's homeostatic status. For a patient with known hypertension, serum electrolyte levels—specifically sodium and potassium levels—can help identify complications arising from hyper-

Estimating systolic blood pressure

If you're taking your patient's blood pressure for the first time, you'll need to estimate his systolic blood pressure and obtain a target measurement for future cuff inflations. First, make sure the center of the cuff bladder is aligned with his brachial artery and that his arm is level with his heart. Then palpate the radial pulse while inflating the cuff. When the radial pulse disappears, note the measurement on the manometer: This is the patient's estimated systolic pressure. To obtain the target for subsequent inflations, add 30 mm Hg.

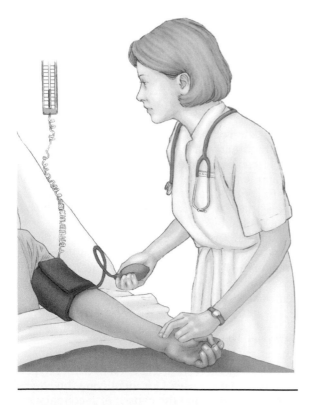

tension and its treatment. Serum electrolyte testing may also help identify disorders causing secondary hypertension, such as hyperaldosteronism, which is characterized by low serum potassium levels.

In many cases, physicians prescribe diuretics and angiotensin-converting enzyme (ACE) inhibitors to treat hypertension. If your patient's treat-

ment plan will include these drugs as well as a sodium-restricted diet, electrolyte testing should be performed before therapy begins. Also, you should monitor the patient's electrolyte levels during therapy to help identify abnormal levels that can result in a life-threatening complication.

If a patient is scheduled for serum electrolyte testing, explain the reasons for the test and the importance of the findings. This will increase his knowledge of his hypertensive condition and help promote compliance with his medical regimen.

Test implications
Normally, serum sodium levels range from 135 to 145 mEq/L, and serum potassium levels range from 3.5 to 5.0 mEq/L. If you note abnormal levels, verify that the patient is adhering to his medical regimen. If he's complying, notify his physician, who may change the regimen—perhaps by adding a potassium supplement.

Abnormally high potassium levels may indicate changes in renal blood flow and electrolyte exchange in the renal tubules, requiring an adjustment in the patient's ACE inhibitor dosage. High potassium levels also may result from treatment with potassium sparing diuretics.

Fasting lipid profile
The fasting serum lipid profile measures total cholesterol, triglyceride, high-density lipoprotein (HDL) cholesterol, and low-density lipoprotein (LDL) cholesterol levels. This test helps in the overall assessment of hypertension and in identifying a patient's risk of developing coronary artery disease (CAD).

Hyperlipidemia commonly results from hypertension. Hypertension injures the endothelial lining of the arterial wall. And this damage promotes platelet aggregation and lipid deposits, leading to intracoronary atherosclerosis and plaque formation.

Patient preparation
To obtain accurate test results, tell the patient to fast for 14 hours before the test. He may drink water during the fast, but he should abstain from drinking alcoholic beverages before the test. Also, he should avoid exercising immediately before the test.

The patient should maintain a stable diet and lifestyle for 2 weeks before this test. An acute illness or an exacerbation of a chronic illness can cause inaccurate test results. Also, certain drugs—such as antilipemics, oral contraceptives, cortico-

What the cold pressor test can tell you

In the cold pressor test, as you may know, an examiner takes two blood pressure readings—one before and one after a patient immerses his hand in ice-cold water for 2 minutes. Normally, the systolic blood pressure increases 10 to 15 mm Hg.

Recently, researchers found interesting links between the results of this test and the type of hypertension a patient has. Here are the key findings:

- The rise in diastolic pressure between the two readings is greatest in patients with severe hypertension.
- Diastolic pressure rises significantly higher in patients with arteriosclerotic hypertension than in those with primary hypertension.
- Patients with left ventricular hypertrophy have particularly high diastolic pressure increases.

- Systolic pressure rises the most in patients with arteriosclerotic hypertension, somewhat less in those with primary hypertension, and somewhat less again in those with renal hypertension.

If you're asked to perform this test, remember these points:

- Make sure the patient hasn't taken a hypertensive drug for a month before the test.
- Tell the patient not to smoke the day of the test.
- Warn the patient that the immersed hand will probably become numb.
- Make sure the water is truly ice cold—41° F (5° C).
- Perform the test in a quiet room without noise or interruptions.
- Leave the blood pressure cuff on the patient throughout the test.

steroids, and diuretics—can interfere with the test results.

Test implications

High levels of total cholesterol and LDL cholesterol can indicate the development of CAD, as can low levels of HDL cholesterol. A patient's risk of CAD also increases when elevated triglyceride levels appear in conjunction with high LDL and low HDL cholesterol levels.

Serum creatinine and blood urea nitrogen tests

Serum creatinine and blood urea nitrogen (BUN) tests can help detect kidney damage resulting from hypertension. The increased systemic vascular resistance caused by hypertension promotes renal vascular changes and decreases renal blood flow. Diminished blood flow through the glomeruli triggers the release of renin, further increasing vasoconstriction and systemic vascular resistance. The glomeruli atrophy, and the kidneys shrink, inhibiting the excretion of creatinine and BUN.

Normally, the kidneys excrete creatinine—a waste product of muscle metabolism. Usually, serum creatinine levels range from 0.8 to 1.2 mg/dl in men and from 0.6 to 0.9 mg/dl in women. But when reduced blood flow through the glomeruli

hinders renal excretion, serum creatinine levels are elevated.

The kidneys also filter and excrete the nitrogen fraction of urea—a waste product of protein metabolism. Normal BUN levels range from 8 to 26 mg/dl.

Test implications

Elevated BUN levels alone don't indicate renal dysfunction because infection, trauma, GI bleeding, diet, and dehydration can also increase BUN levels. But when a patient has elevated BUN and serum creatinine levels, he probably has reduced glomerular blood flow and kidney dysfunction.

If a patient is taking a diuretic or an ACE inhibitor to treat his hypertension, closely monitor his BUN and creatinine test results. Diuretics generally increase water and sodium excretion, which lowers circulating intravascular volume. As circulating volume decreases, so does renal blood flow, causing a rise in BUN and creatinine levels.

Other drugs can also influence a patient's test results. For example, aminoglycosides can increase creatinine levels. Drugs such as allopurinol, furosemide, and indomethacin can increase BUN levels. And chloramphenicol can decrease BUN levels.

Changes in the patient's protein intake and

overhydration and underhydration can also affect the test results.

Fasting blood glucose test

Though not used to diagnose hypertension, fasting blood glucose levels can help in detecting causes of secondary hypertension. For example, if your patient's hypertension results from Cushing's syndrome or pheochromocytoma, he may have hyperglycemia.

If a patient uses an oral antidiabetic drug or insulin, monitor his blood glucose levels to assess the effectiveness of his therapy and any complications resulting from it.

After fasting 8 to 16 hours, a patient's blood glucose levels should range from 70 to 115 mg/dl. However, diuretic therapy can elevate blood glucose levels.

Patient preparation

Tell the patient to fast for 8 to 16 hours before the test. However, the fast should never exceed 16 hours because he may starve his body, causing an artificial rise in blood glucose levels.

The patient can have water during the fasting period. But he may need to have medications withheld before the test, particularly oral antidiabetic drugs or insulin, which can affect the test results. Check with the patient's physician to find out if the patient's medications should be withheld.

Uric acid test

The uric acid test can be used to detect and monitor complications of hypertension such as gouty arthritis of the joints. Normally, the kidneys excrete uric acid, the major end product of purine catabolism. But when hypertension impairs renal function, hyperuricemia—elevated serum uric acid levels—commonly results.

Normally, serum uric acid levels range from 2.1 to 8.5 mg/dl in men and from 2.0 to 6.6 mg/dl in women. However, certain factors that artificially elevate uric acid levels, such as loop or thiazide diuretics and low-dose aspirin, can affect the test results. Poor nutrition, a high-purine diet, and excessive alcohol intake can also elevate uric acid levels.

When a patient is taking a diuretic to treat hypertension, you should monitor his serum uric acid levels. However, elevated levels may not require treatment if he's asymptomatic.

Calcium test

The serum calcium test can be used to monitor a patient's response to treatment with calcium channel blockers such as amlodipine, diltiazem, felodipine, nifedipine, and verapamil. These drugs work by inhibiting the flow of calcium into the cells, promoting arterial relaxation and decreasing peripheral vascular resistance.

About half of the body's calcium is found in its ionized or free form, while the other half is bound to albumin. Calcium testing results in two measurements: the serum calcium level, which is a total of both forms of calcium, and the ionized calcium level.

Normally, blood levels of total calcium range from 9.0 to 10.5 mg/dl, and blood levels of ionized calcium range from 4.4 to 5.0 mg/dl.

Certain factors can affect the results of calcium testing. Thiazide diuretics can cause hypercalcemia. Also, prolonged use of a tourniquet when performing the venipuncture can increase the calcium level by decreasing blood pH.

Plasma renin activity test

Although about 50% of hypertensive patients have normal plasma renin activity, hypertension can cause fluctuations in plasma renin levels. Measurement of plasma renin activity can help in diagnosing renal causes of secondary hypertension, such as primary aldosteronism or renal vascular disease resulting from renal artery stenosis. The test can also be used to monitor renal function during therapy. Patients with renal failure and those taking diuretics and antihypertensive drugs have increased plasma renin activity.

The level of plasma renin activity is tested by two methods. In one, the patient follows a sodium-restricted diet for 3 days; then he's placed upright for 2 to 4 hours, after which a blood sample is taken. In the other, less time-consuming method, the patient doesn't need to follow a sodium-restricted diet. He's given 40 mg of furosemide I.V. and placed upright for a half hour, after which a blood sample is obtained.

Normal plasma renin activity levels vary depending on the patient's age and diet. For patients ages 20 and older on a normal-sodium diet, plasma renin activity levels should range from 0.1 to 4.3 ng/ml/hour. However, patients ages 20 to 39 on a sodium-restricted diet should have plasma renin activity levels ranging from 2.9 to

24.0 ng/ml/hour, and patients ages 40 and older on a sodium-restricted diet should have levels ranging from 2.9 to 10.8 ng/ml/hour. If a patient has been placed on a sodium-restricted diet before the test, he must comply with it to obtain accurate test results.

Nursing considerations

For a test using furosemide, anticipate the need for an indwelling urinary catheter. To obtain accurate results for either test, collect the blood sample using a tube preserved with ethylenediaminetetraacetic acid (EDTA), not heparin: EDTA helps preserve angiotensin I, whereas heparin doesn't. Fill the tube to the appropriate level and immediately chill it to prevent renin breakdown.

Plasma cortisol test

Levels of plasma cortisol—the main glucocorticoid secreted by the adrenal cortex—are used to evaluate adrenal gland function. Plasma cortisol levels can also help in diagnosing causes of secondary hypertension such as Cushing's syndrome. In Cushing's syndrome, adrenocortical hyperfunction elevates plasma cortisol levels.

A patient undergoing plasma cortisol testing will have two blood samples taken, one at 8 A.M. and another at 4 P.M. Normally, the earlier test results should fall between 6 and 18 µ/dl, and the later test results should fall between 2 and 12 µ/dl.

Cortisol levels are usually highest between 6 and 8 A.M., gradually fall during the day, and are lowest at midnight. Of course, if the patient works nights and sleeps during the day, these times and levels will be reversed.

Patient preparation

To obtain accurate results from plasma cortisol testing, tell the patient to follow a daily diet of 2 to 3 grams of sodium for 3 days before the test. The patient will have to limit his physical activity and fast for 12 hours before the test. Finally, for about 30 minutes before the test, the patient should relax completely.

Urine tests

Hypertensive patients almost always have some degree of renal dysfunction, and as blood pressure increases, renal dysfunction progresses. A couple of urine tests can help detect kidney damage related to hypertension.

Urinalysis

Routine urinalysis can help in detecting renal complications from hypertension and identifying coexisting disorders, such as diabetes mellitus. Urinalysis also helps in monitoring the patient's response to treatment for a hypertensive complication or the progress of an underlying cause.

Test implications

Routine urinalysis should be performed at the start of hypertension treatment to provide a baseline for future testing. Normally, a random urine specimen is negative for protein, glucose, and ketones (see *Urinalysis: Normal findings,* page 136).

If the specimen contains glucose, protein, or RBCs, the patient may have hypertensive renal dysfunction resulting from a series of changes in the kidney. Vasoconstriction from hypertension reduces blood flow to the kidney, and endothelial changes occur in the renal arteries, causing increased capillary membrane permeability. This results in a loss of the normal filtration and reabsorption functions of the renal tubules. Consequently, protein and RBCs leak into the filtrate passing through the tubules and are excreted in the urine.

Urine vanillylmandelic acid test

Used to evaluate the function of the adrenal medulla, the urine vanillylmandelic acid test can also help identify pheochromocytoma as a cause of secondary hypertension. Pheochromocytoma, a tumor secreting high levels of epinephrine and norepinephrine, causes peripheral artery vasoconstriction that results in hypertension.

Normally, urine vanillylmandelic acid levels range from 2 to 7 mg per 24 hours. However, with pheochromocytoma, excess catecholamine levels and the hepatic conversion of epinephrine and norepinephrine that produces vanillylmandelic acid result in abnormally high urine levels.

Patient preparation

Tell the patient to restrict his dietary intake of phenolic acid for 3 days before the test. Explain that foods such as coffee, bananas, citrus fruits, chocolate, and vanilla contain phenolic acid.

Urinalysis: Normal findings

Use this chart as a guide when evaluating the results of your patient's urinalysis.

Characteristic or element	Normal finding
Appearance	Clear
Color	Amber, yellow
Odor	Similar to ammonia
pH	4.6–8.0
Protein	0–8 mg/dl
Specific gravity	1.005–1.030
Leukocyte esterase	None
Nitrites	None
Glucose	None
Ketones	None
Crystals	None
Casts	None
Red blood cells	0–2 per high-power field
White blood cells	0–5 per high-power field
Bilirubin	None
Casts	None; few hyaline casts
Bacteria	< 1,000 colonies/ml
Parasites	None

Tell the patient to save all the urine collected in the specially prepared collection bottle. Have him keep the urine specimen cold by placing the collection bottle in the refrigerator. And tell him to avoid strenuous physical activity during the collection period.

Nursing considerations
Before the test, review the patient's drug regimen with his physician to determine if one or more of the drugs will interfere with the test results. If the physician discontinues an antihypertensive drug, monitor the patient's blood pressure closely during the test.

Also, check if the patient has had X-rays recently. The use of X-ray contrast media within a few days of the test can produce falsely low results.

If the patient is collecting his urine at home, suggest that he place a sign in the bathroom as a reminder to collect all urine. Make arrangements for pickup of his collection bottle soon after the 24-hour period.

Other tests

Various other tests, such as chest X-ray, electrocardiogram (ECG), and echocardiogram, can help to evaluate the structure and function of the heart and vessels. These tests can also indicate any changes caused by hypertension.

Chest X-ray
A chest X-ray can help in detecting a hypertensive disorder, particularly left ventricular hypertrophy, and in following its progress. If a patient has left ventricular hypertrophy, an anteroposterior X-ray may show rounding and increased convexity of a patient's lateral cardiac shadow. A lateral view may reveal the posterior border of the heart overlapping the spine.

If a patient has heart failure, his X-ray may show an enlarged cardiac silhouette. Or if he has left ventricular heart failure, his X-ray may reveal pulmonary effusion and an enlarged left atrium and ventricle. For patients with right ventricular heart failure, chest X-ray findings include an enlarged right atrium and ventricle.

Usually, treating heart failure in a hypertensive patient includes administering a diuretic and a vasodilator. As a patient's blood pressure decreases and excessive volume diminishes with diuresis, the enlarged heart chambers decrease in size. These improvements can also be monitored by chest X-ray.

Electrocardiogram
A 12-lead ECG, which records the electrical activity of the heart, may help in diagnosing cardiac complications of hypertension such as left ventricular hypertrophy, myocardial ischemia, an MI, and arrhythmias.

Detecting left ventricular hypertrophy

The lead V_5 waveform on the left shows a normal electrocardiogram (ECG). Compare it to the lead V_5 waveform on the right, which shows the characteristic ECG changes in left ventricular hypertrophy—a complication of long-standing, poorly controlled hypertension.

Normal ECG waveform

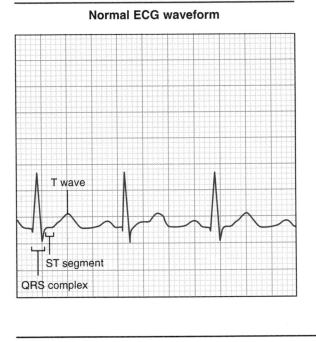

ECG changes in left ventricular hypertrophy

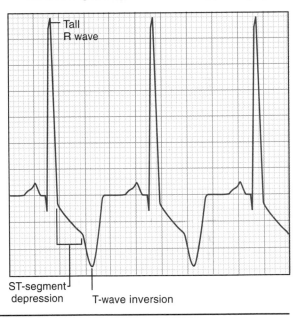

Nursing considerations

Before obtaining a 12-lead ECG, document any antihypertensive drugs your patient is taking. Some of these drugs produce effects that show up on the ECG such as sinus bradycardia or tachycardia, heart block, or a prolonged QT interval. Diuretics in particular may cause electrolyte abnormalities that alter the ECG.

If a hypertensive patient complains of chest pain, evaluate his 12-lead ECG for ischemic changes. Perform the ECG before administering pain-relieving drugs so that you'll have a baseline ECG. If the patient is using antianginal drugs, repeat the ECG as appropriate to assess his response to therapy.

Test implications

If the patient has left ventricular hypertrophy, the ECG shows some characteristic changes:

- The QRS complex shows left-axis deviation.
- The R and S waves of the QRS complex increase in amplitude or depth.
- The ST segment is depressed.
- The T wave is inverted in certain leads (see *Detecting left ventricular hypertrophy*).

If the patient has myocardial ischemia, you'll note ST-segment and T-wave changes. The ST segment, which represents repolarization (the period of recovery after ventricular activation), normally appears flat on the ECG tracing. When coronary blood flow to the myocardium diminishes, however, the ST segment becomes depressed, and the normally upright T wave becomes inverted. Less commonly, ischemia causes an ST-segment elevation.

If a hypertensive patient is taking a diuretic, he may be at risk for developing electrolyte imbalances, which can precipitate arrhythmias. Thiazide diuretics can produce hypercalcemia, which may cause shortening of the ST segment and QT interval. Diuretics also cause hypokalemia, which can lead to ventricular ectopy. ECG abnormalities caused by hypokalemia include ST-segment depression, which can make assessment of ischemic changes difficult; decreased T-wave amplitude; and, occasionally, T-wave inversion.

Echocardiogram

Echocardiography uses sound waves to evaluate the heart's structure and function. In this test, a transducer is positioned on various areas of the chest. The transducer emits sound waves, which make contact with the heart and are then recorded on a monitor as moving images of it. Using this test, a physician can observe a patient's systolic and diastolic function, calculate the sizes of the cardiac chambers, measure left ventricular wall thickness, and measure valve areas.

An echocardiogram can accurately detect ischemia or left ventricular hypertrophy resulting from hypertension. On an echocardiogram, ischemic changes appear as wall-motion abnormalities. However, standard echocardiography may not detect ischemia of the left ventricle.

To detect such ischemia, a physician may order stress echocardiography. This test is performed immediately after the patient exercises. Patients who can't exercise are tested by pharmacologic stress echocardiography. Dobutamine, an inotropic agent, is administered I.V. as the patient lies in bed. The examiner gradually increases the dose until the patient's heart rate mimics an exercise heart rate. Then, echocardiography is performed to evaluate the heart wall for motion abnormalities.

Echocardiography also helps in evaluating a patient's response to hypertensive therapy. For instance, calcium channel blockers can decrease left ventricular hypertrophy and the occurrence of arrhythmias; follow-up echocardiographic testing can verify this response to therapy.

Stress or pharmacologic stress echocardiograms are usually performed when cardiac isoenzymes have returned to normal 7 to 10 days after surgery or an acute MI. And some patients then have these tests performed several months later so that the physician can evaluate therapy and progress.

Nursing considerations

When preparing a patient for an echocardiogram, advise him that he may feel some discomfort during the test because the technician must place the transducer firmly between the ribs to enhance sound-wave transmission and diminish interference. Also, advise your patient that he'll have to lie quietly for 30 to 45 minutes, depending on the technical quality of sound-wave transmission and the cardiac images.

8

Treatment

Whether a patient has primary or secondary hypertension, the goal of therapy is the same: to quickly and safely reduce his blood pressure. Treatment of primary hypertension begins with the patient changing his lifestyle—eating properly, exercising regularly, and the like. If these changes don't lower his blood pressure sufficiently, a physician typically prescribes antihypertensive drug therapy and encourages the patient to continue with his lifestyle changes. Treatment of secondary hypertension, of course, focuses on correcting the underlying cause.

Step-care therapy

The National Committee on the Detection, Evaluation, and Treatment of High Blood Pressure designed step-care therapy specifically to treat primary hypertension. The goal of this therapy is to maintain arterial blood pressure below 140/90 mm Hg.

With this four-step plan, a physician begins with the most conservative therapeutic approach. If that doesn't control the patient's blood pressure, the physician moves on to step 2, prescribing an antihypertensive drug.

If the patient doesn't respond sufficiently to the drug prescribed in step 2, his physician will advance him to step 3. In this step, a physician may add a second drug from another class. Or he may increase the dosage of the first drug or simply substitute a different drug for the first one.

If the patient doesn't respond to these interventions, his physician will begin step 4 treatment by adding a third drug from a different class, substituting a new drug for the second one, or substituting a diuretic, if one hasn't already been tried (see *Step-care therapy for primary hypertension,* page 140).

Lifestyle modifications

Step 1 consists of nonpharmacologic approaches to reducing a patient's blood pressure. These approaches include controlling or reducing weight; moderating alcohol, caffeine, and sodium intake; quitting smoking; and exercising.

Weight control

By controlling or reducing his weight, a hypertensive patient may reduce his blood pressure. Also, by reducing his fat intake, he'll decrease his risk of developing complications from atherosclerosis such as coronary, cerebral, and renal vascular disease.

Recommended foods
To control or reduce his weight, your patient may need to change his eating habits. His diet should include appropriate portions of low-fat foods. He should also avoid high-fat snacks and reduce his total daily caloric intake.

The American Heart Association Healthy Heart diet identifies foods to avoid and foods to include to achieve weight control or reduction.

Step-care therapy for primary hypertension

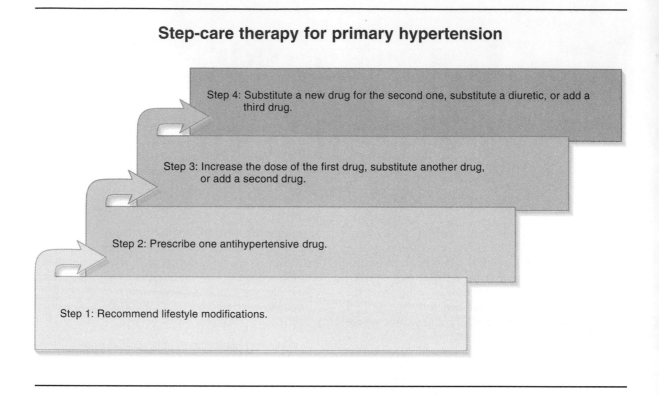

Step 4: Substitute a new drug for the second one, substitute a diuretic, or add a third drug.

Step 3: Increase the dose of the first drug, substitute another drug, or add a second drug.

Step 2: Prescribe one antihypertensive drug.

Step 1: Recommend lifestyle modifications.

Hypertensive patients should avoid these foods:
- animal products—large portions of meat (beef, lamb, pork, or veal), liver or organ meats, bacon, sausage, and luncheon meats
- dairy products—egg yolks, whole milk, ice cream, cheese, and butter
- oil products—beef lard, salad dressings, cream sauces, and gravies
- simple carbohydrates—sweets, candy, sugar, cake, cookies, and jellies.

Hypertensive patients should include daily allowances of the following:
- protein—4 to 6 ounces of fish, skinless poultry, or lean red meat with all visible fat removed
- grains and starches—a minimum of four servings of whole-grain, high-fiber cereals, breads, potatoes, rice, or starchy vegetables
- vegetables—a minimum of two servings of deep green or orange vegetables
- fruit and juice—a minimum of two servings, one of which is citrus
- dairy—a minimum of two servings of skim or low-fat milk, skim cheese, nonfat yogurt, or ice milk.

Nutrition plan

You can estimate the daily caloric intake your patient needs for normal body functioning and weight control by multiplying his ideal body weight by 10. Thus, a patient whose ideal body weight is 180 pounds should have a daily caloric intake of 1,800 calories.

Although some weight-reduction diets severely limit the total daily caloric intake to as little as 800 calories or less, low-calorie diets usually range from 1,000 to 1,500 calories per day. A diet that's lower than 1,000 calories per day may cause muscle loss instead of fat loss. The body also compensates for large reductions in caloric intake by decreasing the metabolic rate.

After you've estimated your patient's total daily caloric intake, you can develop his nutrition plan. Talk with him about his goals for weight reduction or control and make sure they're realistic. Develop these goals with the patient to improve his compliance. Also, teach the family members who are responsible for meal preparation or who will support your patient in his efforts (see *Improving your patient's compliance*).

HEALTH PROMOTION

Improving your patient's compliance

To prevent life-threatening, chronic complications, your hypertensive patient must comply with his prescribed treatment plan. Unfortunately, many hypertensive patients don't comply.

If your patient isn't following his treatment plan, identify the reasons and then take corrective action. Here are some common causes of noncompliance, along with proven intervention strategies.

Patient isn't involved in decision making

Many times, the health care team makes the mistake of deciding what's best for the patient and then telling him what to do. But patients who aren't involved in the planning tend to not get involved in the plan. So be sure to include the patient in discussions about his treatment.

Encourage him to identify problems he might have in complying with the options under discussion. Remember, he'll be more likely to comply with a treatment plan he feels he can realistically follow.

Patient thinks his blood pressure is normal

Patients who feel well may assume that their blood pressure isn't a problem. Teach your patient how to measure his own blood pressure at home and advise him to record how he feels at the time he takes each measurement. Doing so will help him realize that regardless of how he feels, his blood pressure will begin to climb if he forgets to take his antihypertensive drug, cheats on his diet, or fails to reduce his stress.

Patient doesn't integrate treatment into everyday life

The complexity of treatment is inversely related to the degree of patient compliance. This poses a major problem in managing hypertension because several treatments—lifestyle changes and drugs—are usually needed to maintain normal blood pressure.

Anything you can suggest to simplify your patient's treatment plan may help foster compliance. For example, if your patient must take a drug several times a day, ask his physician to substitute one that requires less frequent dosing. Or if the patient must take several different drugs, ask the physician to prescribe a combination product to simplify the patient's drug regimen.

Patient can't afford drugs and foods

Many patients with limited incomes are embarrassed to reveal that they have difficulty purchasing the drugs and foods required for their treatment. To identify this problem early on, explore your patient's ability to pay when you discuss the treatment plan with him. If you identify a problem, call the social worker to make alternative arrangements for your patient.

Nursing considerations

In helping a hypertensive patient control his weight, your primary responsibilities include educating him about his prescribed diet and monitoring his weight reduction. You'll also need to regularly measure his blood pressure.

Review the elements of the weight-reduction diet with your patient. If appropriate, obtain a referral for a dietitian to assist him and his family with planning appropriate meals. Provide him with suggestions to help him comply with the prescribed diet, keeping in mind his food preferences and ethnic background. Also, recommend alternative food choices for patients with poor dentition, food intolerances, and limited physical mobility. And stress the importance of reducing weight to reduce blood pressure.

When teaching your patient, tell him to eat regularly planned meals and to not skip meals. Teach him to measure his foods to determine the correct portions. Also, tell him to avoid foods that are high in fat and sugars and to reduce the amount of fat he uses in cooking. Suggest baking, broiling, or steaming food as a way to eliminate all fried foods from his diet. Also, recommend he reduce fat by removing the skin on poultry before cooking and have him increase his daily intake of fruits and vegetables. And warn your patient to avoid fad and crash diets, which reduce weight only temporarily.

Monitor the success of your patient's weight reduction by recording weekly weights. Don't measure daily weights because they reflect the body's fluid status and don't usually indicate total body weight reduction.

Use ongoing blood pressure measurement to evaluate his body's response to weight reduction. Blood pressure readings don't immediately show dramatic decrease. However, some reduction in blood pressure may occur with a weight loss of as little as 10 pounds. Reinforce the success of weight and blood pressure reductions with your patient to encourage ongoing compliance with the prescribed regimen.

Alcohol restriction

When obtaining your patient's health history, ask him how much alcohol he drinks. If appropriate, advise him to reduce his intake to less than 1 ounce per day.

The exact mechanism by which alcohol raises blood pressure isn't known, but alcohol may increase renin or aldosterone release. Chronic alcohol abuse can also increase blood cortisol levels, which can aggravate hypertension.

Alcohol consumption also affects weight reduction. Alcohol provides empty calories. Plus, one or two drinks a day can slow a person's metabolism by as much as 25%. Drinking three or more alcoholic drinks a day also increases a person's risk of hypertension.

Caffeine restriction

By constricting the peripheral blood vessels, caffeine increases the heart rate and blood pressure. Therefore, you should encourage your hypertensive patient to reduce his intake of caffeinated beverages. Tell him that most drinks such as coffee, tea, and soda are now available in caffeine-free preparations. Also, teach him that many other products contain caffeine, including foods such as chocolate and over-the-counter (OTC) drugs used for the treatment of headaches.

Sodium restriction

You should advise your patient to limit his sodium intake, especially if he's sodium sensitive. Restricting sodium intake may reduce extracellular fluid and total circulating blood volume, thus decreasing the heart's workload.

Sodium may interfere with the effectiveness of certain antihypertensive drugs. Thus, by limiting his sodium intake, the patient may be able to control his blood pressure with lower doses of antihypertensive drugs. And by using lower dosages, he will have less risk of developing adverse effects from the drugs.

Usually, sodium is restricted to 2 grams of sodium or 5 grams of salt per day. A patient can achieve this restriction by not adding table salt to food and by avoiding foods that are high in sodium (see *Teaching your patient to adopt a sodium-restricted diet*).

Smoking cessation

Quitting smoking reduces a patient's risk of developing hypertension and hypertension-related conditions. Nicotine constricts the peripheral blood vessels, reducing blood flow and oxygenation throughout the body and increasing blood pressure. And smoking adds carbon monoxide to the bloodstream and injures the lungs. Although the effects of nicotine on the vasculature aren't completely understood, tobacco use may be linked to peripheral vascular, cerebrovascular, and cardiovascular disease.

Many prescription and OTC drugs are available to help your patient quit smoking. However, be aware that these drugs contain chemicals that either supplement or mimic the effects of nicotine on the body and can keep blood pressure elevated.

To help your patient quit smoking, encourage him to plan ahead, set realistic goals, and seek support from family, friends, or a smoking-cessation group. After your patient has stopped smoking, he may need counseling about his diet. Food may smell and taste more appealing, and he may be tempted eat high-calorie snacks.

Exercise

Regular isotonic exercise—such as walking, jogging, and swimming—can help control blood pressure. Generally, hypertensive patients should participate in a moderate amount of exercise at regular intervals, rather than vigorous exercise at irregular intervals.

HOME CARE

Teaching your patient to adopt a sodium-restricted diet

Many patients with hypertension are sodium sensitive, meaning their blood pressure increases after they consume excessive amounts of sodium and decreases after they reduce their sodium intake. Such patients may be prescribed a sodium-restricted diet, which usually limits sodium consumption to 2 grams a day.

If your patient must comply with such a diet, help him make the change. Along with his dietitian, provide nutritional counseling soon after his hypertension is diagnosed. Include the family or caregiver in your teaching, especially if she prepares the patient's food at home.

Sources of sodium

Your patient must understand which foods and drugs contain sodium. Explain that the most common sources of sodium are table salt, processed foods, drugs, and softened water.

Table salt

Advise your patient to avoid using table salt during food preparation and tell him not to add salt to his food. Common table salt consists of 40% sodium and 60% chloride, so if he takes in 6 grams of salt, he's actually consuming 2.4 grams of sodium.

Foods

Explain that some foods, such as beef and dairy products, naturally contain sodium. Other foods are processed with sodium to enhance the flavor or prolong the shelf life. Preserved or processed foods include pickles, canned vegetables, soups, and gravy. Tell him to be alert for products that list sodium ingredients such as sodium benzoate and sodium citrate.

Also, teach your hypertensive patient how to read food labels for sodium content. To reduce confusion and regulate what manufacturers put on food labels, the Food and Drug Administration has defined the terms used in sodium labeling:

- *Sodium-free:* less than 5 mg of sodium per serving.
- *Very low sodium:* 35 mg or less per serving.
- *Low sodium:* 140 mg or less per serving.
- *Reduced sodium:* sodium content reduced by at least 25% of usual level.
- *Light sodium:* sodium content reduced by at least 50% of usual level.

- *Without added salt, unsalted,* or *no added salt:* foods once processed with salt and now processed without it. (These foods must list the amount of sodium per serving.)

Caution your patient about foods that claim to be low in sodium. If the sodium content is less than 5 mg per serving, he can eat the food without concern. If it's higher than 5 mg, he'll need to include the amount in his calculation of sodium intake for the day.

Drugs

Show your patient how to check labels for the sodium content of over-the-counter drugs such as antacids, cough syrups, and laxatives. For other drugs, advise him to check with his pharmacist. If necessary, he should ask his physician or pharmacist to recommend alternative drugs with little or no sodium.

Water

Natural and softened water can be high in sodium. A patient following a severely sodium-restricted diet should investigate the sodium content of his drinking water by contacting his water company or local public health department. Then he should discuss this information with his physician. Depending on how much sodium is in the water, he may be advised to drink and cook with distilled water.

Other helpful tips

As part of teaching your patient about a sodium-restricted diet, you should also do the following:

- Provide your patient and his family with sample menus to help plan appropriate meals.
- Refer him to community organizations, such as the American Heart Association, for educational materials on hypertension and dietary choices for a sodium-restricted diet.
- Suggest that he use garlic powder and onion powder instead of salt or products containing salt.
- Teach him that other high-sodium sources include baking powder, baking soda, bouillon cubes, some cereals, and soy sauce.
- Explain that using low-sodium salt substitutes containing potassium may lead to electrolyte imbalances if he's taking such antihypertensive drugs as diuretics and angiotensin-converting enzyme inhibitors.

Developing a walking exercise plan

Use this guide to help your hypertensive patient develop a walking exercise plan. Explain that he should exercise three or four times a week.

Week 1
• Walk for 15 minutes at a pace of 3 miles per hour.

Week 2
• Walk for 20 minutes at a pace of 3 miles per hour.

Weeks 3 and 4
• Walk for 20 minutes at a pace of 4 miles per hour.

Week 5 and beyond
• Walk for 30 minutes at a pace of 4 miles per hour.

The short-term benefits of exercise include stress reduction and appetite suppression. Over time, exercise promotes effective blood flow, increases oxygen consumption, and strengthens the cardiac muscle. With stronger muscle, the heart beats more efficiently. Also, blood flows more easily through the vessels and at a lower pressure, thereby reducing systolic blood pressure.

Isotonic exercises, which are recommended for hypertensive patients, don't put unnecessary strain on the heart. However, isometric exercises such as weight lifting significantly raise blood pressure. And participating in isometric exercises increases a hypertensive patient's risk of sustaining an acute myocardial infarction (MI) or cerebrovascular accident.

Isometric exercises are not recommended because they also increase muscle tension and demand more oxygen. In hypertensive patients, the heart contracts with greater force than normal, so blood flows through the vessels with greater force. Hypertension also causes the arterioles and capillaries to be rigid. Therefore, blood flow through these vessels to the muscles may not

meet the increased oxygen demands of isometric exercise. As exercise tolerance decreases, the muscles cramp, and a hypertensive patient may faint from lack of oxygen to the tissues.

Exercise plan
Patients with known cardiac disease or other health problems need a thorough examination, including stress testing monitored by electrocardiography (ECG), before beginning an exercise plan. Also, the patient's physician should approve the program.

Walking is the ideal exercise for the hypertensive patient. The amount of walking should be increased gradually to establish exercise tolerance and to reduce the effects of overexercise (see *Developing a walking exercise plan*).

Nursing considerations
When your hypertensive patient begins an exercise program, teach him about the prescribed exercise. Monitor his exercise tolerance and continue to regularly measure his blood pressure.

During your patient teaching, tell him to exercise at the same time every day. Instruct him to wear loose-fitting clothing and to wear shoes that properly support his feet. If his exercise consists of walking, tell him to walk at a comfortable pace on level ground. Also, urge him to carry identification and a list of the drugs he's taking.

Hypertensive patients with other health problems may need special devices, such as braces or splints, to assist them in an exercise program. Assess your patient's overall physical status and consult with a physical therapist or cardiac rehabilitation specialist for exercise suggestions.

To help your patient adapt his exercise program to his needs and tolerance level, advise him to measure his pulse rate before and immediately after he exercises. He can use his pulse as a guide to increasing or decreasing his activity. Also, tell him to assess himself after 5 minutes of exercise. He should feel warm, not hot and sweating.

Until the patient knows his exercise tolerance, he should exercise with someone else. Instruct him to stop exercising if he becomes extremely tired, short of breath, dizzy, or light-headed. If he develops chest pain, palpitations, or tingling, numbness, or pain in his arms or legs, he should stop exercising and contact his physician. Tell him to seek emergency care if any of these symptoms persists for more than 15 minutes after the exercise activity is stopped.

Review the key elements of the exercise program with your patient. Provide suggestions to help him comply with the plan and stress the importance of exercise for managing his hypertension. Encourage him to do exercises that he enjoys so that he'll be more likely to do them regularly.

Advise your patient to set realistic goals and advance his exercise program at his own pace. To ensure compliance, suggest that he join a walking group such as one that walks in malls.

Monitor the success of your patient's exercise program by checking his blood pressure and resting heart rate weekly. If his blood pressure decreases, emphasize the success of the exercise program to encourage continued compliance.

Antihypertensive drugs

If nonpharmacologic approaches don't sufficiently reduce your patient's blood pressure, his physician will begin drug therapy to reduce blood pressure and to maintain it at less than 140/90 mm Hg. Drug therapy usually begins with a diuretic or a beta-blocker. However, if these drugs are contraindicated or ineffective, the physician may prescribe an alpha-blocker, alpha agonist, angiotensin-converting enzyme (ACE) inhibitor, angiotensin II receptor blocker, calcium channel blocker, or direct vasodilator.

Several factors determine which drug the physician prescribes in step 2. The drug, of course, should be safe for your patient to take, so always check that he doesn't have a documented sensitivity to the prescribed drug. Also, consider the patient's condition in relation to the prescribed drug. For instance, hypertension commonly occurs with pregnancy. However, some antihypertensive drugs can cause fetal abnormalities.

No matter which antihypertensive drug is prescribed for your patient, your initial tasks are the same. Before therapy begins, assess and record your patient's baseline information, including blood pressure, pulse, and serum test results. Also, review his history for any conditions that would contraindicate the drug or require cautious use.

Whenever a patient begins drug therapy, teach him about the drug. Patient education can in-

HOME CARE

Teaching your patient about antihypertensive drugs

No matter which antihypertensive drug your patient takes, he'll need to know some basic facts about hypertension and drug therapy. First, teach him how to monitor his blood pressure. Advise him to measure his blood pressure and pulse at regular intervals at least once a week. Tell him to notify his physician of any sudden changes, especially if his pulse is less than 50 beats per minute or if his blood pressure is less than 90/60 mm Hg.

Emphasize the importance of taking his prescribed drugs at the same time every day, even on days when he feels good. Warn him about the risks of abrupt withdrawal, such as life-threatening arrhythmias.

Explain that most antihypertensives begin to work within 1 to 2 hours of taking a dose and that their effects peak in 6 to 8 hours and last for 12 to 24 hours. Drugs taken once a day are most effective in the first 12 hours. Advise the patient that the best time of day to take his drugs is when he's most active.

Instruct your patient not to chew or crush extended-release tablets or capsules because doing so can destroy their sustained action. Also, make sure he understands the risks of taking over-the-counter medications, especially cold and allergy preparations, which can react adversely with antihypertensives.

After you've explained these general points, talk with your patient about the specific antihypertensives he's taking. Be sure to discuss his drug dosage, possible adverse effects, and appropriate specific considerations.

crease patient compliance (see *Teaching your patient about antihypertensive drugs*).

Diuretics

Diuretics promote renal excretion of water and electrolytes by increasing the glomerular filtration rate. They can also decrease sodium reab-

Diuretics at work

Different types of diuretics act at different sites along the nephron to promote diuresis.

Loop diuretics (1) act primarily on the ascending loop of Henle to increase sodium, chloride, and water secretion. Potassium sparing diuretics (2), thiazide diuretics (3), and thiazide-like diuretics (4) act along the distal tubule. Potassium sparing diuretics inhibit sodium and water reabsorption and increase potassium retention. Thiazide and thiazide-like diuretics increase water, sodium, chloride, and potassium excretion.

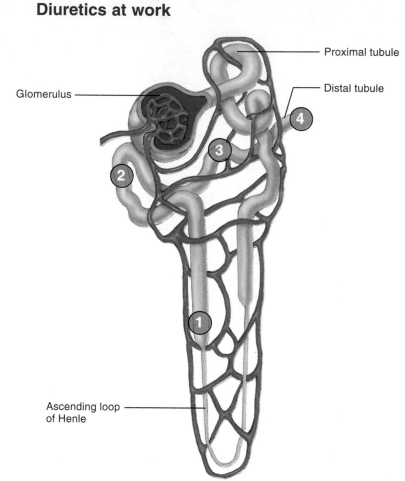

sorption and increase the rate of sodium excretion (see *Diuretics at work*).

Diuretics are divided into several classes: loop, potassium sparing, thiazide, and thiazide-like. Each of these classes has a single mechanism of action. Combination diuretics contain two different classes of diuretic (see *What's in combination diuretics?*).

Loop diuretics
Acting primarily on the ascending loop of Henle, loop diuretics can either inhibit the reabsorption or increase the secretion of sodium, chloride, and water. These drugs include the sulfonamide derivatives bumetanide, furosemide, and torsemide and the ketone derivatives ethacrynate sodium and ethacrynic acid.

Indications and contraindications
As well as being used to treat hypertension, loop diuretics are given to patients with edema caused by heart failure, liver disease, renal disease, pulmonary edema, ascites, and anasarca.

These drugs shouldn't be used in patients who have sulfonamide sensitivity. Nor should they be used in breast-feeding patients or patients with anuria, electrolyte abnormalities, volume depletion, or hepatic coma.

Use loop diuretics cautiously in patients with dehydration, ascites, severe renal disease, or hepatic cirrhosis. Loop diuretics have a potent potassium-excreting effect and may increase your patient's risk of cardiac arrhythmias. Also, use furosemide and torsemide cautiously in diabetic patients. If your patient is using oral antidiabetic drugs or insulin, monitor him for the development of hyperglycemia and assess him regularly for glycosuria.

Adverse effects and interactions

The adverse effects of loop diuretics may be severe because of their potent diuretic effect. The most severe effects include hypokalemia, hypochloremic alkalosis, hypomagnesemia, hyperuricemia, hypocalcemia, hyponatremia, hyperglycemia, and metabolic alkalosis. Other adverse effects include transient hearing loss, impaired glucose tolerance, dermatitis, abdominal pain, diarrhea, and thrombocytopenia.

Loop diuretics may also cause ototoxic effects such as hearing impairment and tinnitus. Usually, these effects result from a rapid I.V. injection of large doses in patients with decreased renal function.

Loop diuretics may interact with several drugs. When given with indomethacin or nonsteroidal anti-inflammatory drugs (NSAIDs), loop diuretics have a decreased diuretic effect. Ototoxicity can develop when loop diuretics are given with cisplatin, aminoglycosides, or vancomycin. Also, the risk of toxicity increases when loop diuretics are given with lithium, nondepolarizing skeletal muscle relaxants, and digitalis glycosides.

Increased anticoagulant effects occur when loop diuretics are given with warfarin. When used with oral antidiabetic drugs or insulin, loop diuretics may decrease the hypoglycemic effect and trigger hyperglycemia.

Loop diuretics are incompatible with dobutamine and milrinone. And furosemide and torsemide shouldn't be taken with vitamin C, corticosteroids, diphenhydramine, epinephrine, gentamicin, meperidine, reserpine, spironolactone, and tetracyclines.

Potassium sparing diuretics

Potassium sparing diuretics have weaker diuretic and antihypertensive effects than loop diuretics. However, by acting on the distal tubule to in-

What's in combination diuretics?

This chart shows the contents of the most commonly used combination diuretics. When administering a combination diuretic, be sure to monitor your patient for the adverse effects associated with both drugs.

Combination diuretic	Drugs
Aldactazide	spironolactone 25 mg and hydrochlorothiazide 25 mg
Aldactazide 50/50	spironolactone 50 mg and hydrochlorothiazide 50 mg
Dyazide	triamterene 50 mg and hydrochlorothiazide 50 mg
Maxzide	triamterene 75 mg and hydrochlorothiazide 50 mg
Maxzide-25	triamterene 37.5 mg and hydrochlorothiazide 25 mg
Moduretic	amiloride hydrochloride 5 mg and hydrochlorothiazide 50 mg
Spirozide	spironolactone 25 mg and hydrochlorothiazide 25 mg

hibit the reabsorption of sodium and water, these drugs increase potassium retention. The potassium sparing diuretics include amiloride, spironolactone, and triamterene.

Indications and contraindications

Physicians prescribe potassium sparing diuretics to treat patients with hypertension or with edema from heart failure. These drugs are also used in combination with other classes of diuretics to maintain a patient's serum potassium levels.

Potassium sparing diuretics shouldn't be used to treat patients with anuria, hyperkalemia, or impaired renal function. Amiloride should be used cautiously in those with dehydration, diabetes, or acidosis. And spironolactone should be given cautiously to patients with hepatic disease. Use triamterene cautiously in patients with heart failure, renal disease, and cirrhosis. When administering any potassium sparing diuretics, monitor your patient's serum chemistry levels for early indications of electrolyte imbalance and increasing renal or hepatic failure.

Adverse effects and interactions
These drugs produce fewer adverse effects than other diuretics. However, a patient taking a potassium sparing diuretic has a greater risk of hyperkalemia, especially if he's also taking potassium supplements.

Dose-related adverse effects include megaloblastic anemia, arrhythmias, headache, dizziness, and orthostatic hypotension. Spironolactone may cause amenorrhea, a deeper voice, gynecomastia, hirsutism, irregular menses, and postmenopausal bleeding. Triamterene may cause a bluish discoloration of the urine.

Your patient may experience hyperkalemia if he takes one of these drugs with another potassium sparing diuretic, an ACE inhibitor, or a salt substitute. If given with lithium, a potassium sparing diuretic may provoke lithium toxicity. Nephrotoxicity may increase if a patient takes triamterene with indomethacin. Also, aspirin decreases the effects of spironolactone.

Thiazide and thiazide-like diuretics
Thiazide diuretics act on the distal tubule by increasing the excretion of water, sodium, chloride, and potassium. Their antihypertensive effect may result from reduced plasma volume and sodium levels, direct relaxation of arteriolar smooth muscle, and decreased reactivity of vascular smooth muscle.

Thiazide-like diuretics differ slightly in their chemical structure from thiazide diuretics, but they have comparable pharmacologic and toxicologic properties. Thiazide-like diuretics act on the distal tubule by increasing the excretion of water, sodium, chloride, potassium, magnesium, and bicarbonate. Indapamide, a thiazide-like diuretic, slows the reabsorption of sodium and inhibits direct vasodilation by blocking the calcium channel.

The thiazide diuretics include chlorothiazide and hydrochlorothiazide. The thiazide-like diuretics include chlorthalidone, indapamide, and metolazone.

Indications and contraindications
Thiazide and thiazide-like diuretics are used to treat patients with mild to moderate hyperten-

sion, edema, and heart failure. Thiazide diuretics are also used for edema associated with corticosteroid or estrogen therapy. And thiazide-like diuretics are used to treat patients with nephrotic syndrome.

Neither thiazide nor thiazide-like diuretics should be given to patients with hypersensitivity to sulfonamides or thiazides. Also, don't administer these diuretics to patients with anuria or renal decompensation.

Thiazide diuretics shouldn't be given to patients with hypomagnesemia, and thiazide-like diuretics shouldn't be given to breast-feeding patients. Use both types cautiously in patients with hypokalemia, renal disease, hepatic disease, gout, and diabetes mellitus. Also, use thiazide diuretics cautiously in patients with chronic obstructive pulmonary disease (COPD) and lupus erythematosus, who may be receiving concomitant corticosteroid therapy. Check serum potassium levels and monitor for hypokalemia when those two drugs are used together.

Adverse effects and interactions
Adverse effects of thiazide and thiazide-like diuretics include volume depletion, orthostatic hypotension, and electrolyte imbalances. Dose-related adverse effects include glucose intolerance, anorexia, nausea, pancreatitis, hypersensitivity reactions, and blood disorders such as agranulocytosis, aplastic anemia, hemolytic anemia, leukopenia, neutropenia, and thrombocytopenia. Monitor your patient's caloric intake and check his complete blood count for signs of malnutrition or anemia.

Thiazide diuretics aren't compatible with amikacin, chlorpromazine, codeine, hydralazine, insulin, morphine, streptomycin, tetracycline, vancomycin, vitamins B and C, and warfarin. These diuretics have an increased risk of toxicity when they're given with lithium, nondepolarizing skeletal muscle relaxants, and digoxin. Also, an increased hypotensive effect may result when a patient takes either type with another antihypertensive or alcohol.

If you give these diuretics with oral antidiabetic drugs or insulin, hyperglycemia, hyponatremia, or thiazide resistance may develop. If you give them with cholestyramine or colestipol, your patient may experience decreased absorption of the diuretic. And if you give them with indomethacin or an NSAID, the hypotensive response decreases.

If you give these diuretics with ticarcillin, glucocorticoids, amphotericin, mezlocillin, or piperacillin, hypokalemia can result. If you give them with diazoxide, hyperglycemia, hyperuricemia, or hypotension can result. Metolazone given with furosemide enhances the hypotensive effect.

Nursing considerations

Administer a diuretic in the morning so that your patient's sleep isn't interrupted by nighttime diuresis. To prevent nausea (a possible adverse effect of diuretics), have the patient take the drug with food.

For intermittent I.V. administration of a loop diuretic, give the drug undiluted at a rate not to exceed 4 mg per minute through a Y-connector, a three-way stopcock, or an intermittent I.V. access device. For a continuous infusion of furosemide, give the drug in normal saline solution or dextrose 5% in water (D$_5$W) at a rate of 5 to 40 mg per hour, using an infusion pump. Remember to protect the solution from light. Make dose adjustments based on the patient's response. And monitor his urine output, blood pressure, and cardiac status frequently.

When administering an I.V. infusion of a thiazide or thiazide-like diuretic, dilute the drug in sterile water or Ringer's, lactated Ringer's, 0.45% normal saline, 0.9% normal saline, D$_5$W, or dextrose 10% in water.

During the course of therapy, monitor your patient's fluid status, including his daily weights, intake, and output. Also, check his blood pressure in the sitting, lying, and standing positions and note any changes that indicate orthostatic hypotension. Monitor his serum electrolytes, including potassium, sodium, chloride, calcium, and magnesium.

Pay particular attention to your patient's potassium level. If it's less than 3 mEq/L, he may need a potassium replacement. If your patient is receiving a potassium sparing diuretic, instruct him to avoid potassium-rich foods such as oranges, bananas, salt substitutes, dried apricots, and dates. Also, if he's receiving triamterene, monitor his liver function studies.

When administering any diuretic, watch for dehydration by checking the patient's mucous membranes and by assessing for skin turgor. Dehydrated patients may also complain of excessive thirst.

Watch for signs of metabolic alkalosis, including drowsiness and restlessness, and for signs of hypokalemia, including malaise, fatigue, tachycardia, leg cramps, and weakness. Monitor the elderly patient for signs of confusion.

MULTISYSTEM ALERT

Loop diuretics and digitalis toxicity

A hypertensive patient taking a loop diuretic has an increased risk of developing electrolyte imbalances, particularly hypokalemia. If your patient also has heart failure and is taking a digitalis glycoside, such as digoxin, and a loop diuretic, he has an increased risk of developing digitalis toxicity.

Be alert for the following signs and symptoms of digitalis toxicity:

- anorexia, nausea, vomiting, diarrhea, and abdominal pain
- headache, restlessness, irritability, depression, personality changes, lethargy, confusion, disorientation, insomnia, psychosis, and seizures
- atrial or ventricular arrhythmias, heart block, accelerated junctional rhythms, and atrial tachycardia with atrioventricular block
- blurred vision, flickering lights, white borders around dark objects, and colored dots.

Also, obtain your patient's baseline serum potassium level and monitor his serum potassium and digitalis levels. To ensure the accuracy of his serum digitalis level, obtain the sample at least 8 hours after the last dose, preferably before administering a daily oral maintenance dose.

Be alert for signs of hearing changes. Large bolus doses may cause ototoxicity. And if your patient is taking digoxin, along with a loop diuretic, look for signs of digitalis toxicity (see *Loop diuretics and digitalis toxicity*).

After you administer the drug, the patient should change position slowly and sit a few minutes before standing to minimize orthostatic hypotension. If he has any adverse reactions, such as muscle cramps, weakness, nausea, and dizziness, report them to his physician.

Instruct your patient to weigh himself daily and report increases of 2 pounds or more over 48 hours or less. Usually, a patient should increase his fluid intake while taking the drug. He should eat foods that are high in potassium and take any prescribed potassium supplements to prevent hypokalemia. He should also check with his physician before taking any other drugs, including OTC drugs, and herbal supplements during the course of his treatment.

Beta-blockers

Beta-blockers are divided into selective and nonselective types. Each has a specific mechanism of action.

Selective beta-blockers

Selective beta-blockers inhibit the stimulation of beta$_1$-adrenergic receptors in cardiac smooth muscle, producing chronotropic and inotropic effects. And by blocking the stimulation of beta-adrenergic receptors, these drugs have the same effects in vascular smooth muscle. Selective beta-blockers also reduce renin release, thus decreasing angiotensin production and aldosterone secretion.

Selective beta-blockers include acebutolol, atenolol, esmolol hydrochloride, and metoprolol.

Indications and contraindications

Selective beta-blockers are used to treat mild to moderately hypertensive patients and patients with cardiac arrhythmias. Esmolol hydrochloride is used in hypertensive crisis.

Don't administer these drugs to patients with cardiogenic shock, heart block, sinus bradycardia, or heart failure. Use them cautiously in patients with diabetes mellitus, renal disease, thyroid disease, COPD, asthma, well-compensated heart failure, and aortic or mitral valve disease. Also, use them cautiously in patients scheduled for major surgery. In particular, use esmolol, a selective beta$_1$ antagonist, carefully in patients with peripheral vascular disease. Because of its negative inotropic effects, monitor your patient's peripheral vascular status for changes in color, temperature, and strength of distal pulses.

Adverse effects and interactions

Because selective beta-blockers can penetrate the blood-brain barrier, these drugs typically produce central nervous system (CNS) effects such as sedation, drowsiness, and depression. Your patient may complain of difficulty concentrating and forgetfulness.

Cardiovascular reactions include bradycardia, hypotension, heart failure, and exacerbation of peripheral vascular disease. Selective beta-blockers can also reduce high-density lipoprotein cholesterol levels and increase serum triglyceride, total cholesterol, low-density lipoprotein cholesterol, and very-low-density lipoprotein cholesterol levels.

Other adverse effects include nausea, vomiting, diarrhea, nightmares, insomnia, hallucinations, dry eyes, paresthesia, transient thrombocytopenia, sore throat, difficulty breathing, and impotence. Patients with peripheral vascular disease may also have increased symptoms of arterial insufficiency.

The warning signs of hypoglycemia—confusion and lethargy—may be overlooked in elderly patients with diabetes mellitus who are taking oral antidiabetic drugs or receiving insulin therapy. Selective beta-blockers may cause hypoglycemia in these patients while masking the symptoms. Notify the physician if you suspect the possibility of a hypoglycemic reaction in your patient. These drugs also may alter test results for serum alkaline phosphatase, blood urea nitrogen (BUN), creatinine, potassium, transaminase, and uric acid levels.

Increased hypotension and reflex bradycardia may occur when selective beta-blockers are used with reserpine, hydralazine, methyldopa, prazosin, or anticholinergics. Also, the antihypertensive effect can decrease when they are used with indomethacin or salicylates.

If atenolol is used with clonidine, hypertension can result. Both atenolol and metoprolol are incompatible with other drugs in solution or syringe. When esmolol is used with digoxin, serum digitalis levels may increase. And the effects of esmolol are reversed when used with isoproterenol, norepinephrine, dopamine, and dobutamine. Esmolol increases the effects of lidocaine. Also, esmolol is incompatible with sodium bicarbonate and furosemide.

Nonselective beta-blockers

Through the combination of sympathomimetic activity with alpha-blocking and beta-blocking effects, nonselective beta-blockers decrease blood pressure without associated reflex tachycardia or reduced heart rate. One drug, pindolol, also decreases stimulation of the renin-angiotensin-aldosterone system.

Nonselective beta-blockers include carteolol, nadolol, pindolol, propranolol, and timolol.

Indications and contraindications

A physician prescribes nonselective beta-blockers to treat patients with mild to moderate hypertension. However, these drugs should not be used in patients with cardiogenic shock, heart block, sinus bradycardia, or heart failure.

Nadolol is contraindicated in patients with heart failure, cardiogenic shock, or COPD. Also, use nadolol cautiously in patients with hyperthyroidism, peripheral vascular disease, or myasthenia gravis.

Use all nonselective beta-blockers cautiously in patients scheduled for major surgery and in those with diabetes mellitus, renal disease, thyroid disease, COPD, heart failure, or nonallergic bronchospasm. Monitor your patient for bradycardia and signs of peripheral vasoconstriction. Check the rate and strength of his peripheral pulses and note changes in extremity temperature or color. Report any adverse findings to the physician.

Adverse effects and interactions

The adverse effects of nonselective beta-blockers are similar to those of selective beta-blockers. Effects on the CNS include sedation, depression, difficulty concentrating, and forgetfulness. Cardiovascular reactions can include bradycardia, hypotension, heart failure, and exacerbation of peripheral vascular disease.

Undesirable changes can occur in serum triglycerides, cholesterol, and lipoprotein levels. Your patient may have gastrointestinal (GI) distress, diarrhea, nightmares, difficulty sleeping, hallucinations, dry eyes, paresthesia, transient thrombocytopenia, sore throat, difficulty breathing, worsened arterial insufficiency, and impotence. In diabetic patients taking oral antidiabetic drugs or receiving insulin therapy, signs of hypoglycemia may be difficult to detect. Nonselective beta-blockers can also alter the serum levels of electrolytes, alkaline phosphatase, BUN, creatinine, transaminase, and uric acid.

Adverse effects specific to nadolol include peripheral ischemia, flushing, edema, laryngospasm, vasodilation, heart conduction disturbances, abdominal cramps, and hepatomegaly. Pindolol may cause claudication, tachycardia, ischemic colitis, abdominal pain, frequent urination, and mesenteric arterial thrombosis. Pindolol and propranolol can cause hallucinations. Propranolol can also cause acute pancreatitis, decreased libido, and bronchospasm.

When nonselective beta-blockers are used with diuretics, other antihypertensive agents, halothane, nitroglycerin, or prazosin, drug interactions include increased hypotensive effects. When they are used with sympathomimetics, NSAIDs, or salicylates, decreased beta-blocking effects occur.

If nonselective beta-blockers are taken with oral antidiabetic drugs or insulin, hypoglycemic effects increase. Nonselective beta-blockers enhance the effect of lidocaine. Also, nadolol enhances the effects of reserpine, digitalis glycosides, ergots, neuromuscular blockers, and calcium channel blockers.

When pindolol is used with reserpine, hydralazine, methyldopa, or anticholinergics, an increased hypotensive effect occurs. Atrioventricular block occurs when propranolol is used with digitalis glycosides and calcium channel blockers. And negative inotropic effects increase when propranolol is used with verapamil and disopyramide. A patient receiving propranolol after an MI has an increased risk of sudden death and reinfarction. If your patient has a known cardiac history, you may want to suggest that the physician choose an alternative therapy.

Propranolol's effects decrease when it's used with norepinephrine, barbiturates, rifampin, dopamine, and dobutamine. Also, its effects decrease if the patient smokes. However, propranolol's effects increase when it's used with cimetidine. Propranolol is incompatible with any drug in solution or syringe.

Nursing considerations

Before you administer selective beta-blockers, measure your patient's apical and radial pulses. When using a nonselective beta-blocker, obtain his baseline pulse rate and blood pressure before each administration. Also, if he has impaired renal function, anticipate a reduced dosage.

Administer atenolol by slow I.V. push, not to exceed 5 mg over 5 minutes, or dilute it in 10 to 50 ml of D_5W, dextrose 5% in normal saline, or normal saline. To administer esmolol, begin with an I.V. bolus dose of 0.5 to 1.0 mg/kg followed by an infusion. Dilute it in D_5W, Ringer's solution, or sodium chloride, and administer it at a rate of 50 to 100 µg/kg/minute with an infusion pump. Also, if your patient's blood pressure is less than 100/60 mm Hg, notify the physician before giving esmolol.

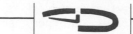

DANGEROUS COMPLICATIONS

Beta-blocker therapy: No sudden stops

If your patient suddenly stops taking a beta-blocker, he may experience angina, arrhythmias, myocardial infarction, or life-threatening hypertension. To prevent these risks, make sure he understands that he should never abruptly stop taking his drug.

Tell your patient to continue his therapy exactly as prescribed, even if he's feeling well. Warn him that abrupt discontinuation of this drug could be fatal.

Teach him the signs and symptoms of beta-blocker withdrawal, including chest pain, palpitations, extreme weakness, and shortness of breath. Tell him to report these signs and symptoms to his physician.

If his physician discontinues the drug, the doses will probably be tapered over a period of several weeks. Advise the patient to use a calendar to plot his drug dosages according to the prescribed tapering schedule.

Usually, oral forms of selective and nonselective beta-blockers can be given before meals and at bedtime, as prescribed. They can be taken with food to reduce GI upset. Also, the tablets can be crushed or swallowed whole.

However, the patient should take pindolol with or immediately after meals. If orthostatic hypotension is severe, he should take this drug at bedtime.

Administer nadolol with at least 8 ounces of water. Propranolol should also be administered with 8 ounces of water but on an empty stomach. And don't give propranolol with aluminum-containing antacids because they decrease the drug's absorption in the intestine.

When using either selective or nonselective beta-blockers, frequently measure your patient's blood pressure for hypotension. Depending on his status, monitor his pulse rate, rhythm, and quality at least every 4 hours. Also, watch for signs of heart failure.

If your patient has diabetes, monitor his blood glucose levels. Also, monitor his fluid balance by measuring intake and output and by obtaining daily weights. Report any significant changes to his physician.

Check the patient's skin turgor and mucous membranes for signs of dehydration, especially if he's elderly. If he develops any CNS effects such as confusion, institute safety precautions.

Instruct your patient to take his drug exactly as prescribed. Also, tell him to avoid using OTC nasal decongestants or cold preparations because they contain alpha-adrenergic stimulants and can cause adverse reactions such as arrhythmias.

Teach the patient how to take his own blood pressure and pulse and tell him to notify his physician about abnormal findings. He should report difficulty breathing, night coughing, or swelling of the legs. Tell him to also report any complaints of dizziness, confusion, depression, and fever. If he's experiencing dizziness, instruct him to avoid activities such as driving. And warn him against abruptly discontinuing his beta-blocker therapy because he may develop life-threatening adverse effects (see *Beta-blocker therapy: No sudden stops*).

Alpha-blockers

Alpha-blockers prevent epinephrine and norepinephrine from activating the sympathetic nervous system's alpha-adrenergic receptors. These drugs can selectively block alpha$_1$-adrenergic receptors or act nonselectively.

Selective alpha-blockers interfere with sympathetic stimulation by relaxing arteriolar smooth muscle. But nonselective alpha-blockers competitively block all alpha-adrenergic receptors, causing vasodilation and lowering blood pressure.

Selective alpha-blockers include doxazosin mesylate, prazosin, and terazosin. Nonselective alpha-blockers include phenoxybenzamine hydrochloride and phentolamine mesylate.

Indications and contraindications
Prazosin is commonly given in reduced dosages with a thiazide diuretic or beta-blocker to reduce blood pressure. In patients with pheochromocytoma, nonselective alpha-blockers are used to prevent or control episodes of hypertension that may occur as a result of stress or manipulation of the tumor.

Don't give selective alpha-blockers to breast-feeding patients. Give these drugs cautiously to patients with heart failure or renal failure. Nonselective alpha-blockers shouldn't be given to patients with coronary artery disease (CAD).

Adverse effects and interactions

Selective alpha-blockers can cause dizziness, headache, nausea, palpitations, dyspnea, orthostatic hypotension, and sexual dysfunction. The first dose of prazosin and doxazosin can cause syncope.

Nonselective alpha-blockers can cause weakness, dizziness, orthostatic hypotension, tachycardia, and nasal congestion. Phentolamine can cause anginal attacks from rebound tachycardia.

After the first dose of prazosin, the severity and duration of hypotension may be greater in patients also receiving beta-blockers. When doxazosin is given with alcohol, nitrates, or other antihypertensive drugs, increased hypotensive effects may occur. Phentolamine decreases the vasoconstrictive and hypertensive effects of epinephrine and ephedrine. Also, phentolamine is incompatible with iron salts.

Nursing considerations

When administering alpha-blockers, remember that initial therapy usually involves low doses, which are increased gradually to minimize adverse effects. Administer these drugs with food or milk to minimize the GI effects.

Phentolamine mesylate is given I.V. or intramuscularly. If severe hypotension develops, use a vasopressor such as norepinephrine.

After administering the drug, have your patient change positions slowly and sit for a few minutes before rising to minimize orthostatic hypotension. Monitor him by frequently checking his blood pressure while he is sitting, lying, and standing. Also, ask him about adverse effects.

When giving prazosin, monitor the patient for signs and symptoms of syncope after the first dose. When giving phentolamine, assess his 12-lead ECG to detect arrhythmias. Also, enforce bed rest for 1 hour after giving the drug.

Tell your patient to take his drugs as prescribed. Warn him to avoid all OTC drugs unless otherwise directed by his physician. And tell him to avoid alcoholic beverages.

Teach the patient to take his own blood pressure and tell him to notify his physician about abnormal readings. Also, warn him about adverse effects that can be caused by the drug, such as dizziness, palpitations, and fainting.

Alpha agonists

Alpha agonists—sympatholytic drugs that decrease arteriolar vasoconstriction—inhibit the sympathetic vasomotor center within the CNS, thereby decreasing blood pressure, pulse rate, and cardiac output (CO). One drug, methyldopa, stimulates central inhibitory alpha-adrenergic receptors or acts as a false transmitter, resulting in reduced blood pressure.

Alpha agonists include clonidine hydrochloride, guanabenz acetate, guanfacine hydrochloride, and methyldopa.

Indications and contraindications

A physician prescribes an alpha agonist to treat a patient with mild to moderate hypertension. Guanfacine is commonly used in combination with thiazide diuretics.

Don't use methyldopa in patients with active hepatic disease and blood dyscrasia. Use guanabenz acetate cautiously in patients with cerebrovascular disease. And use all alpha agonists cautiously in patients with a recent myocardial infarction, diabetes mellitus, chronic renal failure, Raynaud's disease, thyroid disease, depression, COPD, or asthma. Monitor your patient's neurovascular and peripheral vascular status closely to detect signs of circulatory compromise or decreased perfusion. Check the strength and rate of his peripheral pulses. Note the development of edema and the degree of pitting.

Adverse effects and interactions

Alpha agonists typically produce CNS effects such as sedation, drowsiness, and depression. Common effects also include forgetfulness, inability to concentrate, and vivid dreams. These drugs may cause sodium and water retention, edema, hepatic dysfunction, vertigo, paresthesia, weakness, fever, and nasal congestion. They may also cause impotence.

Guanfacine may cause bradycardia, rhinitis, urinary incontinence, dermatitis, purpura, and dyspnea. Methyldopa can cause weight gain, systemic lupus erythematosus–like syndrome, eczema, and myocarditis. Guanabenz may alter taste sensation and cause backache. And clonidine patches may cause skin irritation and excoriation.

When alpha agonists are used with narcotics, sedatives, hypnotics, anesthetics, and alcohol, drug interactions include increased depression of the CNS. If you use alpha agonists with tricyclic antidepressants, monoamine oxidase inhibitors, appetite suppressants, or amphetamines, the hypotensive effects may decrease. When they are used with beta-blockers and digitalis glycosides, the risk of bradycardia increases.

When methyldopa is used with norepinephrine and phenylpropanolamine, vasopressor effects increase. When methyldopa is used with levodopa, hypotension increases. And sedation is aggravated when methyldopa and haloperidol are used together.

Nursing considerations
When administering oral alpha agonists, you'll usually give the last dose at bedtime. However, you can administer guanabenz in the morning or at bedtime. Obtain the patient's baseline blood pressure and pulse before each dose of this drug.

When using clonidine patches, apply one patch per week to a site with minimal hair. The best absorption occurs at the chest or upper arm. Rotate the sites with each application of the patch, and clean the site before applying.

During therapy, frequently measure your patient's blood pressure while he's sitting, lying, and standing. If he's taking methyldopa, monitor his hepatic function by measuring his lactate dehydrogenase levels, especially during the first 6 to 12 weeks of therapy.

If your patient is using a clonidine patch, monitor the application site for signs of an allergic reaction and notify his physician of a rash, urticaria, or angioedema.

Advise your patient to take his drug 1 hour before meals. Suggest that he use mouthwash or eat hard candy to avoid mouth dryness. Also, tell him to avoid using OTC drugs unless prescribed by his physician.

Teach him to measure his own blood pressure at home and tell him to notify his physician if the results are abnormal. Tell him to also notify his physician if he develops mouth sores, sore throat, swelling of the feet or hands, palpitations, irregular pulse, or chest pain.

Warn him that if he abruptly discontinues the alpha agonist, he may develop anxiety, increased blood pressure, headache, insomnia, increased pulse, tremors, nausea, and sweating. Also, warn him to avoid activities such as driving if he becomes drowsy after taking the drug.

Angiotensin-converting enzyme inhibitors

Oral drugs that may be used alone or in combination with other antihypertensives, ACE inhibitors selectively suppress the renin-angiotensin-aldosterone system. This inhibits ACE and prevents the conversion of angiotensin I to angiotensin II, resulting in dilation of the arterial and venous vessels.

The ACE inhibitors include benazepril hydrochloride, captopril, enalapril, fosinopril, quinapril hydrochloride, ramipril, and spirapril.

Indications and contraindications
Used to treat patients with hypertension, ACE inhibitors are commonly prescribed in combination with thiazide diuretics. One drug, enalapril, is also used to treat heart failure.

Administer ACE inhibitors cautiously to patients with hypovolemia, blood dyscrasia, impaired renal and liver function, heart failure, COPD, asthma, and bilateral renal artery stenosis. Also, administer them cautiously to patients receiving dialysis.

Adverse effects and interactions
Adverse effects caused by ACE inhibitors include proteinuria, neutropenia, agranulocytosis, rash, and loss of taste. These commonly occur when a patient takes captopril. You may observe CNS reactions including headache, dizziness, fatigue, and syncope. And GI effects include nausea, vomiting, and diarrhea.

An ACE inhibitor can cause transient elevations of BUN and serum creatinine levels, especially with hypertension resulting from volume depletion or renal or cardiovascular disease. Serum potassium levels commonly increase with ACE inhibitor use, especially in patients with impaired renal function. These drugs can produce tickling of the throat and a dry, nonproductive cough. Angioedema can also occur, resulting in flushing, pallor, and swelling of the face, lips, tongue, glottis, larynx, arms, and legs. When ACE inhibitors are administered with diuretics, other antihypertensives, ganglionic blockers, or alpha-blockers, their hypotensive effects increase. When ACE inhibitors are administered with indomethacin, their antihypertensive effects decrease.

When ACE inhibitors are used with vasodilators, hydralazine, prazosin, potassium sparing diuretics, sympathomimetics, and potassium supplements, the risk of toxicity increases. And simultaneous use of ACE inhibitors and antacids can decrease GI absorption.

Aspirin decreases the effects of enalapril. But phenothiazines, diuretics, phenytoin, quinidine, and nifedipine increase its effects. Enalapril increases the effects of ergots, neuromuscular blockers, antihypertensives, antidiabetic drugs, barbiturates, reserpine, and levodopa. And tetracycline absorption decreases when enalapril is given with quinapril.

Nursing considerations

Before starting therapy with an ACE inhibitor, obtain the patient's blood pressure and pulse rate. After therapy begins, frequently check his blood pressure while he is sitting, lying, and standing to detect orthostatic hypotension or syncope.

Remember that I.V. enalapril should be given undiluted over 5 minutes. Administer quinapril 1 hour before meals. And don't administer antacids for up to 2 hours after giving quinapril because they interfere with its absorption.

Watch for excessive hypotension caused by drug interactions (see *Preventing hypotension from angiotensin-converting enzyme inhibitors*). If your patient develops severe hypotension, administer normal saline I.V. and place him in the modified shock position (see *Treating severe hypotension,* page 156).

Monitor your patient's fluid status including intake, output, and daily weight. Check for proteinuria every 2 to 4 weeks during the first 3 months of therapy to detect decreased renal function. Also, check for polyuria, oliguria, urine frequency, angioedema, and dysuria.

Warn him to avoid salt substitutes containing potassium unless prescribed by his physician. Also, advise him that these drugs can cause dizziness, fainting, and light-headedness, especially during the first few days of therapy.

Teach your patient to monitor his blood pressure at home and to use safety measures to minimize orthostatic hypotension. Advise him to call

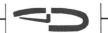

DANGEROUS COMPLICATIONS

Preventing hypotension from angiotensin-converting enzyme inhibitors

When starting therapy with an angiotensin-converting enzyme inhibitor in a patient who already takes another antihypertensive drug—such as a diuretic, an alpha-blocker, or a beta-blocker—frequently check his blood pressure to detect hypotension.

Be alert for hypotension if the patient experiences excessive perspiration, vomiting, diarrhea, or dehydration.

Be particularly alert for hypotension in patients who have severe sodium or volume depletion, such as those with severe heart failure who are taking a diuretic.

his physician if he develops mouth sores, sore throat, fever, edema of the hands or feet, irregular heartbeat, chest pain, excessive sweating, vomiting, or diarrhea.

Angiotensin II receptor blocker

This relatively new class of antihypertensive drug interferes with the renin-angiotensin-aldosterone system to reduce blood pressure. The one drug in this class, losartan, selectively blocks the binding of angiotensin II to specific tissue receptors in the vascular smooth muscle and adrenal gland, inhibiting the release of aldosterone and the vasoconstrictive effect of the renin-angiotensin-aldosterone system.

Indications and contraindications

An angiotensin II receptor blocker is used alone or in combination with other drugs to treat patients with hypertension. It should be used cautiously in those with hypovolemia or hepatic or renal dysfunction.

Adverse effects and interactions

Common adverse effects include headache, dizziness, syncope, diarrhea, abdominal pain, nausea,

Treating severe hypotension

To treat severe hypotension, administer normal saline solution I.V. while the patient is in the modified shock position with his feet elevated and his head down, as shown.

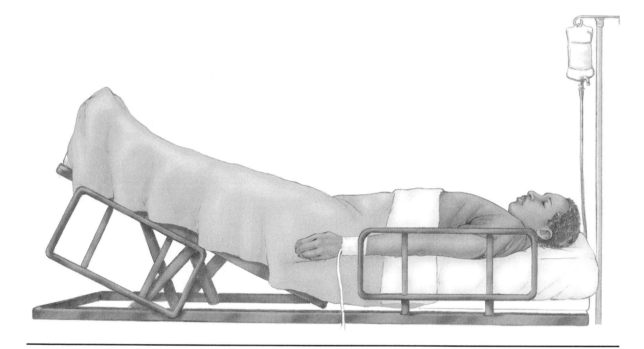

and cough. This drug can also cause symptoms resembling those of an upper respiratory tract infection. When losartan is administered with phenobarbital, its blood levels and its effectiveness decrease.

Nursing considerations

When administering an angiotensin II receptor blocker, obtain your patient's blood pressure before each dose. Once therapy has begun, frequently monitor him for decreased blood pressure caused by fluid loss from heavy perspiration, dehydration, vomiting, or diarrhea. Also, watch for signs of dizziness and syncope and institute safety precautions to prevent injury.

Teach the patient to measure his blood pressure at home and advise him to notify his physician of any abnormal results. Also, teach him how to minimize orthostatic hypotension and ad-

vise him to notify his physician if he develops excessive sweating, vomiting, or diarrhea. Explain that losartan may increase his blood levels of potassium. And remind him not to take dietary potassium supplements without his physician's approval.

Calcium channel blockers

By interfering with calcium ion influx across the cell membrane, calcium channel blockers inhibit calcium-dependent contraction of vascular smooth muscle. This decreases total peripheral vascular resistance and afterload, which reduces blood pressure.

Calcium channel blockers include diltiazem hydrochloride, felodipine, nicardipine, nifedipine, and verapamil.

Indications and contraindications

Physicians commonly prescribe these drugs to treat patients with angina pectoris. However, several oral forms are used to treat vasospasm and mild to moderate hypertension. Parenteral forms are used to treat hypertension, atrial fibrillation, atrial flutter, and paroxysmal supraventricular tachycardia. But sustained-release nifedipine is only used to treat hypertension.

Use calcium channel blockers cautiously in patients with heart failure, hypotension, hepatic injury, and renal disease. Do not administer a calcium channel blocker to patients with sick sinus syndrome, second-degree or third-degree heart block, hypotension, acute MI, or pulmonary congestion. Do not administer verapamil to patients with cardiogenic shock or severe heart failure, and administer it cautiously to patients taking beta-blockers.

Adverse effects and interactions

The most serious adverse effects of calcium channel blockers include cardiovascular changes such as hypotension, arrhythmias, and worsened heart failure. Other common effects include headache, dizziness, flushing, weakness, and persistent peripheral edema. Your patient may also experience nausea, vomiting, diarrhea, muscle fatigue, cramps, worsened angina, skin eruptions, photosensitivity, pruritus, nasal congestion, and mood changes.

Calcium channel blockers can interact with beta-blockers, causing heart block and heart failure. When diltiazem is taken with cimetidine, its effect increases. And when it's administered with cimetidine or ranitidine, felodipine levels increase. Nicardipine increases the effects of digitalis glycosides, neuromuscular blockers, and theophylline. And when nifedipine is administered in combination with theophylline, beta-blockers, other antihypertensives, or digitalis glycosides, it increases their effects.

Quinidine decreases the effects of nifedipine. The hypotensive effects of verapamil increase when the drug is given with prazosin and quinidine. Verapamil also decreases the effects of lithium and increases the blood levels of digoxin, theophylline, cyclosporine, and carbamazepine. Verapamil is incompatible with albumin, amphotericin B, ampicillin, dobutamine, hydralazine, mezlocillin, nafcillin, oxacillin, and sodium bicarbonate.

Nursing considerations

Before administering calcium channel blockers, obtain your patient's baseline pulse rate and blood pressure. If his pulse is less than 60 beats per minute or if his systolic blood pressure is below 90 mm Hg, withhold the dose and notify his physician.

To reduce GI distress, administer oral forms before meals and at bedtime, as prescribed. Give sustained-release verapamil with food. And have your patient swallow felodipine tablets whole.

Administer I.V. felodipine undiluted over 2 minutes or diluted in D_5W, normal saline, or dextrose 5% in 0.45% normal saline. Infuse I.V. doses at a rate of 10 mg/hour, increasing the dosage by 5 mg/hour up to 15 mg/hour.

During therapy, frequently monitor the patient's vital signs. Check for signs of fluid retention by auscultating his breath sounds and by checking for persistent peripheral edema. Also, look for jugular vein distention.

Monitor his 12-lead ECG or ECG tracing for arrhythmias, especially when administering nicardipine or nifedipine.

Teach your patient to monitor his pulse and blood pressure at home. Warn him to avoid hazardous activities until he's stabilized on the drug and dizziness is not a problem. Also, teach him about the adverse effects of calcium channel blockers and advise him to report any dizziness, shortness of breath, palpitations, swelling of the hands or feet, constipation, nausea, hypotension, and severe ataxia.

Advise him to limit his caffeine consumption and to check with his physician before taking OTC drugs. Also, tell him to abstain from drinking alcohol, especially if he's taking nicardipine or nifedipine.

Direct vasodilators

Direct vasodilators act on arteries and veins. They dilate arteriolar smooth muscle by direct relaxation, reducing systolic and diastolic blood pressure while increasing heart rate and CO.

Direct vasodilators include diazoxide, hydralazine hydrochloride, minoxidil, and nitroprusside.

Indications and contraindications

A physician prescribes diazoxide and nitroprusside to treat patients in hypertensive crisis when an urgent decrease in diastolic blood pressure is needed. Oral hydralazine is used to treat patients with primary hypertension; parenteral hydralazine is used in patients with severe primary hypertension and heart failure. Minoxidil is prescribed when severe hypertension is unresponsive to other therapy.

Don't administer hydralazine to patients with CAD or rheumatic heart disease. Do not use minoxidil in patients with acute MI, dissecting aortic aneurysm, or pheochromocytoma. And do not administer nitroprusside to patients with compensatory hypertension.

Don't use diazoxide in patients with hypersensitivity to thiazides or sulfonamide or in patients whose hypertension is caused by coarctation of the aorta, dissecting aortic aneurysm, atrioventricular shunt, or pheochromocytoma. And use it cautiously in patients with tachycardia, fluid and electrolyte imbalances, or impaired cerebral or cardiac circulation.

Adverse effects and interactions

Direct vasodilators commonly produce adverse effects related to reflex activation of the sympathetic nervous system, such as palpitations, angina, tachycardia, ECG changes, edema, rash, breast tenderness, fatigue, and headache. Severe pericardial effusions can develop. And alkaline phosphatase, BUN, and creatinine levels may increase.

Diazoxide commonly causes headache, anorexia, nausea, and diaphoresis. It can also cause excessive hypotension, and in diabetic patients, it may cause hyperglycemia. If more serious effects occur, such as rash, urticaria, polyneuritis, GI hemorrhage, anemia, and pancytopenia, diazoxide should be discontinued.

Hydralazine commonly causes headache, diarrhea, constipation, dizziness, orthostatic hypotension, facial flushing, shortness of breath, nasal congestion, urinary hesitancy, edema, tremors, and muscle cramps. It may also cause impotence.

Minoxidil commonly produces hair growth on the face, arms, and back. It also causes reflex tachycardia and fluid retention. When minoxidil is taken with guanethidine, orthostatic hypotension can occur.

Nitroprusside causes headache, dizziness, nausea, vomiting, abdominal pain, and thiocyanate or cyanide toxicity (see *Responding to the adverse effects of nitroprusside*). Severe hypotension occurs when nitroprusside is administered with ganglionic blockers, volatile liquid anesthetics, halothane,

enflurane, and circulatory depressants. Nitroprusside is incompatible with any drug in syringe or solution.

When diazoxide is administered with a thiazide diuretic, another antihypertensive drug, warfarin, guanethidine, or a sympathomimetic, its effects increase. It's incompatible with other drugs in a syringe or solution. Hyperglycemia and hyperuricemia can result when diazoxide is combined with thiazides and other diuretics. The effects of both diazoxide and sulfonylureas decrease when the drugs are given together.

When hydralazine is used with epinephrine or norepinephrine, tachycardia and angina increase. Hydralazine increases the effects of beta-blockers. And it is incompatible with aminophylline, ampicillin, edetate calcium disodium, chlorothiazide, ethacrynic acid, hydrocortisone, mephentermine, methohexital sodium, nitroglycerin, phenobarbital, verapamil, fructose 10%, dextrose 10%, and lactated Ringer's solution.

Nursing considerations

Before giving each dose of a direct vasodilator, obtain your patient's blood pressure and pulse rate. Hydralazine, especially in high doses, can cause lupus-like syndrome. So before therapy begins, expect to obtain blood samples for a lupus erythematosus preparation and an antinuclear antibody titer to establish a baseline. Throughout therapy, monitor the test results, as ordered, and assess your patient for lupus-like symptoms, including myalgias, arthralgias, and chest pain. Be sure to administer I.V. hydralazine undiluted and keep your patient supine for 1 hour afterward.

Administer diazoxide rapidly as an I.V. bolus of 1 to 3 mg/kg, up to a maximum dose of 150 mg. You can repeat this dose at 5-minute to 15-minute intervals until the desired diastolic pressure is achieved. Keep your patient in the supine position for up to 1 hour after I.V. administration.

Give nitroprusside as a continuous infusion until the desired blood pressure is achieved. Dilute nitroprusside in D_5W and use an infusion pump. Wrap the nitroprusside solution with aluminum foil to protect it from light. If it turns blue, green, or dark red, discard it (see *How to administer nitroprusside safely,* page 160).

Orally administer hydralazine and minoxidil with meals to enhance absorption. And give minoxidil with a beta-blocker or diuretic to maximize its antihypertensive effects.

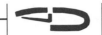

DANGEROUS COMPLICATIONS

Responding to the adverse effects of nitroprusside

If your patient is receiving nitroprusside I.V., he's at risk for developing serious adverse effects, including life-threatening hypotension, cyanide toxicity, and thiocyanate toxicity.

Hypotension
Excessive hypotension—generally a systolic blood pressure of 80 mm Hg or less—causes decreased blood perfusion to vital organs, which can result in death. If your patient is conscious and alert, he may complain of feeling light-headed, lethargic, or confused. He may see spots before his eyes. He may also develop cardiac arrhythmias.

If your patient develops life-threatening hypotension, immediately stop the nitroprusside infusion and notify the physician. Place the patient in the modified shock position to maximize venous blood return to the heart.

Nitroprusside-induced hypotension usually resolves within 1 to 10 minutes after the infusion is stopped. If your patient's hypotension persists for more than 10 minutes after the infusion is discontinued, nitroprusside is not the reason for the crisis, and other causes must be investigated and treated.

Cyanide and thiocyanate toxicity
When the ferrous iron in the nitroprusside molecule reacts with sulfhydryl components in the red blood cells, cyanide forms. The cyanide is metabolized in the liver into thiocyanate, which is eliminated from the body in urine.

Usually, cyanide and thiocyanate toxicity develop when nitroprusside is administered faster than 2 µg/kg/minute, producing cyanide faster than the patient can eliminate it. A prolonged nitroprusside infusion or renal impairment can also result in accumulations of cyanide and thiocyanate in the patient's blood. Thiocyanate toxicity becomes life-threatening when a patient's blood level reaches 200 mg/L or more.

When administering nitroprusside, monitor your patient for the signs and symptoms of cyanide toxicity, including ataxia, dizziness, vomiting, headache, loss of consciousness, metabolic acidosis, dyspnea, tachycardia, and hyperoxia.

Also, watch for the signs and symptoms of thiocyanate toxicity: miosis, blurred vision, dizziness, altered mental status, lethargy, rash, weakness, dyspnea, excessive hypotension, hyperreflexia, and tinnitus.

If you suspect cyanide or thiocyanate toxicity in your patient, immediately stop the nitroprusside infusion and notify his physician. As directed by the physician, administer sodium nitrite to buffer the cyanide and to convert as much hemoglobin into methemoglobin as the patient can safely tolerate. If sodium nitrite administration must be delayed, give amyl nitrite by inhalation every 15 to 30 seconds until a sodium nitrite solution is available.

The physician may direct you to infuse the sodium nitrite 3% solution at 4 to 6 mg/kg (about 0.2 ml/kg) over 2 to 4 minutes. This dose converts about 10% of the patient's hemoglobin to methemoglobin. But be aware that the sodium nitrite infusion may cause transient vasodilation and hypotension.

Infusing sodium thiosulfate helps convert cyanide to thiocyanate, but this treatment doesn't raise thiocyanate to dangerous levels. Sodium thiosulfate is available as 10% and 25% solutions. It should be infused at 150 to 200 mg/kg. A typical adult dose is 50 ml of the 25% solution given over 10 minutes.

If necessary, you may have to repeat the sodium nitrite and sodium thiosulfate regimen after 2 hours at half the initial doses.

After administering an I.V. dose of a direct vasodilator, check your patient's blood pressure every 5 to 15 minutes until it's stable. After administering a direct vasodilator orally, check his blood pressure at least every 3 to 4 hours.

When giving nitroprusside I.V., track your patient's blood pressure by intra-arterial monitoring and watch for signs of an overdose. If he's receiving long-term nitroprusside therapy, obtain thiocyanate levels daily.

Evaluate your patient for orthostatic hypotension by checking his blood pressure while lying, sitting, and standing. Also, monitor his serum electrolyte and glucose levels. If he's receiving hy-

How to administer nitroprusside safely

For a continuous I.V. infusion of nitroprusside, reconstitute each 50 mg with 2 to 3 ml of dextrose 5% in water (D_5W) for injection. Further dilute the solution with 250 to 1,000 ml of D_5W. Don't use other diluents.

Promptly wrap the bag with aluminum foil or another opaque material to protect it from light. If properly protected, the solution will remain stable for 24 hours. Change the solution every 24 hours.

Usually, nitroprusside therapy starts at a low dosage because some patients become dangerously hypotensive even at doses of 3 µg/kg/minute. To be safe, begin the infusion at a rate of 0.3 µg/kg/minute. Gradually titrate it upward every few minutes until the patient's blood pressure reaches the desired level or you reach the maximum recommended infusion rate of 10 µg/kg/minute.

Don't infuse the maximum rate for more than 10 minutes. Because of the potential serious adverse effects, nitroprusside is usually administered only for short durations.

Because the hypotensive effects of nitroprusside have a rapid onset and rate of dissipation, even the smallest change in the infusion rate can lead to wide variations in blood pressure. So use a volumetric infusion pump and monitor your patient's blood pressure with an intra-arterial monitoring system or automatic inflatable blood pressure monitoring device. If you change the concentration of the nitroprusside solution, you must also change the administration tubing because it will be filled with the previous concentration.

Remember that elderly patients are more sensitive to the hypotensive effects of this drug.

---

dralazine, watch for fever, joint pain, and changes in affect, mood, behavior, and personality.

After giving the drug, tell your patient to remain lying down. Tell him to report adverse effects such as a cough, difficulty breathing, dizziness, chest pain, and headache. Teach him the signs and symptoms of cyanide toxicity and tell him to report them.

If the patient is taking minoxidil, tell him to notify his physician if he experiences chest pain, severe fatigue, muscle or joint pain, edema, weight gain, shortness of breath, bruising, bleeding, severe indigestion, panting, or exacerbated angina.

Complementary therapies

Stress reduction and management help reduce blood pressure. Therefore, you should urge your patient to identify the stressors in his life and help him develop and implement methods to cope with them.

Relaxation techniques—exercises that reduce stress by decreasing sympathetic nervous system activity—can reduce blood pressure. In combination with drug therapy, these techniques have even been effectively used for patients with severe hypertension. Relaxation techniques include yoga, meditation, physical relaxation, and physical exercise.

Psychotherapy has also been used successfully as a method of lowering blood pressure. It helps patients deal with anxiety and constructively handle hostile and aggressive impulses. Counseling can also help increase patient compliance with the prescribed drug regimen.

Another therapy, biofeedback, uses specialized equipment to give the patient feedback about his bodily processes. The patient learns to achieve relaxation by self-regulating the autonomic nervous system. Biofeedback can decrease blood pressure; however, the long-term effects of biofeedback and its success in controlling hypertension aren't known.

Nursing considerations

Teach your patient about the various therapies that can work in conjunction with drug therapy and lifestyle modifications. If necessary, refer him to local community agencies for classes taught by qualified instructors. And advise him that patient participation in stress-reducing activities is an important adjunct to medical treatment.

9

HYPERTENSION

Acute Complications

In a hypertensive crisis, a patient's blood pressure rises to extreme levels. Typically, the patient who experiences such a crisis already knows he has hypertension. But the crisis is triggered by another condition, a drug, or the patient's noncompliance with his regimen for hypertension. Sometimes, however, a hypertensive crisis is the first signal that a patient has hypertension.

Actually, a patient may have one of two types of hypertensive crisis—an urgent hypertensive crisis, also called urgent hypertension, or an emergent hypertensive crisis, also called emergency hypertension. Urgent hypertension, as its name suggests, develops more slowly than emergency hypertension, and it isn't life threatening. But if untreated, urgent hypertension can lead to emergency hypertension, a condition that produces serious, fast-developing complications, of which the most common are encephalopathy and aortic dissection.

When a patient is in either type of hypertensive crisis, you'll need to assess him quickly and treat him appropriately to prevent or minimize organ damage. And after the crisis has passed, of course, you'll need to teach your patient how to prevent a future episode by complying with his prescribed regimen or taking other appropriate action.

Urgent hypertension

When a patient has a sustained diastolic blood pressure greater than 120 mm Hg but doesn't develop complications, he has urgent hypertension. This condition can develop quickly over several days or take as long as several weeks. It can result from noncompliance with the prescribed antihypertensive regimen, stress, or drugs that stimulate the sympathetic nervous system, such as cough and cold preparations and anesthetic agents.

Because blood pressure rises less rapidly with urgent hypertension than with emergency hypertension, the body adapts to the gradual increase in pressure. Thus, the organs tend to be spared.

Signs and symptoms

If your patient reports any warning signs of hypertension, suspect urgent hypertension. He may experience a mild headache in the occipital area that's more severe in the morning. He also may experience dizziness, light-headedness, numbness, weakness, and vision changes. These cerebrovascular signs and symptoms may result from hypertension alone or from hypertension and atherosclerosis. He also may report nosebleeds, which occur as a natural safety mechanism to relieve severe hypertension and prevent cerebral hemorrhage.

Your patient with urgent hypertension may experience chest pain, palpitations, dyspnea, paroxysmal nocturnal dyspnea, orthopnea, and edema. These cardiovascular signs and symptoms may develop when his hypertension results from coronary artery disease.

Renal signs and symptoms of urgent hypertension include nocturia, polyuria, hematuria, urinary tract infection, excessive urinary sediment, fatigue, weakness, and muscle cramps. However, these signs and symptoms also may result from kidney damage. If a patient has kidney damage, his condition has worsened from urgent hypertension to emergency hypertension.

Diagnostic tests

To distinguish urgent hypertension from emergency hypertension, a physician may order electrocardiography (ECG) and various blood, urine, and imaging tests (see *Hypertensive crisis: What the tests can tell*). If your patient has urgent hypertension, the tests will reveal no organ damage; however, they may indicate minor changes in cardiac, cerebrovascular, and renal function.

Treatment

The goal of treatment is to decrease blood pressure slowly over days or weeks. The gradual drop in blood pressure is intended to avoid systemic hypotension and rebound hypertension.

Typically, a physician prescribes one of the following oral antihypertensive drugs based on the patient's other medical problems:

- captopril—an angiotensin-converting enzyme (ACE) inhibitor that dilates the arteries and veins and lowers systemic vascular resistance
- clonidine—a centrally acting alpha-blocker that inhibits nerve impulses from the sympathetic nervous system, resulting in peripheral arteriole and vein dilation
- hydrochlorothiazide—a thiazide diuretic that increases water and sodium excretion
- metoprolol—a beta-blocker that prevents sympathetic nervous system stimulation
- minoxidil—a vasodilator that dilates arteries without affecting veins
- nifedipine—a calcium antagonist that dilates peripheral arterioles, resulting in decreased systemic vascular resistance.

Nursing considerations

Before starting antihypertensive drug therapy, obtain a baseline blood pressure reading from each arm. Then, administer the drug, as prescribed. Use caution when administering it so that your patient's blood pressure doesn't fall below the limit

of autoregulation. For example, assess your patient for dizziness and light-headedness. If they occur, withhold the drug and notify the physician.

Monitor a hospitalized patient's blood pressure every 1 to 2 hours after administering the first dose. And continue to monitor his blood pressure every 2 to 4 hours, even after it begins to stabilize. Teach an outpatient how to check his blood pressure and when to call the physician. Also, instruct him to check his blood pressure at least once a day until it's stable, and then to check it once a week.

Monitor your patient for adverse effects of the drug. As prescribed, administer an analgesic for headache and monitor its effectiveness.

Following the physician's guidelines, adjust the antihypertensive drug dosage as your patient's blood pressure drops to the target level. Also, assess your patient's cardiovascular, neurologic, retinal, and renal status after 1 to 4 weeks of drug therapy to evaluate its adverse and therapeutic effects.

Patient teaching

After your patient's urgent hypertension has subsided, instruct him to adhere to his antihypertensive drug regimen to reduce the risk of future episodes. Teach him the names of all his prescribed drugs and their dosages, expected effects, and adverse effects.

Warn your patient about orthostatic hypotension, a common adverse effect of antihypertensive drugs. Tell him to rise slowly from a sitting position to a standing position and to dangle his feet over the side of the bed for several minutes before getting up. If he becomes dizzy, he should sit or lie down until the feeling passes.

Tell your patient about lifestyle changes that can help prevent a recurrence of urgent hypertension. These changes include avoiding alcohol, stopping smoking, increasing his amount of exercise, doing different types of exercise, performing relaxation and other stress-reduction techniques, and following a low-fat, low-sodium diet. As appropriate, refer him to other health care professionals, such as a dietitian.

Make sure your patient knows the signs and symptoms of hypertension, including headache,

Hypertensive crisis: What the tests can tell

Tests	Findings	Implications
Blood tests		
Fasting glucose level	• > 120 mg/dl	• diabetes mellitus or other endocrine disorder, such as Cushing's syndrome
Blood urea nitrogen level	• elevated	• emergency hypertension
Cholesterol and triglyceride levels	• elevated	• atherosclerosis
Creatinine level	• elevated	• acute hypertensive nephropathy
Hemoglobin level and hematocrit	• elevated	• dehydration
	• severe anemia	• chronic renal disease
Potassium level	• decreased	• increased renin level
Sodium level	• decreased	• urgent hypertension or emergency hypertension
Urine tests		
24-hour catecholamine level	• elevated epinephrine or norepinephrine	• pheochromocytoma
Urinalysis	• granular or red cell casts or hematuria	• acute glomerulonephritis and renal-induced hypertension
	• proteinuria and low specific gravity	• renal impairment caused by hypertension
Electrocardiography and imaging tests		
Electrocardiography	• increased voltage in leads V_5 and V_6	• left ventricular hypertrophy
	• ST-segment depression and T-wave inversion	• repolarization abnormalities caused by endocardial fibrosis accompanying hypertrophy
Chest X-ray	• enlarged heart	• left ventricular hypertrophy
	• widened silhouette of thoracic aorta or widened mediastinum	• aortic dissection
Echocardiography	• increased thickness of left ventricle	• left ventricular hypertrophy
Renal ultrasonography and renal arteriography	• abnormal results	• renal disease or renal artery stenosis

dizziness, light-headedness, weakness, vision changes, and chest discomfort. Also, spell out the signs and symptoms of altered organ functioning, such as headache, dizziness, and weakness in cerebrovascular dysfunction; chest pain, palpitations, dyspnea, and peripheral edema in cardiovascular dysfunction; and nocturia, polyuria, and hematuria in renal dysfunction. Instruct the patient to promptly report such signs and symptoms to his physician.

Explain that hypertension can be dangerous even without obvious symptoms. Stress the importance of taking his antihypertensive drug even if he feels well. Tell him to report unpleasant adverse effects, such as beta-blocker–induced fatigue, nightmares, and sexual dysfunction, because the physician may be able to change the prescription.

Discuss the need to have his blood pressure evaluated frequently so that appropriate adjustments can be made in his drug regimen. Confirm that he knows the date and time of the follow-up appointment with his physician and, if appropriate, the date and time of diagnostic testing to evaluate organ function.

After discharge, your patient may need follow-up care by a home care nurse. Explain that the home care nurse will monitor his blood pressure daily for the first few days after therapy begins.

The home care nurse will perform a physical assessment to obtain baseline blood pressure readings. Then she'll monitor the patient's blood pressure and report values outside the limits prescribed by the physician.

The home care nurse will confirm that the patient has a follow-up appointment with his physician and ensure that he's making lifestyle changes, as needed. She'll also note whether he's taking his antihypertensive drugs as prescribed. If necessary, she'll teach him to take his blood pressure. And she'll remind him to report signs and symptoms of hypertension to his physician.

Emergency hypertension

Emergency hypertension is characterized by a sudden, sustained elevation of diastolic blood pressure. About 1% of patients diagnosed with hypertension experience this complication. It's most common in African-Americans ages 40 to 50 with primary hypertension.

The speed at which blood pressure rises during emergency hypertension causes more destruction than the elevated pressure itself. So treatment must be initiated as quickly as possible to prevent the complication from becoming life threatening.

If untreated, emergency hypertension results in significant damage to organs such as the heart, brain, kidneys, and eyes. It can also damage the peripheral vascular system. And a patient not treated for his emergency hypertension has a 90% risk of dying within 2 years of its onset. However, if the complication is treated swiftly, the chances of survival improve dramatically.

Many conditions can cause emergency hypertension to develop in a patient with primary hypertension (see *What causes emergency hypertension*). However, because increased public awareness of hypertension has resulted in improved blood pressure control, emergency hypertension is seen in fewer patients with primary hypertension.

If emergency hypertension occurs in a patient under age 30 or over age 60 who isn't known to have hypertension, consider a secondary cause. Many cases of emergency hypertension result from the use of phencyclidine, lysergic acid diethylamide, amphetamines, cocaine, or crack-cocaine.

Complications of emergency hypertension include acute pulmonary edema, chest pain, dissecting aortic aneurysm, hypertensive encephalopathy, renal failure, and intracerebral hemorrhage.

Pathophysiology

Usually, emergency hypertension is caused by arteriolar constriction that results from increased vascular reactivity, increased angiotensin II or norepinephrine levels, decreased circulating vasodilator levels, or decreased cholinergic tone. In many instances, these causes are interrelated.

When emergency hypertension results from increased levels of angiotensin II and other vasoactive substances, the kidneys produce large volumes of urine, resulting in sodium and water loss. Hypovolemia produces a further release of vasoactive substances, which, in turn, worsens the hypovolemia.

When systemic blood pressure rises, autoregulation in the organs triggers local vasoconstriction as the body attempts to maintain tissue perfusion. If the emergency hypertension goes untreated, overregulation can cause arteriolar spasm and decreased tissue perfusion.

Severely elevated systemic pressures may cause the autoregulatory mechanism to fail. This can decrease tissue perfusion, resulting in necrosis and vascular damage, which can lead to edema, hemorrhage, and infarction (see *What happens in emergency hypertension,* pages 166 and 167).

Ultimately, emergency hypertension leads to damage in the cardiovascular, cerebrovascular, and renal systems. It also can cause damage to the retina.

Cardiovascular complications include:
- left ventricular hypertrophy
- heart failure
- myocardial ischemia
- myocardial infarction (MI)
- aortic dissection.

Cerebrovascular complications include:
- encephalopathy
- cerebral edema
- aneurysm
- cerebrovascular accident (CVA).

Renal complications include:
- renal parenchymal damage
- nephrosclerosis
- renal failure.

Retinal damage can include:
- hemorrhage
- papilledema
- other retinal changes, such as vessel narrowing and tortuosity.

Health history

Because emergency hypertension requires immediate treatment, quickly obtain a complete health history to help determine the cause of the condition. Ask your patient about any family history of hypertension and underlying diseases, such as heart failure, aortic dissection, ischemic heart disease, and renal failure.

Determine if your patient has diabetes. If he does, keep in mind that you won't be able to tell whether renal or retinal damage results from diabetes or from emergency hypertension.

Ask which drugs he takes, including antihypertensive and other prescription, over-the-counter, and illicit drugs.

What causes emergency hypertension

Emergency hypertension can result from several disorders, drugs, and procedures. Be alert for any of the following in your patient's history.

Cardiovascular disorders
- acute left ventricular failure
- acute myocardial infarction
- dissecting aortic aneurysm
- unstable angina pectoris
- worsening of chronic hypertension

Neurologic disorders
- cerebrovascular accident
- head trauma
- hypertensive encephalopathy
- intracranial hemorrhage
- spinal cord disease
- subarachnoid hemorrhage

Renal disorders
- acute glomerulonephritis
- renal parenchymatous disease
- renovascular hypertension

Other disorders
- eclampsia
- necrotizing vasculitis
- pheochromocytoma
- preeclampsia
- scleroderma crisis
- vasculitis

Drugs
- amphetamines
- clonidine (withdrawal syndrome)
- cocaine
- lysergic acid diethylamide
- monoamine oxidase inhibitors taken with foods containing tyramine
- oral contraceptives
- phencyclidine
- sympathomimetic drugs

Medical and surgical procedures
- carotid artery manipulation
- coronary artery bypass surgery

What happens in emergency hypertension

Emergency hypertension begins with increased vascular reactivity, increased angiotensin II levels, increased norepinephrine levels, decreased circulating vasodilator levels, or decreased cholinergic tone. When one of these factors triggers arteriole constriction, it starts a vicious circle that keeps elevating blood pressure.

How emergency hypertension develops

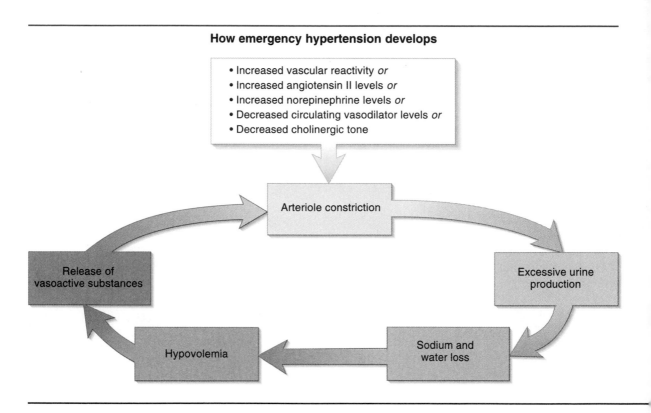

• Increased vascular reactivity *or*
• Increased angiotensin II levels *or*
• Increased norepinephrine levels *or*
• Decreased circulating vasodilator levels *or*
• Decreased cholinergic tone

Arteriole constriction

Excessive urine production

Release of vasoactive substances

Sodium and water loss

Hypovolemia

Signs and symptoms

The signs and symptoms of emergency hypertension include an abrupt rise in diastolic blood pressure to greater than 120 mm Hg and a persistent headache accompanied by nausea, vomiting, fatigue, dizziness, and restlessness. As with urgent hypertension, the headache usually affects the occipital region and is more intense in the morning. Other signs and symptoms include altered cognitive status, confusion, ataxia, irritability, drowsiness, increased fatigue, and decreased responsiveness.

Your patient may exhibit signs and symptoms of heart failure resulting from left ventricular dysfunction or volume retention caused by renal dysfunction. In a patient with heart failure, you may note these signs and symptoms:
• chest pain
• tachycardia
• S_3 and S_4 heart sounds
• ischemic ECG changes
• dizziness
• crackles
• shortness of breath
• dyspnea with exertion
• pedal edema with unequal or absent pulses
• jugular vein distention.

The body compensates for the increased blood pressure by causing further vasoconstriction to improve tissue perfusion. Eventually, autoregulation fails, and the resulting decreased perfusion can lead to edema, hemorrhage, or infarction.

How the body tries to compensate

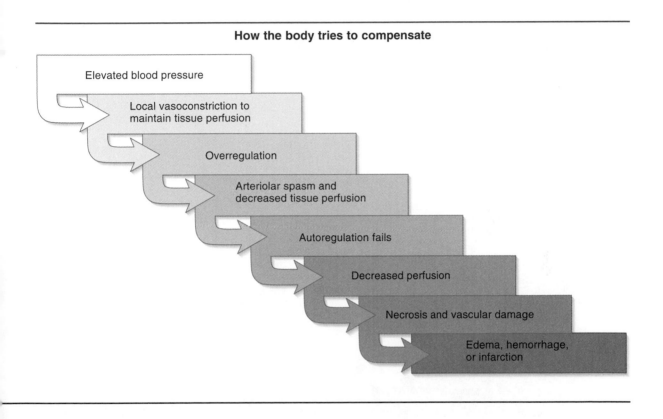

Elevated blood pressure

Local vasoconstriction to maintain tissue perfusion

Overregulation

Arteriolar spasm and decreased tissue perfusion

Autoregulation fails

Decreased perfusion

Necrosis and vascular damage

Edema, hemorrhage, or infarction

The neurologic signs and symptoms of emergency hypertension commonly mimic those of a CVA. However, the focal signs of a CVA that signal neurologic problems, such as speech difficulties and weakness on one side of the body, won't appear with emergency hypertension.

If emergency hypertension has affected your patient's renal system, he may have hematuria, nocturia, and elevated blood urea nitrogen (BUN) and creatinine levels. If he has retinal damage, he may experience vision changes, transient blurred vision, or temporary blindness. An ophthalmic examination may reveal signs of acute retinopathy, such as hemorrhages, exudates, and papilledema.

Diagnostic tests

A physician diagnoses emergency hypertension when the patient's diastolic blood pressure reaches 120 mm Hg or higher. Further diagnostic testing focuses on identifying organ damage, preventing it from becoming irreversible, and ruling out secondary causes of the hypertension.

As with urgent hypertension, the tests for emergency hypertension include chest X-ray, ECG, echocardiography, renal ultrasonography, renal arteriography, and various blood and urine tests. If the test results indicate organ damage, your patient will need immediate aggressive treatment.

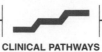

CLINICAL PATHWAYS

Caring for a patient with emergency hypertension

	History and physical examination	Diagnostic tests	Discharge planning	
Day 1	• history of hypertension with sudden rise of diastolic pressure above 120 mm Hg • history of heart failure, dissecting aortic aneurysm, ischemic heart disease, or renal failure • signs and symptoms, such as headache, dizziness, nausea, vomiting, and vision changes • continuous blood pressure monitoring to assess effectiveness of drug therapy • ophthalmic examination for hemorrhages, exudates, papilledema, vision changes, or acute retinopathy • hourly neurologic assessment for mental status changes • hourly cardiovascular assessment for evidence of heart failure • renal assessment every 2–4 hours for evidence of nocturia and hematuria	• none specific to hypertension • chest X-ray • electrocardiography (ECG) • electrolyte levels • blood glucose level • urinalysis • serum creatinine and blood urea nitrogen levels • hemoglobin level and hematocrit	• Determine cause of emergency hypertension. • Determine support systems.	
Day 2	• continuous blood pressure measurements • systems review every 2–4 hours	• echocardiography • urine catecholamine levels • renal ultrasonography and renal arteriography • studies, such as ECG and electrolyte levels	• Initiate review of hypertension management. • Consult dietitian.	
Day 3	• blood pressure measurements every 1–2 hours • systems review every 4–8 hours	• serum cholesterol and triglyceride levels • studies, such as ECG and electrolyte levels	• Participate in interdisciplinary review of patient's anticipated home needs. • Meet with patient and family to review home care management.	
Day 4	• blood pressure measurements every 4–8 hours • systems review each shift	• studies, such as ECG and electrolyte levels	• Schedule follow-up care. • Make referrals, as needed.	

Treatment

Understanding cerebral autoregulation provides a basis for treating a patient with emergency hypertension. Normally, cerebral autoregulation maintains a consistent blood flow to the brain and keeps cerebral perfusion pressure within normal limits despite variations in systemic arterial pressure. Normally, a mean arterial pressure (MAP) of 60 mm Hg is the lower limit at which cerebral autoregulation is effective. But in patients with chronic hypertension, the lower limit of effective autoregulation is a MAP of about 120 mm Hg. The upper limit of effective autoregula-

Drugs	Interventions	Patient teaching
• continuous sodium nitroprusside I.V. drip at 0.3–10 µg/kg/minute • other parenteral antihypertensives as indicated • supportive drug therapy for complications	• Maintain bed rest. • Change patient's position slowly. • Maintain safe environment, especially for neurologically impaired patient. • Maintain quiet environment. • Monitor fluid intake and output hourly. • Begin sodium and fluid restrictions, as prescribed.	• Explain all procedures and treatments to allay anxiety. • Orient patient to unit.
• continued titration of nitroprusside or other parenteral antihypertensive dosages according to blood pressure response • continued supportive drug therapy for complications	• Allow patient to sit in chair for short intervals. • Continue to maintain quiet environment. • Monitor fluid intake and output every 2–4 hours. • Maintain sodium and fluid restrictions, as prescribed.	• Explain causes and risks of hypertensive emergency and measures to take to prevent recurrence. • Assess knowledge of hypertensive management regimen.
• preparation for switch from parenteral to oral antihypertensive drugs when blood pressure has stabilized • continued supportive drug therapy for complications	• Prepare patient for transfer from intensive care unit to step-down unit or medical-surgical unit. • Maintain sodium and fluid restrictions, as prescribed.	• Provide instructions on prescribed antihypertensive drugs.
• continued oral antihypertensive therapy • continued supportive drug therapy for complications	• Maintain sodium and fluid restrictions, as prescribed.	• Provide instructions on dietary and other lifestyle changes for blood pressure control. • Ensure understanding of follow-up care.

tion is 160 mm Hg. And cerebral edema occurs when MAP is greater than 160 mm Hg.

So the goal of treatment for a patient with emergency hypertension is to lower MAP by 25% and to reduce diastolic blood pressure to 100 to 110 mm Hg over several hours, while maintaining cardiovascular, cerebral, retinal, and renal function (see *Caring for a patient with emergency hypertension*). If the blood pressure drops too low or too quickly, the central nervous system's autoregulatory mechanism may not be able to respond fast enough. Cerebral perfusion may become inadequate, and emergency hypertension may be compounded by cerebral ischemia or a CVA.

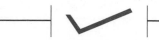

Administering sodium nitroprusside for emergency hypertension

Sodium nitroprusside—the most effective and potent treatment for emergency hypertension—has a fast onset and short duration of action, permitting minute-by-minute regulation and tight control. The drug relaxes the arteries and veins, decreases arterial and venous pressures, and decreases systemic vascular resistance.

Usually, a patient with emergency hypertension receives an I.V. infusion of 0.3 to 10 µg/kg/minute. Remember that administering sodium nitroprusside requires careful monitoring. When the drug is administered for more than 2 days, it can cause thiocyanate and cyanide toxicity in patients with hepatic and renal insufficiency.

Signs and symptoms of thiocyanate and cyanide toxicity include fatigue, nausea, anorexia, rash, headache, disorientation, and psychotic behavior. These signs and symptoms tend to occur when thiocyanate blood levels reach 60 mg/L. Thiocyanate levels above 200 mg/L can be life threatening.

Further treatment should focus on slowly reducing the patient's blood pressure to a normal level over several days to several weeks.

However, if your patient has an aortic dissection, take steps to lower his blood pressure as quickly as possible to stop the progressive dissection. But remember that aggressive antihypertensive therapy is contraindicated for a patient with a cerebral infarction, intracerebral hemorrhage, or subarachnoid hemorrhage because of the risk of cerebral hypoperfusion.

Drug therapy
Treatment usually begins in the emergency department and continues in the intensive care unit (ICU).

The vasodilator of choice for emergency hypertension is sodium nitroprusside administered at 0.3 to 10 µg/kg/minute (see *Administering sodium nitroprusside for emergency hypertension*). By working directly on the vessels, this drug immediately lowers the patient's blood pressure. After his blood pressure has been stabilized and he has begun taking an oral antihypertensive drug, sodium nitroprusside can be discontinued.

Several other antihypertensive drugs also are commonly used to treat emergency hypertension. Drugs with a short duration of action are preferred because hypotensive effects can be reversed quickly by reducing the dose or stopping the drug.

A physician prescribes the drug regimen based in part on the complications the patient has. Depending on the complication, a physician may need to prescribe a vasodilator other than nitroprusside (nitroglycerin, diazoxide, or hydralazine), an adrenergic blocker (phentolamine mesylate or labetalol), an ACE inhibitor (enalapril), a ganglionic blocker (trimethaphan), or a calcium channel blocker (nicardipine). See *Drug therapy for emergency hypertension and its complications.*

Nitroglycerin
Nitroglycerin dilates veins and arterioles. It also decreases preload and afterload.

To treat emergency hypertension, you'll administer nitroglycerin at a rate of 5 to 10 µg/minute and increase the rate by 5 µg/minute every 3 to 5 minutes, as ordered. If the patient's blood pressure doesn't decrease by the time he's receiving 20 µg/minute, increase the rate by 10 to 20 µg/minute, as prescribed, until the desired blood pressure is reached. Typically, nitroglycerin begins working in 5 minutes.

A patient receiving nitroglycerin may experience orthostatic hypotension, tachycardia, flushing, and headache. Also, he may develop a tolerance to the drug over time.

Diazoxide
Diazoxide dilates arteriolar smooth muscle. It's administered to treat emergency hypertension in doses of 50 to 150 mg every 5 minutes as an I.V. bolus or 7.5 to 30 mg/minute as an I.V. infusion. Diazoxide begins working 1 to 5 minutes after administration.

A patient receiving diazoxide may experience nausea, vomiting, abdominal discomfort, hyperglycemia, tachycardia, hypotension, sodium retention, fluid retention, and angina. Diazoxide may exacerbate an MI, heart failure, and an aortic dissection. It also may trigger cerebral ischemia.

MULTISYSTEM ALERT

Drug therapy for emergency hypertension and its complications

When choosing a drug to treat a patient with emergency hypertension, a physician must consider any complications caused by the condition.

Complication	Drugs that produce desirable effects	Drugs that produce undesirable effects
Unstable angina or acute myocardial infarction	• *calcium channel blockers and labetalol:* lower blood pressure and improve coronary perfusion • *nitrates:* decrease systemic vascular resistance and improve coronary perfusion	• *diazoxide and hydralazine:* increase myocardial oxygen demand and heart rate • *nitroprusside:* may divert blood flow from ischemic areas
Left ventricular failure	• *diuretics:* reduce pulmonary edema • *sodium nitroprusside:* reduces preload and afterload	• *beta-blockers:* reduce myocardial contractility • *diazoxide and hydralazine:* can trigger reflex tachycardia
Dissecting aortic aneurysm	• *sodium nitroprusside with a betablocker:* produces negative inotropic effect that reduces blood pressure rapidly • *trimethaphan:* reduces blood pressure and sharpness of pulse wave produced by ventricular contractions	• *diazoxide and hydralazine:* increase shearing stress and worsen the dissection
Renal failure	• *calcium channel blockers and labetalol:* don't compromise renal perfusion	• *sodium nitroprusside:* increases the risk of developing thiocyanate toxicity
Cerebral infarction or cerebral hemorrhage	• *sodium nitroprusside:* allows quick reversal of effects because of short duration of action	• *clonidine:* produces drowsiness and sedation, making neurologic evaluation difficult

When administering diazoxide, don't mix it with other drugs. Protect the drug from light. And inject it rapidly, in less than 30 seconds, to overcome protein binding.

During and after administration, monitor your patient's blood glucose level. Also, monitor him for sodium and fluid retention. If he's retaining sodium and fluid, he may need a diuretic.

Hydralazine
Typically, a physician prescribes hydralazine, which dilates arteriolar smooth muscle, for patients with renal insufficiency because it doesn't compromise renal function. For emergency hypertension, the drug usually is administered as an I.V. bolus of 5 to 20 mg. It begins to work in 5 to 20 minutes.

A patient receiving hydralazine may experience tachycardia, palpitations, headache, fluid retention, nasal congestion, gastrointestinal (GI) symptoms, angina, and an MI. If the patient shows signs and symptoms of lupus-like syndrome, discontinue the drug.

Phentolamine mesylate
A physician may prescribe phentolamine mesylate, an alpha-blocker, for emergency hypertension resulting from elevated catecholamine levels, clonidine withdrawal, and interactions between monoamine oxidase inhibitors and tyramine.

Phentolamine mesylate is administered as an I.V. bolus dose of 2.5 mg. You can also give a subsequent I.V. bolus of 5 mg, as ordered. Usually, the drug begins working within seconds.

A patient receiving phentolamine mesylate may experience tachycardia, dry mouth, flushing, nausea, vomiting, MI, arrhythmias, angina, and hypotension.

Labetalol

Labetalol, an alpha-blocker and beta-blocker, is prescribed for emergency hypertension resulting from elevated catecholamine levels and antihypertensive drug withdrawal. It's prescribed for patients with emergency hypertension who have had an MI and for those with an aortic dissection. It also is prescribed for emergency hypertension in patients with renal failure because the drug doesn't compromise renal perfusion.

For emergency hypertension, labetalol is administered as an I.V. infusion at a rate of 0.5 to 2 mg/minute or as an I.V. bolus in doses of 20 to 80 mg every 10 minutes. The maximum cumulative dose for the drug is 300 mg. Usually, it begins to work in 5 minutes.

A patient receiving labetalol may experience orthostatic hypotension, bronchospasm, nausea, vomiting, heart failure, and arrhythmias. When administering the drug, monitor the patient for heart failure and heart block.

Enalapril

Enalapril, which suppresses the renin-angiotensin-aldosterone system, is prescribed for emergency hypertension in I.V. doses of 0.625 to 1.25 mg over 5 minutes. You also can give it in subsequent 1.25 mg doses every 6 hours, as ordered. Usually, the drug begins to work in 5 to 15 minutes.

A patient receiving enalapril may experience proteinuria, renal failure, loss of taste, hyperkalemia, tachycardia, neutropenia, and agranulocytosis. If the patient has hypovolemia or is taking a diuretic when enalapril is administered, he also may experience excessive hypotension.

Trimethaphan

Trimethaphan blocks transmission in the autonomic ganglia, exerting a direct peripheral vasodilator effect. A physician prescribes it for patients who have emergency hypertension and acute aortic dissection because it reduces blood pressure and reduces the sharpness of the pulse wave produced by ventricular contractions.

Trimethaphan is administered I.V. in 500 mg doses diluted in 500 ml of dextrose 5% in water or 0.9% normal saline solution and infused at a rate of 0.5 to 5 mg/minute. Then, it's titrated until the desired blood pressure is reached. Usually, the drug begins to work in 1 to 2 minutes.

A patient receiving trimethaphan may experience intestinal and bladder paresis, blurred vision, dry mouth, respiratory arrest, orthostatic hypotension, paralytic ileus, and urticaria.

Nicardipine

Nicardipine, a calcium channel blocker, dilates the arterioles. It's prescribed for emergency hypertension in patients with renal failure because it doesn't compromise renal perfusion.

Nicardipine is administered by I.V. infusion at a rate of 5 to 15 mg/hour. Usually, it begins to work in 1 to 15 minutes.

A patient receiving nicardipine may experience tachycardia, nausea, vomiting, flushing, and headache. The drug is contraindicated in a patient who has aortic stenosis.

Nursing considerations

During treatment and then every hour thereafter, assess your patient's organ functions until his blood pressure stabilizes. Once his blood pressure is stable, continue your assessments every 4 hours. Immediately report any changes to the physician.

Assess your patient's cardiovascular system for signs and symptoms of heart failure, including increased heart rate, arrhythmias, chest pain, shortness of breath, jugular vein distention, edema, crackles, murmurs, and S_3 and S_4 heart sounds. Listen for carotid and abdominal bruits (see *How to auscultate for carotid bruits*). Also, palpate peripheral pulses to determine whether they are of equal strength.

Monitor your patient's neurologic status by determining his level of consciousness, pupil size, reaction to light, limb movement, and reactions to physical stimuli. To determine if his retinal function is impaired, ask him if he has experienced blurred vision, loss of vision, and any other vision changes.

Assess your patient's renal status by measuring fluid intake and output hourly. Oliguria is the first sign of renal impairment, so immediately report urine output of less than 30 ml per hour for 2 consecutive hours. Obtain a urinalysis for proteinuria and hematuria. Also, obtain laboratory studies to detect rising BUN and creatinine levels.

When administering a parenteral drug to initially reduce your patient's blood pressure, be sure to titrate the dosage based on the prescribed target pressure. Following the physician's guidelines, decrease the dosage or discontinue the drug if the patient's blood pressure drops below the target level.

While you titrate the dosage, monitor your patient's blood pressure and MAP every 1 to 5 minutes, using an intra-arterial line. Intra-arterial pressure monitoring reflects systemic vascular resistance, not just blood flow (see *Reading arterial waveforms,* page 174).

When using intra-arterial blood pressure monitoring, remember to immobilize the insertion site and keep it visible. If the line is ejected or the tubing becomes detached, the patient can quickly lose a great deal of blood.

Familiarize yourself with the tubing and stopcock positions. Set the alarm parameters 10 to 20 mm Hg above and below the patient's baseline blood pressure and leave the alarm on at all times.

To ensure accurate readings, level the transducer's air reference point at the phlebostatic axis—an imaginary line between the fourth intercostal space and the anteroposterior chest wall. And compare the arterial line pressure with the cuff pressure at least once per shift.

If direct blood pressure monitoring isn't available, use an automated blood pressure monitoring machine. Monitor blood pressure and MAP every 15 to 30 minutes after your patient's blood pressure stabilizes.

To prevent orthostatic hypotension, a common adverse effect of antihypertensive drugs, keep your patient on bed rest and help him change positions slowly. When his blood pressure stabilizes, administer an oral antihypertensive drug, as ordered, and monitor his blood pressure every 1 to 2 hours.

To relieve your patient's anxiety, explain all procedures, monitoring equipment, and unfamiliar sounds. Also, explain why he must remain in the ICU. Don't overwhelm him with too much in-

How to auscultate for carotid bruits

When auscultating for carotid bruits, hold the bell of the stethoscope over the carotid artery, as shown. Have your patient hold his breath during auscultation.

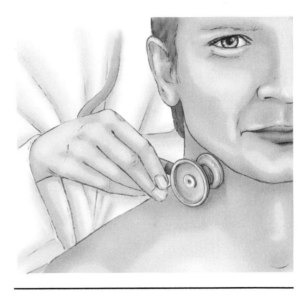

formation, but try to allay his fears by discussing his concerns and by making him as comfortable as possible.

Determine the extent of your patient's pain and the severity of his headaches. Provide analgesics and anxiolytics, as prescribed, and monitor their effectiveness. Maintain a quiet environment and, if possible, place your patient in a private room. Reassure him that efforts are being made to reduce his blood pressure.

Patient teaching

Assure your patient and his family that the prognosis is good after treatment for emergency hypertension. Reinforce the need for him to stay in the ICU to receive I.V. drugs and to have his blood pressure monitored continuously. And tell them that he'll be monitored con-

Reading arterial waveforms

Arterial waveforms reflect ventricular systole and diastole. These waveforms have four components: the anacrotic limb, the systolic peak, the dicrotic notch, and end diastole. Each represents a specific physiologic action.

The anacrotic limb appears as the aortic valve opens and blood is ejected from the ventricle into the aorta. The sharp rise in arterial pressure during ejection causes the systolic peak.

As blood flows into the peripheral vessels, arterial pressure drops, shown on the waveform as a downslope. As pressure continues to fall, the aortic valve closes, producing the dicrotic notch on the waveform.

Once the aortic valve closes, diastole starts. On the waveform, the lowest point of diastolic pressure is referred to as end diastole.

Any variation in an arterial waveform can signal a serious complication. For example, a diminished amplitude on inspiration may indicate a paradoxical pulse, which can result from cardiac tamponade or constrictive pericarditis.

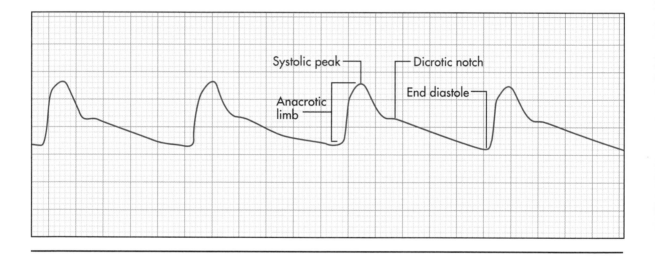

stantly to reduce the risk of long-term organ damage.

After the crisis, teach the patient how to manage his blood pressure and reduce the risk of future episodes of emergency hypertension. Start with a review of lifestyle modifications. Obtain any necessary referrals to other health care professionals, such as a home care nurse, dietitian, or psychologist. And refer the patient to appropriate community resources, support groups, and educational programs.

The physician probably will prescribe antihypertensive drugs to control the patient's blood pressure after he leaves the hospital. So teach your patient the following:
• name of each drug
• prescribed dosage
• relevant information about each drug, such as whether it should be taken with food
• therapeutic effect of each drug
• possible adverse effects of each drug
• possible interactions with other drugs.

Warn the patient not to stop taking his antihypertensive drugs. Reducing his dosage even slightly could cause his blood pressure to rise, provoking a recurrence of emergency hypertension. So explain that because hypertension rarely causes symptoms, he should continue to take his drugs as prescribed—even when he feels well. Instruct him to report unpleasant adverse effects, such as GI distress, lethargy, and sexual dysfunction, to the physician, who may be able to eliminate them by prescribing a different drug or dosage. Also, tell the patient not to take other drugs, including nonprescription drugs, without his physician's permission.

Determine whether your patient can pay for his drugs. If not, consult with your facility's social services department about resources to assist in paying for his treatment.

Although diagnostic testing is performed throughout an episode of emergency hypertension, the full effects of the trauma may not be evident for several days or weeks. Instruct your patient to report any increase or decrease in his urine output. Also, tell him to report urine that is bloody or tea colored or contains white mucous threads. Tell him to notify his physician if he experiences any changes in vision, including cloudiness, blurred vision, or temporary blindness.

Instruct your patient to report any changes in neurologic or cardiovascular function and teach him the signs and symptoms of impaired function. Neurologic changes may include increased drowsiness, fatigue, confusion, forgetfulness, and difficulty waking from sleep. Cardiovascular changes may include palpitations, chest pain, swelling of the legs and feet, decreased tolerance to exercise, shortness of breath, dyspnea on exertion, productive cough, and pink-tinged frothy sputum.

Before your patient is discharged, inform him that he'll need frequent blood pressure monitoring and physical examinations by his physician and that his drug dosage may have to be adjusted. Periodically, he also may be asked for urine and blood specimens for laboratory tests and may have to undergo diagnostic testing to monitor his organ functions. Confirm that he knows the date and time of his follow-up appointment with his physician.

Teach him and his family the basics of home blood pressure monitoring. If a home care nurse will be visiting him after discharge, let him know that she'll routinely monitor his blood pressure and review the readings he has recorded between her visits. She'll monitor his compliance, make sure he takes his antihypertensive drugs properly, reinforce and support his lifestyle modifications, and regularly assess his organ functioning. The home care nurse also will reevaluate his plan of care to determine whether its goals are being met (see *After emergency hypertension: What to tell the home care nurse*).

HOME CARE

After emergency hypertension: What to tell the home care nurse

When your patient is discharged after treatment for emergency hypertension, give this information to his home care nurse:
- systolic and diastolic blood pressures at the time of discharge
- blood pressure abnormalities to report to the patient's physician
- time of the last dose of each drug given in the hospital
- physical assessment findings upon discharge, including cardiovascular, neurologic, retinal, and renal findings
- a list of patient-education topics covered in the hospital and a note indicating which points may need reinforcement
- observations of interactions between the patient and his family
- an assessment of the patient's ability to handle stress and a list of coping mechanisms that worked and didn't work during his hospitalization.

Hypertensive encephalopathy

Hypertensive encephalopathy—profound cerebral edema that disrupts cerebral functioning and causes loss of consciousness—commonly results when a patient's diastolic blood pressure rises rapidly to more than 140 mm Hg. The condition is more common in hypertensive patients with renal dysfunction. But it also can occur when a patient who usually has normal blood pressure experiences an abrupt onset of hypertension. Without treatment, hypertensive encephalopathy can progress to coma and death.

Pathophysiology

Under normal conditions, autoregulation maintains a constant cerebral blood flow despite variations in MAP. When blood pressure rises sharply, the cerebral blood vessels constrict. When blood pressure drops quickly, they dilate to maintain consistent cerebral perfusion.

Hypertensive encephalopathy occurs when autoregulation fails to decrease cerebral blood flow during emergency hypertension. The breakdown in autoregulation leads to heightened vasospasm and vasoconstriction or increased cerebral blood flow. High hydrostatic pressures in the capillaries increase capillary permeability, allowing vascular fluid to leak into the interstitial spaces. This leakage leads to cerebral edema and increased intracranial pressure (ICP).

Signs and symptoms

The signs and symptoms of hypertensive encephalopathy result from a rapid increase in diastolic blood pressure to more than 140 mm Hg and the abrupt onset of hypertension in a patient with no history of hypertension or in one with well-controlled hypertension.

Initially, your patient may complain of a severe, generalized headache and restlessness. This may progress to nausea and projectile vomiting. His neurologic signs and symptoms may include confusion, drowsiness, stupor, and generalized tonic-clonic or focal seizures. Because the encephalopathy results from emergency hypertension, he also may exhibit signs of impaired cardiovascular and renal function, such as myocardial ischemia and a decreased glomerular filtration rate.

Retinal damage also can result from hypertensive encephalopathy. An ophthalmic examination may reveal retinal hemorrhages, exudates, and papilledema—a condition known as grade IV hypertensive retinopathy.

Diagnostic tests

Computed tomography (CT) and magnetic resonance imaging help rule out other causes of your patient's severe headache, such as a CVA. Imaging may reveal areas of hemorrhage ranging in size from pinpoint to massive.

A lumbar puncture is contraindicated because of the patient's high ICP. Introducing a needle into the central canal of his spinal cord would cause cerebrospinal fluid (CSF) to gush, and the sudden and dramatic decrease in CSF could force

delicate brain tissue to herniate into the spinal canal, resulting in immediate death.

Treatment

Usually, a physician prescribes an antihypertensive drug to rapidly reduce ICP and arterial blood pressure and to maintain diastolic blood pressure at about 100 mm Hg. The drugs used to treat hypertensive encephalopathy include vasodilators, beta-blockers, and osmotic diuretics. Most commonly, a physician prescribes the vasodilator nitroprusside. Vasodilators relax vascular smooth muscle, which reduces peripheral artery and vein dilation. Beta-blockers may be used to reduce vascular resistance.

The physician may prescribe mannitol, an osmotic diuretic, if the patient already shows signs and symptoms of cerebral edema. Although osmotic diuretics reduce ICP, they're contraindicated in patients with active cerebral bleeding. The adverse effects of osmotic diuretics—confusion, convulsions, dizziness, disorientation, headache, rebound increased ICP, and syncope—can mimic a worsening neurologic condition (see *Using mannitol to relieve intracranial pressure*).

Although rapidly reducing your patient's blood pressure will dramatically improve the symptoms of hypertensive encephalopathy, he'll require continued close monitoring in an ICU.

Nursing considerations

Monitor your patient's neurologic status frequently. Look for signs and symptoms of worsening neurologic deficits, such as mental status changes, agitation, weakness, unequal pupils, vomiting, and bradycardia. Each time, compare your findings with those of your previous assessment and immediately report any changes to the physician.

If you're administering mannitol, closely monitor your patient's intake and output to assess fluid balance and fluid loss. Include the mannitol as part of his intake.

Monitor his cardiovascular status by taking continuous blood pressure readings using an arterial line or an automatic sphygmomanometer. Be alert for potential cardiac decompensation, such as ectopy or heart block.

Assess the rhythm and depth of the patient's respirations, his respiratory rate, and any changes in his breathing pattern. Cheyne-Stokes respirations—episodes of apnea that last 10 to 60 seconds followed by a gradual increase in respiratory rate and depth—may result from brain stem herniation.

Closely monitor your patient's serum electrolyte levels, including his potassium, sodium, and chloride levels. Also, check his BUN, creatinine, and arterial blood gas (ABG) levels and blood pH. Obtain a complete blood count, as well.

Patient teaching

During the acute phase of your patient's condition, orient him and his family to the unit. Explain the treatment plan, including the diagnostic tests that will be performed.

Before discharge, explain the need for strict compliance with the prescribed antihypertensive drug regimen. Stress the importance of reducing risk factors that can exacerbate his hypertension. Be sure to describe the underlying disorder that led to his severely high blood pressure and subsequent hypertensive encephalopathy.

If your patient will be discharged to his home, the home care nurse should evaluate his compliance with the drug regimen and recommended lifestyle changes. She should monitor his blood pressure and be alert for the recurrence of neurologic deficits, such as localized weakness, agitation, confusion, blurred vision, dizziness, and lightheadedness.

A patient who has had hypertensive encephalopathy may need extensive rehabilitation. His home care nurse should oversee the rehabilitative therapies he'll need, such as exercise and physical therapy. And she should reevaluate his plan of care regularly to determine whether it remains realistic and whether the goals are being met.

Aortic dissection

Aortic dissection—a longitudinal tear of the aorta's medial layer by a column of blood—is a life-threatening emergency. About 70% of patients who develop an aortic dissection have hypertension. Most commonly, it develops as a complication of hypertension in men ages 50 and older. When the condition is untreated, a patient has a 50% risk of death in the first 48 hours.

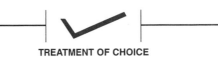

TREATMENT OF CHOICE

Using mannitol to relieve intracranial pressure

Mannitol—a potent osmotic diuretic used to relieve intracranial pressure—increases the osmolarity of glomerular filtrate, thereby raising the osmotic pressure of fluid in the renal tubules. The kidneys respond by decreasing water and electrolyte reabsorption and by increasing sodium and chloride excretion.

Usually, you'll administer mannitol I.V. in dosages of 1.5 to 2 g/kg in a 15%, 20%, or 25% solution over 30 to 60 minutes.

Complications
Mannitol can cause dizziness, headache, and convulsions—the very signs and symptoms it's meant to eliminate. And these signs and symptoms can mimic an acute neurologic event. The drug also increases sodium excretion, which can cause nausea and vomiting. And decreased sodium levels can trigger convulsions and coma.

Nursing considerations
Before administering mannitol, warm the bottle by placing it in hot water to dissolve any crystals that may have formed. Immediately before starting the infusion, shake the bottle vigorously to help eliminate the crystals and always use a filter in the I.V. tubing to prevent any remaining crystals from entering the bloodstream.

Warn the patient against changing position quickly. As his circulating volume decreases, he'll be at risk for orthostatic hypotension.

If possible, monitor his blood pressure directly using an intra-arterial line, as you administer the drug.

If you note urine retention when you're administering mannitol, palpate the patient's abdomen for a full bladder. A urinary drainage catheter probably will be in place during the treatment, so check for kinking or an obstruction.

Measure and record fluid intake and output. Include the mannitol infusion as intake.

Monitor your patient's electrolyte levels and check for hyponatremia in particular. Notify the physician of any signs or symptoms of hyponatremia, including nausea, vomiting, and seizures. Assess the patient's neurologic status and report any changes to the physician.

Pathophysiology

Although the exact causes of an aortic dissection aren't known, it may result when the elastic medial layer of the aorta becomes necrosed and a small tear develops in the intimal lining. The tear, called a dissecting aneurysm, allows blood to flow between the intimal and medial layers, creating a false lumen of flowing blood.

With each cardiac contraction, the systolic pulse increases pressure on the damaged area, widening the dissection. As it extends above and below the initial tear, the dissection may occlude major branches of the aorta, obstructing blood flow to the brain, abdominal organs, spinal cord, arms, and legs.

Weakened by the dissection, the aortic wall may rupture. And if the aortic root is involved, severe aortic regurgitation may occur.

Aortic dissections are classified as one of three types:
- Type I dissections affect the ascending aorta and the aortic arch. They extend into the abdominal aorta.
- Type II dissections affect only the ascending aorta.
- Type III dissections affect the aorta distal to the left subclavian artery. They extend into the thoracic or abdominal aorta.

Signs and symptoms

Typically, the first symptom of an aortic dissection is sudden, severe pain in the back, chest, or abdomen. Many patients describe this pain as "tearing" or "ripping." Your patient also may experience tachycardia, dyspnea, pallor, and sweating. If cerebral vessels are compromised because of aortic arch involvement, he also may have a decreased level of responsiveness, dizziness, and weakened or absent carotid and temporal pulses.

If the dissection affects the ascending aorta, your patient may experience left ventricular failure, orthopnea, and pulmonary edema. When checking his heart sounds, you may hear a diastolic murmur caused by aortic insufficiency. This type of murmur begins after S_2, continues through diastole, and ends before S_1. You also may hear an S_3 or S_4 gallop.

If the dissection affects the subclavian artery, blood pressure and pulses may differ widely between the left and right arms. A dissection of the descending aorta can alter perfusion to the legs. If the spinal cord becomes ischemic, a patient may show signs of impaired motor function.

Diagnostic tests

The diagnostic tests for aortic dissection include chest X-ray, ECG, and CT scan. When a patient has a dissecting aortic aneurysm, a chest X-ray may reveal a left pleural effusion. An ECG helps in differentiating aortic insufficiency from ascending aortic dilation and aortic dissection. A CT scan provides information on the location and severity of the dissection.

Treatment

Usually, treatment of a patient with an aortic dissection involves reducing his blood pressure and decreasing myocardial contractility to reduce the pulsatile force within the aorta. Typically, you'll administer trimethaphan or sodium nitroprusside to rapidly reduce blood pressure and propranolol to reduce myocardial contractility. Many patients with an aortic dissection need long-term drug therapy. A patient also may need blood transfusions and therapy to reduce pain and manage heart failure.

Patients with complications, such as heart failure, a leaking dissection, or an arterial occlusion, may need surgery. For patients with these complications, surgery usually is delayed as long as possible because the aorta is fragile and edematous. The delay allows time for the edema to clear, permits blood to clot in the false lumen, and allows healing to begin. However, a patient with a dissection of the ascending aorta has a high risk of rupture. Thus, surgery should be delayed only long enough to stabilize his condition.

Surgery for an aortic dissection involves removing the segment containing the tear and replacing it with a synthetic graft. The amount of aortic repair depends on the extent of the dissection. If the aortic root is affected, aortic valve repair or replacement may be necessary. Aortic valve replacement usually involves an aortic valve prosthesis, the caged-ball valve (see *Aortic valve replacement with a caged-ball valve*).

Nursing considerations

To prevent increases in blood pressure, maintain your patient on bed rest in a semi-Fowler's position and establish a quiet environment. Administer a continuous I.V. infusion of the prescribed antihypertensive drugs to reduce his blood pressure safely. To reduce his anxiety and pain, provide nursing measures. For example, answer the patient's questions, encourage him to discuss his fears, and administer anxiolytic and analgesic drugs, as prescribed.

Every 2 to 3 minutes, monitor your patient's blood pressure using an intra-arterial line and titrate his drug dosages to achieve the target blood pressure. Monitor his ECG and vital signs and palpate his peripheral pulses. Perform neurologic checks to assess cerebral perfusion.

If your patient undergoes surgery for an aortic dissection, focus on maintaining cardiopulmonary and renal function and graft patency postoperatively. Also, monitor him for complications of surgery, such as hemorrhage; hypovolemia; embolism; renal dysfunction; graft occlusion, dissection, or infection; and GI dysfunction.

To assess cardiopulmonary status, monitor the patient's vital signs, ECG, serum electrolyte levels, and ABG measurements. Assess all peripheral pulses and compare the pulse, warmth, and color in his arms. Monitor his pulmonary artery wedge pressure (PAWP) readings and treat him for low blood volume as needed. Perform neurologic checks every 30 to 60 minutes, assessing his level of consciousness, pupillary reaction to light, arm and leg movement, and hand grasps.

A thrombus or plaque that breaks loose from the aorta may impair renal perfusion. And hypotension can reduce renal perfusion. So monitor your patient's blood pressure and PAWP and administer fluids and volume expanders to ensure adequate renal perfusion. Monitor his urine output. Report an output of less than 30 ml per hour for 2 consecutive hours. Also, assess his BUN and creatinine levels for adequate renal function.

To assess graft patency, palpate the peripheral pulses distal to the graft. Immediately report to the surgeon a decreased or absent pulse accompanied by cool, mottled skin.

Protect graft patency by preventing hypotension and hypertension. Treat hypotension, which

Aortic valve replacement with a caged-ball valve

Usually, when a patient with aortic dissection undergoes aortic valve replacement, he receives a caged-ball valve. This valve is made up of three or four struts that house a silastic ball. Pressure changes in the heart make the ball move back and forth in its cage. As pressure falls, the ball moves back and closes the valve. When pressure rises, the ball moves forward and opens the valve, allowing blood to flow out to the aorta. As blood flows through the open valve, it moves laterally, away from the centrally located ball.

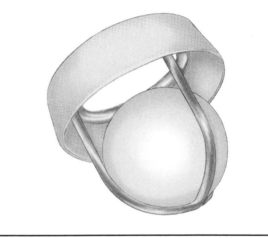

promotes thrombosis, with I.V. fluids, volume expanders, or blood products, as prescribed. Treat hypertension, which puts stress on the graft suture lines, with the prescribed diuretic or other antihypertensive drug.

To monitor your patient for graft infection, check his temperature and white blood cell count every 4 hours. Observe the operative site for signs of local infection, such as warmth, redness, edema, and purulent drainage. Administer a broad-spectrum antibiotic as ordered and encourage coughing and deep breathing.

In the postoperative period, your patient is at risk for paralytic ileus caused by bowel manipulation, anesthesia, pain medication, immobility, and bowel ischemia from thrombus or plaque formation in the mesenteric artery. Auscultate his abdomen for the return of bowel sounds. Monitor him for flatus and record his GI output. Turn and reposition him every 2 hours and encourage early ambulation.

Patient teaching

Before your patient undergoes surgery, explain the procedure and outline what he can expect in the ICU, including cardiac and PAWP monitoring and I.V. fluid administration. Also, tell him that he may need an arterial line, indwelling urinary catheter, and endotracheal tube.

After surgery, explain the need for frequent assessments of vital signs and peripheral pulses to determine the patency of the graft. Also, explain the need for early ambulation to prevent postoperative complications. Instruct the patient on coughing, deep breathing, and splinting the incision and have him perform return demonstrations.

Whether your patient had surgery or was successfully treated with drug therapy, he may be prescribed one or more antihypertensive drugs. Before he goes home, teach him the name of any prescribed drug, the dosage, and its therapeutic and adverse effects. Teach him how to take his blood pressure at home. And demonstrate how to take a pulse.

Discuss the signs and symptoms of a recurring dissection. Stress the pressing need for him to return to a health care facility if the signs and symptoms recur.

10

HYPERTENSION

Chronic Complications

Each year, more than 35,000 Americans die as a direct result of hypertension. And thousands more die as a result of chronic complications that affect the coronary arteries, aorta, heart, brain, kidneys, and eyes.

When atherosclerotic plaques form in the aorta and in the large and medium-sized arteries, the resulting hypertension can cause coronary artery disease (CAD) and peripheral vascular disease. When atherosclerosis of the carotid arteries causes hypertension, cerebral ischemia can result. And if hypertension causes the rupture of an aneurysm in a tiny cerebral artery, it can result in cerebral hemorrhage.

When hypertension affects the vessels of the eyes and kidneys, retinopathy and renal insufficiency may develop. When hypertension results in damage to the aorta's intimal lining, it can cause an aortic dissection.

If your patient has been diagnosed with hypertension, you'll need to teach him that he's at risk for developing these chronic complications. You'll also need to teach him how to prevent them and how to slow their progress.

Coronary artery disease

Hypertension is a major modifiable risk factor for CAD. Normally, CAD takes years to develop, but hypertension accelerates the atherosclerotic process that causes CAD. Then, as CAD progresses, the resulting arterial narrowing worsens the hypertension.

Pathophysiology

In CAD, atherosclerotic plaques collect in the arteries. These deposits, which line the intimal layer, consist of cholesterol and lipids.

In a person with hypertension, the elevated blood pressure causes high shear stress, speeding the atherosclerotic process. As a result, the artery's endothelial lining is injured. Then, platelets begin to accumulate at the site of the damage, resulting in a denuding injury (see *Understanding nondenuding and denuding injuries,* page 182).

Alternatively, hypertension can result when CAD causes a nondenuding injury. After the endothelium is damaged, low-density lipoproteins (LDLs) and growth factor from platelets stimulate smooth-muscle proliferation and arterial-wall thickening. Smooth-muscle cells proliferate, trapping lipids. Over time, the lipids calcify and irritate the endothelium, causing platelets to adhere and aggregate. Thrombin is generated, and fibrin and thrombi form.

With denuding and nondenuding injuries, the thickened walls of atherosclerotic arteries lose their elasticity. Thus, the heart must beat harder to pump blood through the restricted vessels, increasing blood pressure even more.

Signs and symptoms

Usually, CAD progresses for a long time without producing signs or symptoms. However, when CAD reduces blood flow so much that it no longer

Understanding nondenuding and denuding injuries

After the endothelium of an artery becomes damaged, hyperlipidemia can cause a nondenuding injury, resulting in hypertension, or hypertension can cause a denuding injury.

Artery with endothelial damage

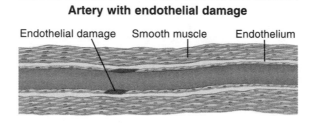

Endothelial damage   Smooth muscle   Endothelium

Nondenuding injury

In a patient who doesn't have hypertension, hyperlipidemia can cause a nondenuding injury, in which smooth muscle proliferates around the endothelial damage.

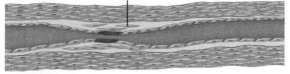

Smooth-muscle proliferation

Then collagen and elastic fibers accumulate.

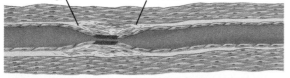

Collagen fibers   Elastic fibers

The lesion grows and becomes calcified, occluding the artery and increasing blood pressure.

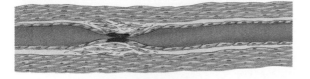

Denuding injury

In a patient with hypertension, the atherosclerotic process accelerates, causing a denuding injury, in which platelets accumulate and adhere around the damaged area.

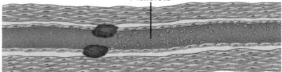

Platelets

Increased blood pressure increases platelet adherence, which leads to thrombus formation and occludes the artery.

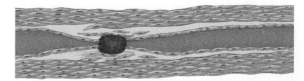

meets the body's need for oxygen, signs and symptoms appear. The most common symptom is angina. Typically, patients with CAD describe this pain as a feeling of tightness, squeezing, burning, or indigestion. The pain may radiate to the jaw, shoulders, arms, or back.

If your patient is experiencing angina, he also may develop nausea, anxiety, sweating, shortness of breath, or numbness of the arms. Angina rarely lasts longer than 15 minutes and usually can be relieved with rest or nitroglycerin.

Although most people with CAD feel pain, those with hypertension also may experience silent ischemia—cardiac ischemia without symptoms. As elevated blood pressure increases afterload, the heart must work harder to pump blood, resulting in an increased myocardial demand for oxygen. Because blockage and narrowing of the coronary arteries prevent the heightened oxygen demand from being met, ischemia develops. Over a prolonged period, the ischemia may trigger angina, or it may progress to a nontransmural myocardial infarction (MI).

A completely occluded coronary artery usually results in an MI. An acute MI causes severe chest pain that can't be relieved with rest or nitroglycerin. If your patient experiences heart failure, you may hear an S_3 heart sound or crackles.

Diagnostic tests

A physician uses certain tests to assess the patient's risk of CAD, others to indicate whether he has CAD, and still others to determine if he has had an MI—a serious complication of CAD.

Blood tests
A physician typically orders a serum lipid profile to assess the patient's risk of CAD. A total blood cholesterol level below 200 mg/dl indicates a relatively low risk of CAD. A level of 200 to 239 mg/dl indicates a moderate risk; one that exceeds 239 mg/dl indicates a serious risk of CAD.

High-density lipoprotein (HDL) and LDL cholesterol levels may help predict the risk of CAD more accurately than total cholesterol levels. An elevated LDL cholesterol level indicates an increased risk of CAD, but a high HDL cholesterol level indicates a lower risk.

A series of cardiac serum enzyme assays can confirm an MI. Total creatine kinase (CK) levels

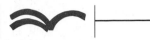

RESEARCH UPDATE

Using cardiac troponin levels to determine myocardial damage

Cardiac troponins, proteins that regulate calcium-dependent interactions between myosin and actin, facilitate cardiac contraction and relaxation. These proteins have three forms: troponin C, troponin I, and troponin T. Troponin C is found in cardiac and skeletal muscle cells. Troponin I and troponin T are specific to cardiac muscle.

Studies of patients with chest pain show that measurements of troponin I and troponin T levels may be more sensitive indicators of myocardial damage than measurements of creatine kinase levels. And measuring cardiac troponin blood levels may more specifically identify patients who are at increased risk for cardiac complications.

In one study of 1,404 patients with unstable angina and non–Q-wave myocardial infarctions (MIs), those with troponin I levels of 0.4 ng/ml or more had a significantly higher short-term risk of death.

In another study, patients with lower troponin T levels had improved long-term outcomes. During the first 4 months of follow-up, the risk of an MI or death increased with higher troponin T levels.

rise within 6 hours after the start of an MI and peak in 12 to 24 hours after cardiac tissue death. When cardiac tissue dies, CK-MB isoenzymes, which are found only in myocardial cells, enter the bloodstream. Measuring their level can help determine the amount of myocardial damage. Cardiac troponin levels may be better indicators of myocardial damage than CK levels (see *Using cardiac troponin levels to determine myocardial damage*).

The lactate dehydrogenase (LD) level also can indicate an MI. The blood's LD level rises 24 to 48 hours after an MI and peaks in 3 to 6 days. Two of the five isoenzymes that make up LD—LD_1 and LD_2—appear primarily in the heart. Normally, the LD_2 level is higher than the LD_1 level. But when a patient has had an MI, the LD_1 level is higher.

Other blood tests, such as aspartate aminotransferase and myoglobin protein levels, also may be used to detect an MI. However, because these tests are not specific for MI, they aren't commonly used. With an MI, the level of serum aspartate aminotransferase, formerly called serum glutamic-oxaloacetic transaminase, rises. But because serum aspartate aminotransferase doesn't contain any heart-specific isoenzymes, the results aren't definitive. The myoglobin protein level is highly sensitive to myocardial injury, but an elevated level doesn't confirm an MI because trauma, inflammation, and ischemia also can increase the myoglobin protein level.

Scans
A thallium scan—a radionuclide study—can help evaluate heart muscle perfusion. The examiner injects thallium I.V. and then performs the scan. Ischemic and infarcted areas of heart muscle don't take up the thallium, and they appear as cold spots on the scan. A physician may order an exercise stress test with a thallium scan to assess a patient for ischemia during exercise. Scans are performed at levels of peak exercise and 2 to 4 hours after exercise.

A physician may use dipyridamole thallium scanning for patients who are physically unable to exercise. Dipyridamole simulates exercise conditions by dilating the coronary arteries. Scans are performed when the arteries are dilated and 2 to 4 hours later.

In a multiple gated acquisition scan, another radionuclide scan, technetium is injected, and the heart is scanned during several cardiac cycles. This test analyzes ventricular wall motion and determines the ejection fraction—the amount of blood ejected from the ventricle during contraction. In a patient with CAD, this test shows abnormal movement and reduced performance of the left ventricular wall and a below-normal ejection fraction.

Electrocardiography and cardiac catheterization
Electrocardiography (ECG) can be used to detect an MI. However, an ECG reading may be normal unless your patient experiences chest pain at the time of the test. During chest pain, ST-segment elevation may appear on the ECG. T-wave inversion, ST-segment elevation, and abnormal Q waves may develop, suggesting an MI. If possible, a physician should compare the patient's current ECG with previous ECGs so that changes can be identified accurately. A physician also may order an exercise stress test to assess ischemic ECG changes and arrhythmias.

Cardiac catheterization, the most invasive method for diagnosing CAD, permits direct visualization of the coronary arteries, helping the physician determine the most appropriate therapy.

Treatment

Treating a patient with CAD involves risk-factor management, drug therapy, and, if needed, invasive procedures or surgery. Treatment has two goals: reducing myocardial oxygen demand and increasing oxygen supply.

Risk factor management
To slow the progression of CAD, a patient needs to change his lifestyle. Be sure you teach your patient the importance of taking the following measures:
• quitting smoking
• controlling his weight
• controlling his lipid levels
• reducing stress
• lowering his elevated blood pressure
• exercising.

Drug therapy
Aspirin, taken in doses of 80 to 325 mg every day or every other day, helps prevent an MI by inhibiting platelet aggregation. Typically, a physician will recommend this approach when CAD is first diagnosed or as soon as possible after an MI occurs. He also may prescribe dipyridamole, an antiplatelet drug, to prevent reinfarction and to manage chronic angina.

A physician may prescribe a beta-blocker to treat a patient with angina or with a history of MI. Of course, beta-blockers also may be used to treat hypertension. These drugs decrease myocardial oxygen consumption by reducing heart rate, blood pressure, and contractility. However, beta-blockers are contraindicated in patients with heart failure, hypotension, bradycardia, or asthma. These drugs also may mask hypoglycemic symptoms in a patient with Type 1 diabetes.

A physician may prescribe a calcium channel blocker to dilate the coronary arteries and reduce afterload, heart rate, and myocardial contractility, thus reducing myocardial oxygen demand. Calcium channel blockers also help lower blood pressure in hypertensive patients.

Nitroglycerin, a vasodilator, reduces venous return to the heart and increases coronary blood flow. It also decreases myocardial oxygen consumption, thus increasing the myocardial oxygen supply. Over time, a patient may develop a tolerance to nitrates. However, scheduling a short nitrate-free period, such as overnight, may lessen this tolerance.

Nitroglycerin in sublingual or spray form may be used to prevent or treat angina attacks. These forms of the drug act quickly and last for 20 to 45 minutes. Transdermal ointment may be used to treat unstable angina; its effects last 3 to 6 hours. Transdermal controlled-release patches deliver nitroglycerin steadily over 24 hours. Nitroglycerin also is available in a long-acting, oral form that's effective for up to 8 hours. This form is used to reduce angina attacks.

A physician may prescribe a thrombolytic drug—such as urokinase, anisoylated plasminogen-streptokinase activator complex, and tissue plasminogen activator (t-PA)—to treat coronary artery occlusions. These drugs are most effective when administered 1 to 4 hours after the onset of acute chest pain from a coronary artery occlusion. As the drugs dissolve thrombi, they restore blood flow. However, thrombolytic drugs are contraindicated in patients who have uncontrolled hypertension because they increase the risk of intracerebral bleeding if the hypertension results in a hemorrhagic stroke.

Streptokinase can be administered peripherally or directly into the coronary arteries. However, it has a long half-life and antigenic properties, which may trigger anaphylaxis. The drug t-PA works only at the site of the clot and doesn't cause generalized lysis. This drug has a short half-life and nonantigenic qualities; however, it's expensive.

Invasive procedures and surgery

In severe cases of CAD, a patient may require an invasive procedure to relieve the signs and symptoms of the disease. Several procedures use a balloon-tip coronary artery catheter to restore blood flow to blocked coronary arteries by enlarging the arterial lumen (see *Clearing coronary arteries,* page 186).

The most common of these procedures is percutaneous transluminal coronary angioplasty, which uses balloon inflation to clear arteries.

Other procedures include intra-coronary stenting, atherectomy, and laser angioplasty.

A physician performs these procedures in a cardiac catheterization laboratory using coronary angiography to evaluate progress. He inserts a femoral artery sheath and threads a catheter with a balloon, rotor blade, or laser tip through the aorta into the affected coronary vessel.

When the procedure is complete, the physician removes the catheter but leaves the sheath in place for up to 8 hours. Most patients receive a heparin infusion during the procedure and for several hours afterward. Some require long-term anticoagulant therapy.

If the procedure fails to remove the blockage, the patient usually will need coronary artery bypass grafting. This surgery involves bypassing the occluded artery with a graft from a saphenous vein or internal mammary artery. The graft is sutured to the aorta and anastomosed to the affected coronary artery.

Nursing considerations

If you're administering a thrombolytic drug, monitor your patient's heart rhythm for reperfusion arrhythmias. Also, monitor him for reocclusion of the coronary artery. Report any chest pain or ischemic changes on the ECG to the physician. To reduce the risk of reocclusion, begin heparin therapy after thrombolytic therapy, as prescribed, and monitor your patient's partial thromboplastin time (PTT). Titrate the heparin to maintain the PTT at twice the control time.

Assess the puncture site for bleeding and hematoma formation. Also, avoid performing venipunctures or a phlebotomy after injecting the thrombolytic drug. Assess the patient's pedal pulses distal to the puncture and immediately report any loss of pulse. Monitor his vital signs for signs of hemorrhage, such as hypotension and tachycardia. If you're administering streptokinase, observe the patient for an allergic reaction.

Coronary artery catheterization

If your patient is scheduled for coronary artery catheterization, explain the procedure to him and answer any questions. Tell him that he'll be awake during the procedure and that he may be asked to assist with catheter placement by taking deep breaths.

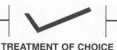

Clearing coronary arteries

A physician may clear an obstructed artery using one of several invasive procedures.

Percutaneous transluminal coronary angioplasty

In this procedure, a physician inserts a balloon-tip coronary artery catheter so that the balloon is positioned at the area of occlusion. The balloon is then inflated, and the plaque is pushed back against the vessel walls, opening the occlusion.

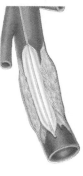

Intra-coronary stent placement

A physician uses a balloon-tip coronary artery catheter to open the occluded artery. Then, he inserts an intra-coronary stent to prevent the artery from closing.

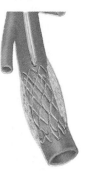

Atherectomy

A physician uses a catheter with a rotor blade to remove atherosclerotic plaque. The rotor blade slices the plaque, which is then collected in a chamber for removal.

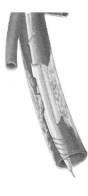

Laser angioplasty

A physician threads a laser catheter over a guide wire and sends brief pulses of energy to the blockage, vaporizing the plaque and creating a passageway for blood flow. In some cases, a balloon is then threaded over the catheter and through the passageway for angioplasty. If intimal tears, cracks, or flaps are created during angioplasty, laser energy can be used to fuse the intimal layers and create a smooth surface.

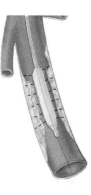

After the procedure, your patient's arterial and venous sheaths may remain in place for up to 8 hours, if he has received a thrombolytic drug. Connect the sheaths to a heparin flush setup to maintain patency. Ask the patient about back pain, a possible indication of retroperitoneal bleeding from the sheath site. And frequently check the insertion site for signs of bleeding.

Instruct your patient to keep the affected leg straight and to stay in bed with the head of the bed at a 45-degree angle or less.

After the sheaths have been removed and hemostasis has been achieved, a pressure dressing will be applied. Frequently assess the circulation of the affected leg by checking its warmth, color, and distal pulses. Watch your patient for signs and symptoms of complications, such as chest pain, shortness of breath, and changes in mental status. Monitor his heart rate and rhythm carefully. Also, monitor him for angina, which could be caused by coronary vasospasm or reocclusion. Report any unusual findings to the physician.

Coronary artery bypass grafting

If your patient is scheduled for coronary artery bypass grafting, thoroughly assess his cardiovascular status before the operation.

After the procedure, monitor your patient's hemodynamic status. Maintain the patency of his chest tube (or tubes) and assess tube drainage. Also, observe the surgical wound for signs and symptoms of infection and provide routine wound care as necessary.

Monitor the patient's fluid balance and serum electrolyte levels. Administer fluids, blood products, or vasoactive infusions, as ordered. Record his fluid intake and output and daily weights.

Monitor the patient's breath sounds and chest X-ray results for signs of atelectasis. Help him increase his activity level gradually, following the guidelines of his cardiac rehabilitation program.

Patient teaching

Help your patient identify his personal risk factors for CAD and develop a realistic risk-reduction plan. Encourage him to enroll in a cardiac rehabilitation program for exercise training to improve his cardiovascular endurance.

Depending on the severity of the patient's disease, tell him that he may need to exercise while attached to an ECG monitor to increase his confidence and allow detection of ischemia and arrhythmias. Tell him that as he progresses, he'll be instructed about home activities that he can perform safely. And explain that cardiac rehabilitation professionals will help determine when he can return to work and resume recreational activities.

A cardiac rehabilitation program also may have classes in which he can learn about the anatomy and physiology of the heart and the pathophysiology of CAD. The program may help him by offering psychosocial support as he makes lifestyle changes to manage his disease.

If your patient is scheduled for an invasive procedure, explain the procedure, the expected outcome, and the care he'll receive afterward. If a surgical procedure will involve a saphenous vein graft, make sure he understands that the physician will make an incision in his leg.

Before he's discharged, instruct your patient and his family about prescription drugs he must take at home. Make sure they know the proper administration route, whether oral, transdermal, or sublingual. In particular, ensure that the patient knows how to use sublingual nitroglycerin for angina. Discuss the therapeutic and adverse effects of each drug. Also, teach him the symptoms that warrant an immediate call to his physician.

Heart failure

Hypertension affects about 75% of all patients with heart failure, a condition in which the heart can't pump enough blood to meet the tissues' metabolic demands. Hypertension causes heart failure by increasing afterload. As a patient's hypertension becomes more severe, his risk of heart failure increases.

Pathophysiology

Hypertension causes the heart to pump blood against increased arterial pressure. Over time, this condition leads to left ventricular hypertrophy, as the heart tries to meet the body's metabolic needs despite the increased pressure. Eventually, the left ventricle develops poor contractility, which inhibits the heart's ability to efficiently empty the ventricle during contraction.

If untreated, left ventricular heart failure causes blood to back up in the pulmonary system. As the pulmonary vessels becomes congested, fluid accumulates in the interstitial spaces in the lungs. Then, the right ventricle must pump against a high pulmonary artery pressure, which eventually leads to right ventricular hypertrophy.

As the right ventricle becomes increasingly unable to empty efficiently during contraction, blood backs up in the venous system. This venous congestion from right ventricular heart failure results in peripheral edema, hepatomegaly, and splenomegaly.

As the complication progresses, the body tries to compensate for the failing heart by activating

Stages of heart failure

Typically, heart failure is categorized by its effect on a patient's activity.

Category	Effect on physical activity
Stage 1	• Disease doesn't limit physical activity. • Ordinary physical activity doesn't cause symptoms.
Stage 2	• Disease slightly limits physical activity. • No symptoms occur at rest. They may occur with ordinary physical activity.
Stage 3	• Disease more severely limits physical activity. • Patient usually is comfortable at rest, but symptoms occur with unusual physical activities, such as dancing or lawn mowing.
Stage 4	• Disease prohibits physical activity. • Symptoms occur during rest and activity.

compensatory mechanisms in the sympathetic nervous system and the renal system.

When the sympathetic nervous system is activated in response to reduced stroke volume and low cardiac output (CO), stimulated baroreceptors increase the release of epinephrine and norepinephrine. The release of these substances triggers vasoconstriction, increases the heart rate, and increases myocardial contractility in an attempt to raise CO. This activity, however, increases the body's demand for myocardial oxygen. The chambers of the heart dilate, and the heart muscle fibers stretch to increase their contractile force. Over time, dilation becomes the primary compensatory mechanism.

When the renal system is activated in response to decreased circulating volume, it stimulates the renin-angiotensin-aldosterone system, causing vasoconstriction and fluid retention. However, vasoconstriction, intended to increase renal blood flow, increases afterload, making the heart work harder.

If heart failure is untreated, the body's compensatory mechanisms eventually will fail to maintain cardiac function. The accelerated heart rate from sympathetic nervous system stimulation exacerbates the oxygen demands of the heart muscle and reduces the filling time of the coronary arteries, resulting in myocardial ischemia. As the kidneys try to increase their perfusion by retaining sodium and water, the extra fluid causes the ventricles to become even more distended, decreasing the force of myocardial contractions and causing further congestion.

Signs and symptoms

During low-level activity, the patient with left ventricular heart failure may experience fatigue, dyspnea, and tachypnea. He may have orthopnea when lying down and paroxysmal nocturnal dyspnea when he tries to sleep. He may have a dry, hacking, or moist cough and produce frothy sputum tinged with blood. His impaired oxygenation can cause restlessness, anxiety, confusion, and memory loss.

With left ventricular heart failure, diminished CO increases the heart rate. As a result, your patient's skin may be cold, clammy, and diaphoretic. He may have S_3 and S_4 heart sounds, alternating strong and weak pulses, and chest pain. Lung congestion may result in tachypnea and dyspnea. And you may hear crackles when auscultating the lungs.

Your patient with right ventricular heart failure may have signs of congestion of the organs and peripheral tissues, including peripheral and dependent edema, sudden weight gain, hepatomegaly, splenomegaly, neck vein distention, and ascites. He may report fatigue, anorexia, abdominal distention, and nausea.

In the early stages of the disease, symptoms may occur only when the patient exerts himself. But as heart failure worsens, they may occur while he rests. Patients with chronic heart failure are categorized by the degree to which their symptoms limit their activity (see *Stages of heart failure*).

Diagnostic tests

Diagnostic testing for heart failure includes chest X-ray, ECG, echocardiography, and pulmonary artery catheterization.

In a patient with heart failure, a chest X-ray reveals an enlarged heart, indicating hypertrophy or dilation. If the patient is in the early stages of heart failure, the chest X-ray may show congested pulmonary veins in the upper lobes. If he is in the late stages, the X-ray may show interstitial pulmonary edema and pulmonary effusion. If the patient has biventricular failure, the chest X-ray may show a pleural effusion.

A physician uses an ECG to detect left ventricular hypertrophy. This condition appears on the ECG as high voltage in leads V_5 and V_6 and deep S waves in leads V_1 and V_2. An ECG also detects signs of arrhythmias, such as irregular QRS complexes and F waves, and signs of myocardial ischemia, such as T-wave inversion and ST-segment elevation.

Used to measure the size of the heart chambers, echocardiography may reveal an enlarged right or left atrium. This test also is used to assess ventricular function and to detect ventricular hypertrophy. With normal ventricular function, echocardiography shows concentric contractility, a lack of abnormal wall movement, and a left ventricular ejection fraction of 55% to 60%. With left ventricular hypertrophy, it displays a ventricular wall thickness that exceeds 1.2 cm during diastole.

Pulmonary artery catheters are used to measure cardiac pressures. In right ventricular heart failure, the patient's right atrial pressure may be elevated. In left ventricular heart failure, his pulmonary artery pressure and pulmonary artery wedge pressure are elevated, and CO is reduced.

Treatment

Treatment of heart failure includes drug therapy and nutritional therapy. Typically, a physician prescribes an inotropic drug with a diuretic and an angiotensin-converting enzyme (ACE) inhibitor for a patient with normal renal function (see *Administering inotropic drugs for heart failure,* pages 190 and 191). The physician may prescribe a digitalis glycoside to increase the strength of cardiac contractions and slow the heart rate. When the ventricles can empty more completely, the blood volume remaining inside during diastole is reduced, and CO is increased.

For short-term management of heart failure, the physician may prescribe a beta-agonist to increase myocardial contractility. Or he may pre-

scribe a phosphodiesterase inhibitor to increase contractility. However, because they're such potent vasodilators, phosphodiesterase inhibitors are only administered parenterally in the intensive care unit (ICU).

Antihypertensive drugs

Many types of diuretics are used to mobilize edematous fluid, reduce pulmonary vein pressure, and reduce preload. Usually, a physician first prescribes a thiazide diuretic. These drugs reduce hypertension and treat edema by inhibiting sodium reabsorption in the distal renal tubule and promoting sodium and water excretion. If your patient has pulmonary edema, his physician also may prescribe morphine to reduce preload and control anxiety.

By acting on the loop of Henle, loop diuretics also promote sodium and water excretion. With thiazide or loop diuretics, the patient may need potassium supplements. Or the physician may prescribe potassium sparing diuretics if the patient is prone to hypokalemia.

The only class of drugs that improves survival in patients with heart failure, vasodilators reduce systemic vascular resistance and pulmonary and peripheral vein pressures, increase left ventricular stroke volume and CO, and enhance myocardial function by reducing myocardial oxygen demand. Sodium nitroprusside, a potent vasodilator, commonly is administered for acute heart failure.

A physician also may prescribe an ACE inhibitor. These drugs prevent the conversion of angiotensin I to angiotensin II, thus increasing CO by reducing systemic vascular resistance.

Sodium restriction

For a patient with heart failure caused by hypertension, a physician may prescribe a sodium-restricted diet. The degree of sodium restriction will depend on the severity of the heart failure and the success of the drug therapy. Usually, a patient with heart failure is limited to 2 grams of sodium per day. However, a patient with severe heart failure may be limited to 500 to 1,000 mg of sodium per day.

Nursing considerations

Monitor your patient's response to drug therapy by assessing his blood pressure, heart rate,

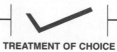

TREATMENT OF CHOICE

Administering inotropic drugs for heart failure

Drug	Dose	Drug interactions	Nursing considerations
Digoxin	• individualized according to age, renal function, and lean body weight • average loading dose over 24 hours: 0.75–1.25 mg orally; 0.5–1.0 mg I.V. • average daily dose: 0.125–0.5 mg orally; 0.125–0.25 mg I.V.	• hypokalemia with diuretics, amphotericin B, carbenicillin, ticarcillin, corticosteroids, and piperacillin • bradycardia with beta-blockers and antiarrhythmics • decreased digoxin level with thyroid agents • increased digoxin level with propantheline bromide, spironolactone, quinidine, verapamil, aminoglycosides, amiodarone, anticholinergics, and quinine	• Take pulse before administration. • Expect physician to order drug withheld if patient's pulse is < 60 beats per minute. • Administer drug orally with or without food. • Administer drug I.V. undiluted or 1 ml diluted with 4 ml sterile water, dextrose 5% in water (D_5W), or normal saline solution over 5 minutes with continuous cardiac monitoring. • Monitor patient for signs and symptoms of toxicity, such as loss of appetite, gastrointestinal discomfort, diarrhea, weakness, drowsiness, headache, blurred or yellow vision, rash, and depression.
Dobutamine	• 2.5–10 µg/kg/minute by continuous infusion	• arrhythmias with general anesthesia • arrhythmias and pressor effect with tricyclic antidepressants and monoamine oxidase (MAO) inhibitors • decreased dobutamine activity with beta-blockers • incompatible with sodium bicarbonate, acyclovir, aminophylline, bretylium, bumetanide, calcium chloride, calcium gluconate, cefamandole, cefazolin, cephalothin, diazepam, digoxin, furosemide, heparin, hydrocortisone, insulins, magnesium sulfate, penicillin, phenytoin, potassium phosphate, and ethacrynate sodium	• Inform patient that drug may cause anxiety. • Administer drug I.V., diluting each 250 mg in 250 ml D_5W or normal saline solution. • Gradually increase dose to achieve desired effect.
Dopamine	• for renal effect: 0.5–2 µg/kg/minute • for inotropic effect: 2–10 µg/kg/minute • for vasopressor effect: > 10 µg/kg/minute	• hypertensive crisis within 2 weeks of using MAO inhibitors, phenytoin, and barbiturates • hypertension with oxytocics • arrhythmias with general anesthesia • increased pressor effect with tricyclic antidepressants and MAO inhibitors • additive effects with diuretics • incompatible with acyclovir, amphotericin B, cephalothin, gentamicin, sodium bicarbonate, and alkaline solutions	• Treat hypovolemia before administration. • Administer drug carefully because extravasation may cause tissue sloughing and gangrene. • Gradually increase dose to achieve desired effect. • Monitor patient for oxygenation-perfusion deficit. • Monitor patient for headache, palpitations, tachycardia, hypertension, ectopic beats, angina, nausea, vomiting, and diarrhea.

Administering inotropic drugs for heart failure (continued)

Drug	Dose	Drug interactions	Nursing considerations
Epinephrine	• initial dose: 1 μg/ minute • subsequent dose: 1–4 μg/minute	• hypotension with methyldopa, mecamylamine, and reserpine • hypertension with MAO inhibitors and beta-blockers	• Note that drug is contraindicated in idiopathic hypertrophic subaortic stenosis, severe hypertension, and narrow-angle glaucoma. • Gradually increase dose to achieve desired effect. • Monitor patient for anxiety, nervousness, nausea, vomiting, urine retention, and palpitations.
Isoproterenol	• 0.5–10 μg/kg/ minute	• increased effects with other sympathomimetics • decreased effects with beta-blockers • incompatible with aminophylline, barbiturates, carbenicillin, diazepam, epinephrine, lidocaine, and sodium bicarbonate	• Dilute drug in normal saline solution or D₅W. • Gradually increase dose to achieve desired effect. • In cardiac emergency, give 1:5,000 undiluted, as ordered. • Monitor patient for tremors, anxiety, cardiac arrest, and bronchospasm.
Milrinone	• loading dose: 50 μg/kg I.V. over 10 minutes • maintenance dose: 0.375–0.75 μg/kg/ minute I.V.	• excessive hypotension with antihypertensives	• Give drug through Y-connector into running dextrose infusion. • Dilute drug with normal saline solution; don't dilute with dextrose for long-term infusion. • Gradually increase dose to achieve desired effect. • Monitor patient for thrombocytopenia and hepatotoxicity.
Amrinone	• loading dose: 0.75 mg/kg I.V. over 2 to 3 minutes, repeated every 30 minutes • maintenance dose: 5–10 μg/kg/minute	• excessive hypotension with antihypertensives • additive effect with digitalis glycosides • incompatible with furosemide and dextrose	• Mix drug only with normal saline solution for direct infusion. • Administer drug through a running dextrose infusion only if using a Y-connector. Never mix drug directly with dextrose because a chemical reaction will occur. • Gradually increase dose to achieve desired effect. • Note that a precipitate forms if drug comes into contact with furosemide. • Monitor patient for thrombocytopenia, nausea, vomiting, anorexia, arrhythmias, hepatotoxicity, and ascites.

heart sounds, ECG results, breath sounds, urine output, and weight. Also, assess him for peripheral edema.

If the physician prescribes a digitalis glycoside, take your patient's apical pulse for a full minute before administering the drug. Withhold the drug if his apical pulse is less than 60 beats per minute.

Begin digitalis glycoside therapy by administering a loading dose to achieve a therapeutic level more quickly. Monitor your patient's serum digoxin level to ensure that it remains in the therapeutic range of 1 to 2 ng/ml. Also, assess him for signs and symptoms of digitalis toxicity. If he's also receiving a thiazide or loop diuretic, monitor his serum potassium level; a low potassium level can lead to digitalis toxicity.

Other drugs that increase the risk of digitalis toxicity include beta-blockers, anticholinergics, quinidine, verapamil, nifedipine, amiodarone, and propafenone. If your patient is receiving one of these drugs during digitalis glycoside therapy, monitor his heart rate and rhythm and assess for signs of digitalis toxicity, such as gastrointestinal, neurologic, or vision disturbances. If he shows evidence of toxicity, discontinue the digitalis glycoside until his level returns to the therapeutic range.

During therapy, reduce your patient's cardiac workload by restricting his activity. Provide oxygen through a face mask or nasal cannula, as prescribed, to support his heart's oxygen demands. If necessary, measure his arterial blood gas (ABG) levels.

After therapy, refer your patient to an occupational therapist to learn how to conserve oxygen and energy while performing daily activities. The therapist also may help your patient modify his environment to reduce cardiac workload. For example, the therapist may suggest moving bedroom furniture to the first floor and obtaining a bedside commode.

Patient teaching

Teach your patient and his family about his prescribed drug therapy. If a digitalis glycoside has been prescribed, instruct him to take his pulse before taking the drug. Tell him to withhold the dose and call the physician if his pulse is lower than 60 beats per minute. Also, teach him the signs and symptoms of digitalis toxicity, such as nausea, vomiting, diarrhea, fatigue, vision changes, and an abnormally slow pulse rate; hypokalemia, such as weakness, fatigue, nausea, abdominal cramps, and diarrhea; and hyperkalemia, such as muscle tenderness, fatigue, and constipation. Tell your patient that he may need potassium supplements with diuretic and digitalis glycoside therapy.

If your patient is taking more than one drug, help him devise a dosage schedule that accommodates his lifestyle. For example, advise him to take twice-daily drugs before breakfast and din-

ner (if not contraindicated) to avoid forgetting to take them during a busy workday.

Instruct the patient to follow a low-sodium diet. If necessary, refer him to a dietitian. Tell him to record his daily weights in a log and to report a weight gain greater than 3 pounds over 2 days or less.

Tell him to conserve his energy by resting frequently. Explain how to obtain and use supplemental oxygen, if prescribed.

Most patients with heart failure benefit from a home care referral. If your patient will have a home care nurse, tell him that she'll perform a complete assessment of his cardiac and respiratory status. She'll answer questions about his drug regimen and monitor his compliance with the drug regimen and dietary restrictions. She'll also instruct him and his family about using home oxygen therapy, if prescribed.

Peripheral vascular disease

Peripheral vascular disease includes various abnormalities that affect the arteries and veins. Hypertension can accelerate the progression of these vascular abnormalities.

Pathophysiology

In chronic peripheral vascular disease, which is caused by atherosclerosis, a vessel's intimal and medial layers thicken gradually. If a patient has hypertension, his increased blood pressure also causes degenerative changes in the vessel's epithelial lining. Platelets begin to adhere to the irregular vessel walls, narrowing the vessel lumen and reducing blood flow to the legs. Usually, diabetic patients are affected in arteries below the knee; nondiabetic patients are affected in the femoral and popliteal arteries.

Eventually, the vessels become occluded. Without treatment, ischemia causes atrophy of the skin and underlying tissue. Eventually, gangrene may develop.

Signs and symptoms

In the early stages of peripheral vascular disease, your patient may experience pain in the calves or buttocks when walking, depending on the level of the vascular occlusion. Usually, this pain, called claudication, disappears with rest.

You can determine the level of the occlusion by palpating the patient's peripheral pulses. If his femoral pulse is diminished, he may have aortoiliac disease. If his popliteal pulse is absent, he may have a femoral-arterial occlusion.

As the disease progresses, the pain will increasingly limit a patient's activity, and he'll feel pain at rest. The pain may disrupt his sleep, causing him to sleep with his legs in a dependent position. However, this position further compromises venous return, decreasing blood flow to his legs.

He also may experience numbness and tingling caused by ischemic nerve tissue in the affected leg. The skin of the affected leg may be hairless, cold to the touch, dry, and shiny. The toenails may be hypertrophied. When the affected leg is elevated, it may be pale. When it's in a dependent position, it may be ruborous (deep red-blue-purple).

If peripheral vascular disease results in severe ischemia, painful ulcers may form at pressure sites and over bony prominences, such as the heel, ankle, toes, and dorsum of the foot. Usually, these ulcers are round, well circumscribed, and pale gray. They also may be covered with black eschar.

Diagnostic tests

Noninvasive tests for peripheral vascular disease include segmental pressure measurements, ankle-brachial indexes, and pulse volume recordings.

For a segmental pressure measurement, blood pressure cuffs are placed at four sites: on the thigh, directly above the knee, directly below the knee, and at the ankle. Then, the pressure cuffs are inflated sequentially. If systolic pressure decreases by 15% or more from one site to another, the patient may have significant lesions.

A physician may order an exercise stress test along with an ankle-brachial index and pulse volume recording. During the test, the patient exercises until he develops significant claudication. Then an ankle-brachial index is performed by taking systolic blood pressures in the ankle and arm simultaneously. Severe claudication causes a significant difference between the ankle and brachial blood pressures during low-level exercise.

Pulse volume recordings are obtained at the same time as the ankle-brachial index. If the pa-

tient has significant occlusions, the volume's amplitude will be reduced, and the height of its contour will be decreased.

Two invasive diagnostic tests, color flow Doppler ultrasonography and angiography, also can detect peripheral vascular disease. These procedures are performed to pinpoint the area of the lesion when surgery or angioplasty is planned. Color flow Doppler ultrasonography allows direct visualization of the major vessels and blood flow. Angiography provides information on the location and extent of the atherosclerotic disease.

Treatment

The treatment of peripheral vascular disease may include drug therapy, surgery, or both. If your patient has peripheral artery occlusive disease, the physician may prescribe pentoxifylline, which is the only effective drug for treating the condition. Pentoxifylline increases erythrocyte flexibility and reduces blood viscosity, thus increasing the oxygenated blood supply to the ischemic muscle.

The physician may prescribe an antihypertensive drug to control your patient's blood pressure. If your patient undergoes arterial bypass surgery for peripheral vascular disease, his physician also may prescribe aspirin and warfarin to maintain graft patency.

To treat peripheral vascular disease, a surgeon may perform patch graft angioplasty. In this procedure, the surgeon opens the occluded artery and removes the atherosclerotic plaque. Then he places a patch over the opening to widen the vessel lumen.

If your patient has atherosclerotic disease of the iliac and femoral arteries, he may need percutaneous transluminal angioplasty. In conjunction with angioplasty, the surgeon may use an atherectomy catheter to slice or pulverize the plaque. Or he may use laser treatment to remove plaque with thermal or acoustic energy. After the plaque has been removed, the surgeon may insert intravascular stents to prevent restenosis.

Usually, a patient with claudication at rest has more severe ischemia that results from occlusions at two or more levels. A patient with such pain may require angiographic evaluation and arterial bypass surgery.

A surgeon also may use bypass grafting to improve ulcer healing by increasing blood flow to the affected area. However, if infection occurs in an ischemic leg with an ulcer that won't heal, amputation may be required.

Nursing considerations

If your patient is receiving drug therapy, monitor the effects of the prescribed drugs. Assess the neurovascular status of his legs and report any deterioration in circulation.

Place lamb's wool between the patient's toes to prevent pressure necrosis. If he has ulcers, provide wound care as needed. Assess the ulcer for signs and symptoms of infection. Cover the ulcer with a dry sterile dressing, topical antibiotic, or other wound care product, as ordered.

If your patient has had surgery for peripheral vascular disease, check his leg for color, temperature, sensation, movement, and pulses during the immediate postoperative period. Report any loss of pulse immediately. Observe the incision site for redness, swelling, and drainage.

Turn and reposition your patient every 2 hours. Tell him to not cross his legs and to avoid severe hip or knee flexion. To aid circulation, add a footboard to the bed, use a sheepskin under his legs, or place him on an air, pressure, or other special mattress.

If the patient has undergone percutaneous transluminal angioplasty or another form of surgical catheterization, assess the site for bleeding, edema, ecchymosis, and hematoma. Monitor his peripheral pulses every 15 to 30 minutes for the first hour, every hour for the next 4 hours, and then once every 4 hours after that. Assess his leg for sudden changes in color and temperature. Also, monitor him for muscle cramping, pain at rest, and changes in motor and sensory function. Administer heparin, monitor his PTT, and adjust the infusion rate, as needed.

Patient teaching

Teach your patient how to promote circulation. Help him devise a progressive exercise program to develop collateral circulation and enhance venous return. Instruct him to stop exercising if he feels pain. Also, tell him to inspect his feet daily for color changes, mottling, scabs, skin texture changes, skin breakdown, and hair growth changes.

Advise the patient to change positions frequently to avoid blood pooling in the feet. Teach him how to promote perfusion by keeping his legs and feet warm and by avoiding vasoconstrictive substances, such as caffeine and nicotine. Tell him that wearing tight, restrictive clothing on the legs can hinder blood flow.

If the physician has prescribed an anticoagulant, review its therapeutic effect, dosage, and adverse effects with your patient. Tell him that he'll have to undergo frequent blood tests that monitor the drug's effectiveness.

If your patient will have a home care nurse, tell him that she'll assess his legs and feet and evaluate any changes. She'll also evaluate wounds and incisions, provide wound care, and assess susceptible areas for infection. She'll reinforce proper foot care and teach him to perform self-care. And she may observe him as he sits and rests so that she can recommend better positions for sitting and for elevating his legs.

Cerebrovascular disease

Cerebrovascular disease includes complications resulting from an inadequate blood supply to the brain, such as a cerebrovascular accident (CVA) and a transient ischemic attack (TIA).

A CVA, the most common form of cerebrovascular disease, results from an interruption of the cerebral blood supply caused by cerebral artery occlusion or rupture. Prolonged interruption of the blood supply leads to permanent damage in the affected area of the brain.

A TIA results from momentary or temporary interruption of the blood supply, which causes reversible neurologic deficits.

Pathophysiology

Hypertension can complicate cerebrovascular disease in a couple of ways. If hypertension causes prolonged elevated blood pressure in the cerebral arteries, the vessels may weaken, increasing the risk of rupture and hemorrhage. Hypertension also accelerates the formation of atherosclerotic plaque within cerebral vessels. The resulting formation of thrombi and emboli increases the risk of TIAs.

Hemorrhage

If hypertension causes prolonged elevated pressure in a cerebral artery already damaged by atherosclerosis, the artery can rupture, causing bleeding into the brain tissue. Blood flowing into the brain tissue forms a mass, displacing the surrounding structures.

With hypertension, the increased force of the blood flow hinders clot formation. The bleeding in the cranium leads to increased intracranial pressure (ICP) and further displacement of cranial structures. Major cerebral hemorrhages can lead to midline displacement, brain stem herniation, coma, and death.

Thrombi

Thrombi—the most common cause of cerebral injury—form from platelets and fibrin that collect on vessel walls. If atherosclerosis narrows the cerebral vessels, a thrombus may form in the narrowed section, occluding the vessel. The resulting ischemia can cause cerebral edema in the occluded area.

Emboli

Emboli—segments of atherosclerotic plaques, fat, or other debris in the bloodstream—typically originate in vessels outside of the brain. An embolus travels through the arterial system until it reaches a vessel too small for it to pass through, causing an embolism. If an embolism in a cerebral vessel is small, it may cause a TIA.

Signs and symptoms

The signs and symptoms of cerebrovascular disease depend on the location of the hemorrhage, thrombus, or embolus and the extent of cerebral tissue affected. General signs and symptoms of a hemorrhagic or ischemic event include motor dysfunction, such as hemiplegia and hemiparesis.

Early in a CVA, the patient may experience flaccid paralysis, followed by increased muscle tone and spasticity. He may lose his gag reflex and ability to cough. He may have communication deficits, such as dysphagia, receptive or expressive aphasia, dysarthria, and apraxia. He also may develop spatial and perceptual deficits, such as the loss of half of his visual field (homonymous hemianopia) and the inability to recognize an object (agnosia).

Other signs and symptoms of a CVA include vomiting, seizures, fever, ECG abnormalities, confusion that leads to a complete loss of consciousness, labored or irregular respirations, apneic periods, increased blood pressure, and bowel and bladder incontinence.

Signs and symptoms specific to a hemorrhagic CVA include abrupt onset of a severe headache, nuchal rigidity, and rapid onset of complete hemiplegia. As the hematoma enlarges, the patient's neurologic deficits worsen from gradual loss of consciousness to coma.

Signs and symptoms of a thrombotic CVA follow the "stroke in evolution" pattern and include the progressive deterioration of motor and sensory function, slow deterioration of speech, and lethargy. These signs and symptoms peak when edema develops, usually about 72 hours after the onset of the thrombotic event.

For a patient with an embolic CVA, signs and symptoms include a sudden onset of motor and sensory deficits, deteriorated speech, and headache on the side of the head where the embolism is occurring. If the embolus breaks into smaller pieces and the occlusion resolves, these signs and symptoms may dissipate.

Diagnostic tests

The diagnostic tests used to detect cerebrovascular disease include computed tomography (CT) scans, magnetic resonance imaging (MRI), cerebral angiography, and digital subtraction angiography.

By using a contrast medium to enhance the view of cerebral vessels, a CT scan helps determine whether a patient's neurologic changes resulted from an ischemic or hemorrhagic CVA. In an ischemic CVA, the CT scan will show areas of decreased absorption or density. In a hemorrhagic CVA, it will show areas of increased absorption or density. If the patient has had an ischemic CVA, a CT scan can help determine the size and location of a thrombus or embolus. A CT scan also can be used to monitor the effects of a patient's treatment.

If the patient has experienced a hemorrhagic CVA, the physician may order an MRI to precisely locate the lesion.

Cerebral angiography helps identify the location of a hemorrhagic or ischemic CVA. This test

Treating an ischemic cerebrovascular accident

Each year, nearly 500,000 people in the United States experience a cerebrovascular accident (CVA), making it the leading cause of adult disability. But for those who have an ischemic CVA, recombinant tissue plasminogen activating factor (t-PA) may reduce the risk of long-term disability. In one study, t-PA given up to 3 hours after the onset of an ischemic CVA increased by 30% the likelihood of a patient having little or no disability 3 months later.

However, t-PA increases the risk of severe bleeding, so before prescribing the drug, a physician must determine that the patient hasn't suffered a hemorrhagic CVA. A physician must also consider these contraindications:
• signs and symptoms of a CVA that improve rapidly
• a seizure during the onset of signs and symptoms
• pregnancy or lactation
• oral coagulant use
• a platelet count less than 100,000/mm³, a prothrombin time greater than 15 seconds,

and, if heparin has been administered within 24 hours, an elevated partial thromboplastin time
• a blood glucose level greater than 400 mg/dl or less than 50 mg/dl
• a lumbar puncture or arterial puncture at a noncompressible site within a week
• major surgery or serious trauma at a site other than the central nervous system within 2 weeks
• gastrointestinal or genitourinary bleeding within 3 weeks
• serious head trauma within 3 months
• intracerebral hemorrhage from a cause that's likely to recur.

Before prescribing t-PA, a physician must rule out conditions that mimic a CVA, such as severe hypoglycemia, subarachnoid hemorrhage, and postictal paralysis. Also, a computed tomography (CT) scan of the head must be performed to rule out intracerebral bleeding. Facilities that can't perform a CT scan can't offer t-PA therapy.

---

also helps determine the extent of damage to the surrounding cerebral tissue, while allowing direct visualization of the cerebral vascular system. However, cerebral angiography may induce a cerebral embolism, cerebral hemorrhage, or spasm.

Digital subtraction angiography commonly is used with cerebral angiography to better visualize the cerebral arteries by computerized fluoroscopy.

Treatment

Treatment of a patient who has had a cerebrovascular event may involve drug therapy and surgery.

If your hypertensive patient has experienced an ischemic or hemorrhagic CVA, the physician may prescribe an antihypertensive drug to lower his blood pressure. However, if elevated ICP results from a hemorrhagic CVA, his blood pressure

shouldn't be reduced too quickly or too much.

The physician may prescribe heparin I.V. to treat TIAs and ischemic CVAs, but not to treat hemorrhagic CVAs because it increases the risk of bleeding. If heparin is administered for a TIA or an ischemic CVA, titrate the drug to maintain the PTT at about twice the normal level. Once your patient's PTT has reached this therapeutic level, the physician may prescribe warfarin, which is taken orally. Typically, heparin therapy continues until the warfarin brings the prothrombin time to a therapeutic level.

If the patient has experienced an ischemic CVA, the physician may prescribe recombinant t-PA to disintegrate the thrombus or embolus that's causing the occlusion (see *Treating an ischemic cerebrovascular accident*).

A physician also may prescribe a drug that prevents platelet aggregation, such as aspirin, dipyridamole, or ticlopidine hydrochloride, to prevent thrombus and embolus formation and to treat an ischemic CVA.

After the patient has been stabilized, the physician may use drug therapy to minimize disability. Typically, he'll prescribe mannitol I.V. to reduce cerebral edema. This drug draws fluid out of the extravascular space and into the vascular system.

If the patient has a large hematoma displacing a considerable amount of surrounding tissue or if drug therapy fails to lower his elevated ICP, he may require a craniotomy to remove the hematoma and relieve pressure.

A surgeon may perform an endarterectomy to reduce the risk of future TIAs or a CVA. This procedure removes atherosclerotic plaque that's obstructing blood flow to the brain. Commonly, endarterectomies are performed on the common carotid bifurcation and the arch of the aorta.

If the surgeon can't remove the obstruction causing an ischemic CVA, he may perform an extracranial-intracranial bypass. This procedure involves bypassing the intracranial artery just beyond the obstruction with an extracranial artery, thus restoring blood flow.

Nursing considerations

Nursing management of your patient with an acute CVA includes maximizing cerebral perfusion, improving cardiopulmonary function, and preventing further motor and sensory deterioration.

Monitor your patient's cerebral perfusion by assessing his neurologic status, including level of consciousness, pupil size and reaction to light, motor response, and vital signs. Report any changes that indicate deteriorating neurologic status to the physician immediately.

Keep the head of the patient's bed at a 30-degree angle. Instruct him to avoid extreme neck and hip flexion. Take seizure precautions by padding the bed's side rails and leaving suction equipment at the bedside.

If t-PA is prescribed, administer the drug, as ordered. The usual dosage is 0.9 mg/kg, initiated by 10% of that amount given as a bolus. The remainder of the drug is infused over 10 minutes. After the drug has been started, closely monitor your patient's blood pressure. If his systolic pressure exceeds 185 mm Hg or his diastolic pressure exceeds 110 mm Hg, report the increased blood pressure immediately.

After your patient has received t-PA, monitor him closely for signs of internal bleeding, including hematuria, hematemesis, epistaxis, and ecchymosis. Also, be alert for signs of a mild reaction to the drug, such as fever, rash, itching, or chills.

Monitor the patient's hemoglobin level and coagulation parameters. Post a sign warning staff not to give him injections and not to take his temperature rectally. If minor bleeding develops at local sites, hold pressure on the site for at least 30 seconds. If an arterial puncture must be performed, hold pressure on the site for 30 minutes, then apply a pressure dressing.

If heparin is prescribed, check your patient's PTT and titrate the drip according to your institution's protocol. Assess him for the signs and symptoms of hemorrhage and avoid any trauma that might cause bleeding, such as intramuscular injections. If an antihypertensive drug is prescribed, monitor your patient's blood pressure frequently to keep it within the target range.

Administer mannitol I.V., if ordered. Monitor your patient for adverse effects, including pulmonary congestion, angina, headache, blurred vision, and fever.

If your patient has had surgery, monitor him for the early signs and symptoms of ICP. If he exhibits any signs or symptoms of this complication, notify the physician immediately. Assist with hyperventilating the patient, as ordered (see *Monitoring your patient for increased intracranial pressure,* page 198).

If the physician prescribes a loop diuretic, administer the drug, as ordered, and monitor your patient's electrolyte levels. If the physician prescribes a neuromuscular blocker and sedative to quiet the patient's physical activity, monitor his mechanical ventilation and sedation level.

If the physician orders an ICP monitor, check your patient's ventriculostomy drainage and open or close the drain based on ICP readings. Also, calculate his cerebral perfusion pressure by subtracting his ICP from his mean arterial pressure. Cerebral perfusion pressure is a rough index of cerebral blood flow and usually should be between 70 and 100 mm Hg.

Monitor your patient's cardiopulmonary function by checking his fluid intake and output, vital signs, breath sounds, and breathing patterns. Maintain fluid restrictions, as needed. Because stress increases the production of antidiuretic

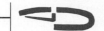

Monitoring your patient for increased intracranial pressure

Increased intracranial pressure, a serious complication of hypertensive cerebrovascular disease, can affect your patient's level of consciousness, pupillary responses, motor and sensory functions, and vital signs.

Left untreated, this condition results in coma, brain stem herniation, and death. The earlier you recognize the signs and symptoms of this dangerous condition and intervene, the better your patient's chances of recovery. By the time late signs and symptoms appear, interventions may not prevent irreversible damage.

Early signs and symptoms
- subtle changes in orientation
- restlessness
- sudden quietness
- unilateral pupillary constriction or dilation, sluggish bilateral pupillary reaction, and unequal pupil size
- sudden weakness
- motor changes on the contralateral side
- positive pronator drift
- intermittent increases in blood pressure

Late signs and symptoms
- nonreactive, fixed, dilated pupils
- papilledema
- profound weakness
- decerebration
- decortication
- increased systolic pressure
- bradycardia
- abnormal respirations

hormone and aldosterone, monitor his electrolyte levels closely. Also, monitor the ECG for rate and rhythm changes. Administer an antiarrhythmic and provide continuous oxygen therapy, as ordered.

Maintain your patient's musculoskeletal function by helping him perform passive range-of-motion exercises. Promote anatomic alignment of his body parts. Turn and position him every 2 hours. Check his pressure points for redness that

doesn't disappear within 15 minutes. Also, check for evidence of skin breakdown. If skin breakdown becomes a problem, he may require a pressure-relief or pressure-reduction mattress.

Before feeding your patient, make sure his gag reflex is working. If it isn't, he may need enteral feedings until he can swallow safely. If needed, obtain a referral for physical therapy to begin a program to stimulate swallowing.

To feed your patient, place his bed in high Fowler's position with his head flexed slightly forward. To reduce the risk of aspiration, keep him upright for at least 30 minutes after each meal.

Check for bowel impaction every 2 days. Administer laxatives and stool softeners, as needed. Ensure adequate fluid intake and offer the bedpan every 2 hours.

To meet the needs of your patient with communication problems, speak clearly and slowly. Use simple, repetitive directions. Allow time for him to understand and respond. You may want to use pictures or a communication board.

Patient teaching

The effects of cerebrovascular disease on your patient and his family can be devastating. A tremendous amount of education and support is needed for optimum recovery.

During the acute phase of a CVA, orient the patient and his family to the unit, to the procedures being performed and the equipment used, and to the treatment plan. Explain the need for rehabilitative therapy after the acute phase has passed.

Once the patient's condition has stabilized and the amount of cerebral tissue damage has been determined, explain the disease, his deficits, and the planned rehabilitation. If necessary, ensure that each rehabilitation team member explains his or her specialty so that the patient and his family fully understand the rehabilitation process.

Teach the patient the signs and symptoms of a CVA and stress the importance of seeking treatment immediately if any of the following occur:
- sudden onset of weakness, numbness, or paralysis of the face, arm, or leg, usually on one side of the body
- sudden blurring or loss of vision in one or both eyes
- loss of speech or trouble talking or understanding speech

HOME CARE

Teaching your patient about anticoagulant therapy

Effective anticoagulant therapy requires strict patient compliance, so give your patient clear, accurate instructions before discharge and encourage him to follow the prescribed regimen.

General instructions
Teach your patient the generic and trade names of the prescribed drug and its dosage, action, and adverse effects. Instruct him to take the anticoagulant at the same time each day, preferably with dinner. Explain that if he misses a dose, he should take it as soon as possible and then return to his regular schedule. However, if he misses a whole day, he should skip the missed dose because taking a double dose may cause bleeding.

Instruct him to maintain regular eating habits. He should consume his usual amount of vegetables and fruits. Tell him not to drink more than two alcoholic beverages per day. Also, tell him to consult his physician before making any changes in his diet.

Advise your patient to check with his physician before taking any over-the-counter drugs. If your patient is taking warfarin, tell him that certain vitamins, such as vitamins C and K, can reduce the drug's effect and that aspirin and nonsteroidal anti-inflammatory drugs can increase its effect.

Tell him to post his physician's name and phone number in prominent places at home and at work so that others can contact the physician quickly in an emergency.

Adverse effects
Instruct your patient to notify his physician if he experiences any of the following adverse effects:

- bruises or purplish marks on his skin
- bleeding gums when he brushes his teeth
- nosebleeds
- heavy bleeding or oozing from cuts or wounds
- blood in the urine or sputum
- bloody or tarry black stools
- diarrhea
- constipation
- vomitus that looks like coffee grounds
- unusual pain or swelling in his joints or stomach
- backaches
- dizziness
- severe or continuing headaches.

Special instructions
Advise your patient to keep all appointments for blood tests because his physician may need to adjust the dose of the anticoagulant based on the test results. If the patient is taking warfarin, tell him to inform other physicians he sees that he's taking it. Also, instruct him to wear a medical alert tag or bracelet that shows he's taking warfarin.

If your patient taking warfarin is a woman, urge her to delay pregnancy because the drug can interfere with fetal development and cause placental bleeding. Tell her to report excessive or unexpected menstrual bleeding to her physician.

Tell your patient to check with his physician before beginning a strenuous exercise program. Also, urge him to avoid activities such as rough play with children or dogs. To help him reduce his risk of injury, instruct him to wear shoes at all times, place a nonskid mat in his bathtub, shave with an electric razor, and use a soft-bristled toothbrush.

- sudden severe headache
- unexplained dizziness or loss of balance, especially if combined with other signs and symptoms.

If the physician prescribes an antihypertensive, anticoagulation, or antiplatelet aggregation drug, teach your patient the name of the drug, its dosage, and its therapeutic and adverse effects. If he must take an anticoagulant, also teach him the signs and symptoms of bleeding that he should

report (see *Teaching your patient about anticoagulant therapy*).

If the physician has prescribed warfarin, tell your patient which drugs interact with it. Instruct him to maintain a diet that provides moderate amounts of vitamin K. Explain that extreme variations in vitamin K intake can cause wide fluctuations in the anticoagulant level. Tell the patient to avoid trauma and to wear a medical alert tag or bracelet at all times. Inform him that he'll need frequent blood tests for his physician to adjust the warfarin dose.

Depending on the amount of cerebral damage, your patient may be transferred to a rehabilitation facility or a skilled nursing facility for further treatment. If he requires a wheelchair or walker, tell him that a home care nurse or other health provider should visit his home to identify physical barriers that would limit their use.

Explain that the home care nurse will monitor his vital signs, check his compliance with antihypertensive drug therapy, and assess his response to the drug. She'll evaluate his bowel and bladder function and provide retraining, if necessary. She'll also assess his response to rehabilitation, determining which assistive devices might be useful to him.

Retinopathy

Hypertensive retinopathy results from chronic primary hypertension, malignant hypertension, or eclampsia. If untreated, it can lead to retinal detachment. Plus, retinal vessel damage suggests that the patient has suffered damage to other organs, as well.

Pathophysiology

With retinopathy, retinal changes are categorized according to the severity of the vessel damage. Retinal arteriolar narrowing and increased diastolic blood pressure are directly related.

Grade I retinal changes may occur when a patient has mildly elevated diastolic blood pressure, about 90 mm Hg. These retinal changes include vascular spasm and arteriolar constriction.

Grade II retinal changes occur when a patient has sustained elevated diastolic blood pressure of more than 100 mm Hg. These retinal changes include localized and generalized arteriole narrowing at arteriovenous junctions.

If the patient's hypertension is left untreated and his diastolic blood pressure remains above 100 mm Hg, he may experience grade III retinal changes. Occlusion of the retinal arterioles may cause superficial, flame-shaped hemorrhages and small, white areas of retinal ischemia called soft exudates or cotton wool spots. Hard, yellow-white exudates may produce a star-shaped figure around the macula.

Further untreated hypertension can lead to grade IV retinal changes. The occluded arterioles cause the optic disk to become congested and edematous, leading to papilledema (swelling of the optic nerve head). Papilledema causes the optic disc margins to become blurred and indistinct. Without treatment, this condition can lead to blindness.

Signs and symptoms

Usually, the early grades of hypertensive retinopathy go undetected. A patient may have no significant signs or symptoms to report nor any apparent reason to seek medical attention.

However, as his diastolic blood pressure remains elevated in grades III and IV, retinal lesions may produce blurred vision and scotomata (blind gaps in his visual field). Papilledema or hemorrhage in the macula can result in blindness.

Diagnostic tests

A physician uses an ophthalmoscopic examination to diagnose hypertensive retinopathy. This examination is used to detect constricted retinal vessels in grades I and II retinopathy and to detect hemorrhages, yellow exudates, and papilledema in grades III and IV retinopathy.

If the patient has papilledema, the ophthalmoscopic examination will reveal engorged, tortuous retinal veins, flame-shaped retinal hemorrhages in the superficial nerve fiber layer, and round hemorrhages in the deeper nerve layers.

Treatment

If your patient has hypertensive retinopathy, a physician may prescribe an antihypertensive drug to regulate his diastolic blood pressure—typically, a beta-blocker or diuretic. If other drugs or disorders contraindicate these antihypertensive drugs, the physician will prescribe another one, such as an ACE inhibitor. Controlling the patient's blood pressure may reduce or eliminate the signs and symptoms of retinopathy. However, if he has experienced optic nerve ischemia, he may have a permanent loss of vision.

Nursing considerations

Focus on controlling your patient's blood pressure. Administer an antihypertensive drug, as ordered. Also, instruct your patient in lifestyle modifications that can help control his hypertension, including limiting his sodium intake, losing weight, and exercising.

If your patient with hypertensive retinopathy is a pregnant woman, monitor her for signs and symptoms of eclampsia and worsening hypertension, which can cause retinal detachment from fluid leaking under the retina. Administer an antihypertensive drug, as ordered. When her hypertension is controlled, the retinal detachment may resolve.

Patient teaching

Instruct your patient in lifestyle modifications to manage his hypertension. Help him develop a diet plan to reduce his sodium intake and reduce his weight. Also, help him develop an exercise program.

If the physician has prescribed an antihypertensive drug, teach your patient the name of the drug, its dosage, and its therapeutic and adverse effects. Explain the relationship between untreated hypertension and chronic complications, such as retinopathy.

Tell the patient that he'll need regular ophthalmic examinations to detect and monitor retinal changes. Teach him the signs and symptoms of retinal detachment, such as dark irregular floaters, flashes of light, blurred vision, and a progressively enlarged dark area in his field of vision. Tell him to report any of these signs and symptoms to the physician immediately.

If your patient can't care for himself because of vision limitations, he may require evaluation for home care assistance. If necessary, refer him to an occupational or physical therapist for suggestions on assistive devices and ways he can adapt his home to meet his needs.

Renal disease

A patient with hypertension has an increased risk of developing renal disease. In stage I renal disease, the patient has a diminished renal reserve

Assessing your hypertensive patient for renal disease

Because your hypertensive patient has an increased risk of developing renal disease, monitor his laboratory results for the following.

Stage I: Diminished renal reserve
- reduced kidney function with no accumulation of metabolic wastes
- mild elevation in blood urea nitrogen (BUN) and creatinine levels

Stage II: Renal insufficiency
- mild accumulation of metabolic wastes
- elevated BUN, creatinine, uric acid, and phosphorus levels
- anemia
- mild hyperkalemia
- reduced ability to concentrate urine

Stage III: End-stage renal disease
- excessive accumulation of metabolic wastes
- severely elevated BUN, creatinine, potassium, and phosphorus levels
- decreased sodium and calcium levels
- decreased hemoglobin level and hematocrit
- fluid retention

but no symptoms of renal disease. If untreated, the condition may progress to stage II renal disease, in which the patient experiences renal insufficiency. He'll have lost over 75% of his glomerular function and will begin to experience the effects of renal disease, such as anemia and mild hyperkalemia. Further uncontrolled hypertension can lead to stage III, end-stage renal disease, in which the patient may develop chronic renal failure (see *Assessing your hypertensive patient for renal disease*).

Pathophysiology

In hypertension, increased vascular resistance of the sclerosed vessels causes blood to enter the glomerulus under high pressure, damaging the glomerular membrane. The impaired membrane loses its ability to filter selectively, leading to necrosis of the tubules.

Hypertension also interferes with the renin-angiotensin-aldosterone system, resulting in ischemia and reduced blood volume to the kidneys. Water and sodium reabsorption are increased in an attempt to increase the glomerular filtration rate, resulting in volume overload and higher vascular pressure, which cause sclerosis of the glomeruli.

Signs and symptoms

The signs and symptoms of renal insufficiency may be similar to those of renal failure, depending on the degree of kidney involvement. If your patient's kidneys lose the ability to concentrate urine, he may develop polyuria and nocturia. If his renal disease is untreated and renal failure progresses, he may develop oliguria. His urine may have a low specific gravity and a high sodium concentration. Also, it may be bloody or tea colored and contain casts and high concentrations of red blood cells (RBCs) and white blood cells (WBCs).

Your patient may have a low serum sodium level because of his kidneys' inability to reabsorb sodium. He also may have a low serum calcium level caused by reduced renal absorption. And his serum potassium and phosphate levels may be elevated because of reduced renal excretion of potassium and phosphate.

If he has elevated blood urea nitrogen (BUN) and creatinine levels, his renal disease may result in azotemia. If his kidneys lose their ability to produce erythropoietin, he may become anemic.

Your patient's renal disease also may cause signs in other body systems. He may have jugular vein distention, a full and bounding pulse, peripheral edema, pulmonary edema, and heart failure. He may show signs of metabolic acidosis, including Kussmaul's respirations. And he may develop anorexia, nausea, vomiting, diarrhea, lethargy, and difficulty concentrating.

Diagnostic tests

A physician uses renal ultrasonography, excretory urography, and renal arteriography to diagnose renal disease. Renal ultrasonography helps the physician visualize renal structures to evaluate the integrity of tissues and vessels. This procedure is safe for patients with renal insufficiency because it doesn't use contrast media.

A physician uses excretory urography to identify the absence or presence of lesions, areas of restricted blood flow, and areas of vascular occlusion. He also may use renal arteriography to evaluate renal blood flow. Excretory urography and renal arteriography require the use of contrast media, placing your patient with renal insufficiency at risk for worsening kidney function.

Treatment

The treatment of renal disease includes drug therapy and nutritional therapy. To prevent renal insufficiency from deteriorating further, the treatment is designed to control hypertension with antihypertensive drugs and sodium and fluid restrictions.

Usually, a physician will prescribe an ACE inhibitor or a calcium channel blocker to control your patient's hypertension. He also may prescribe a diuretic to reduce your patient's fluid overload.

If your patient's phosphate level is elevated, the physician may limit his phosphate intake to 700 to 1,200 mg per day. He also may prescribe an antacid that contains aluminum hydroxide, aluminum carbonate, or a calcium-based phosphate binder. Because high aluminum levels can induce neurologic symptoms, a calcium-based phosphate binder may be preferable. Antacids that contain magnesium are contraindicated because magnesium is excreted by the kidneys.

If your patient is anemic, the physician may prescribe iron supplements and folic acid to increase RBC production. He also may order erythropoietin to be administered I.V. or subcutaneously. However, your patient will need his blood pressure monitored closely, because erythropoietin may worsen his hypertension.

Nutritional therapy may include protein, sodium, potassium, and fluid restrictions. A protein restriction may slow the deterioration of kidney function. Usually, if the physician orders a protein restriction, your patient's daily protein intake will be reduced to 0.6 to 0.8 g/kg of body weight.

A sodium restriction may vary from 1 to 3 grams per day, depending on the ability of the patient's kidneys to excrete sodium as well as the amount of edema and the severity of the hypertension. If the physician orders a potassium restriction, your patient's potassium intake will be reduced to between 2 and 3 grams per day. Be-

HOME CARE

Teaching your patient to calculate his fluid intake and output

If your patient will have to restrict his fluid intake after discharge, teach him to monitor his intake and output accurately. Explain that his fluid intake includes the following:
- everything he drinks, including the liquid in prepared foods
- soups
- everything that melts into liquid at room temperature, such as gelatin, custard, ice cream, and ice cubes
- liquid medications and fluids used to wash down pills or capsules.

Tell him that his fluid output includes everything that leaves his body in fluid form, including urine, wound drainage, watery stool, and vomitus.

Measuring intake
Tell your patient to measure and record the amount of fluid he drinks with each meal, with medicine, and between meals. If he receives nutritive fluids I.V. or through a feeding tube, he should measure and record the amounts.

Suggest that he pour each liquid into a measuring cup and record the amount before drinking it. Instruct him to wash the measuring cup after each use, except after measuring water.

Explain that the labels on cans and bottles will help him determine precise fluid amounts. But tell him to subtract from his total any fluid that he either throws away or saves for future consumption.

Measuring output
Instruct your patient to measure and record the amount of fluid that leaves his body. Tell him to keep a container in his bathroom for measuring urine output and to wash it after each use.

If he's using drainage bags, tell him to measure and record the amount of fluid in each bag before disposing of it.

Converting common measurements
Tell your patient that he may have to convert household measurements (such as ounces and quarts) to metric measurements (such as milliliters). Instruct him to convert fluid ounces to milliliters by multiplying the ounces by 30 and to convert milliliters to ounces by dividing the milliliters by 30.

Give him a copy of the following equivalents to use as a reference:
- 2 tablespoons (1 oz) = 30 ml
- 1 cup (8 oz) = 240 ml
- 1 pint (16 oz) = 480 ml
- 1 quart (32 oz) = 960 ml.

cause most salt substitutes contain potassium, avoid giving them to your patient with renal disease.

If the physician orders a fluid restriction, your patient usually will be limited to an intake equal to his urine output plus 500 to 600 ml.

Nursing considerations

Monitor your hypertensive patient with renal disease for fluid overload. Assess his fluid status by taking his daily weights, checking his fluid intake and output and breath sounds, and checking him for peripheral edema. Maintain fluid restrictions, as ordered, and assess his serum electrolyte levels for hyperkalemia, hyperphosphatemia, hypocalcemia, and hyponatremia. Administer a calcium-based phosphate binder, as necessary. And restrict his potassium intake, as ordered.

Monitor your patient's hemoglobin level and hematocrit for anemia. If the physician prescribes erythropoietin for anemia, administer it I.V. or subcutaneously, as ordered. Because the drug may worsen your patient's hypertension, monitor his blood pressure closely.

If the physician prescribes an antihypertensive drug, administer it, as ordered. Monitor the drug's effectiveness by measuring your patient's blood pressure frequently. For a hospitalized patient, expect to measure it every 4 hours for the first 24 hours. For an outpatient, plan to measure it two or three times a day for the first day or two.

Cautiously administer drugs excreted by the kidneys. Such drugs include digitalis glycosides, aminoglycosides, penicillin, tetracyclines, and narcotics. If the physician has prescribed any of these drugs, he may have to modify your patient's dosage. Do not administer meperidine to your hypertensive patient with renal disease because its metabolite is cleared by the kidneys and can cause seizures as it accumulates.

Patient teaching

If the physician has prescribed dietary restrictions, help your patient design a diet plan for maintaining the restrictions or refer him to a dietitian, as needed. If the physician has prescribed a fluid restriction, tell your patient to comply with the restriction by calculating his intake and output (see *Teaching your patient to calculate his fluid intake and output,* page 203).

Teach him the name of each prescribed drug and its dosage and therapeutic and adverse effects. If the physician has prescribed a calcium-based phosphate binder, tell your patient not to take iron because aluminum and calcium bind the iron. Tell him to avoid over-the-counter drugs, such as laxatives and antacids, that contain magnesium.

Instruct your patient on self-care measures, such as taking his daily weights and measuring his blood pressure. Teach him to identify edema and electrolyte imbalances, such as hyperkalemia. Tell him to report either of these to his physician.

If your patient will have a home care nurse, tell him that she'll perform physical assessments, including measuring his daily weights and urine output, checking his breath sounds, and checking for edema. She'll also assess him for signs and symptoms of electrolyte imbalances and evaluate his compliance with the drug regimen and dietary restrictions.

Tell the patient that she'll provide assistance as he adapts to his illness and its accompanying restrictions. She may suggest support groups and counseling, if needed. She'll provide emotional support and encourage him and his family to participate actively in the treatment program.

Aortic aneurysm

Aortic aneurysms—dilated segments of the aorta—are more common in men ages 50 to 70. Hypertension increases the risk of a patient developing an aortic aneurysm by accelerating atherosclerosis in peripheral blood vessels. If an aortic aneurysm is larger than 6 cm in diameter, it has a 50% chance of rupturing within a year.

Pathophysiology

An aortic aneurysm results from atherosclerotic plaque formation on the aorta's walls. These plaques, consisting of lipids, cholesterol, fibrin, and other debris, cause degenerative changes in the aorta's medial layer. The aorta loses elasticity and becomes weak. The pulsatile flow of the blood places additional stress on the weakened aorta, causing it to dilate, thus forming an aneurysm.

The growth rate of an aortic aneurysm can't be determined, but the larger the aneurysm, the greater the risk of rupture. An aneurysm can form anywhere along the aorta. But the most common location is the abdominal aorta below the renal arteries. Typically, an abdominal aortic aneurysm involves the iliac arteries at the point of bifurcation.

Aneurysms are divided into two classifications: true aneurysms and false aneurysms. In a true aneurysm, at least one layer of the aorta remains intact. One-fourth of true aneurysms occur in the thoracic region and three-fourths occur in the abdominal region. A true aneurysm may be a fusiform or saccular dilation (see *Aneurysms: True and false*).

A false aneurysm is a disruption of all three layers of the aorta. This condition results in blood leakage into a contained area.

The rupture of an aortic aneurysm is a life-threatening complication. If the rupture causes bleeding into the retroperitoneal space, it may be stopped by compression from the nearby organs. Bleeding into the abdominal cavity is fatal.

Signs and symptoms

Aneurysms in the thoracic aorta may be asymptomatic. But if signs and symptoms appear, they may include deep, diffuse chest pain; hemoptysis; orthopnea; and dyspnea.

Aneurysms within the ascending aorta and aortic arch can cause hoarseness, stridor, or a weak voice because of pressure on the laryngeal nerve. Pressure on the esophagus can result in dysphagia. Pressure on the superior vena cava may result in neck vein distention and edema of the head and arms. Pressure on pulmonary structures may cause coughing, dyspnea, and airway obstruction.

Aneurysms: True and false

A true aneurysm involves all three layers of the arterial wall: the intima, media, and adventitia. Weakening of the elastic medial layer causes the other layers to stretch and bulge, forming a fusiform or saccular aneurysm.

A *fusiform aneurysm,* the most common type, circles the aorta in a spindle shape.

A *saccular aneurysm* is a balloon-shaped bulge with a narrow neck. This type of aneurysm is more likely to rupture than a fusiform aneurysm.

A *false aneurysm* results from blood leaking and clotting between the disrupted arterial layers. A bulge, formed by fibrous tissue enclosing the blood clot, can be seen on an X-ray, but the arterial lumen looks normal or almost normal on angiography.

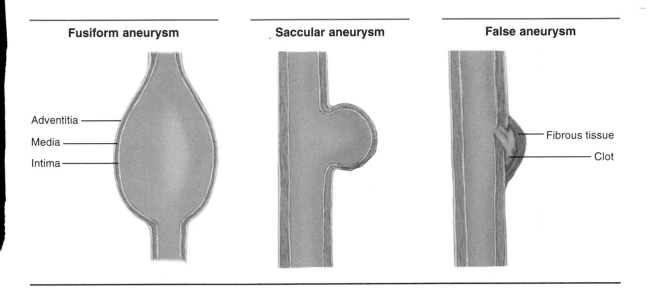

Fusiform aneurysm   **Saccular aneurysm**   **False aneurysm**

Adventitia
Media
Intima

Fibrous tissue
Clot

Usually, abdominal aortic aneurysms are asymptomatic. They're commonly detected during a routine physical examination as a pulsatile mass palpated in the periumbilical region left of the midline, with audible bruits auscultated over the mass. An abdominal aortic aneurysm may cause epigastric discomfort from intestinal obstruction caused by bowel compression. It may cause a feeling of throbbing in the abdomen. And lower back pain may result from pressure on the lumbar nerve. In a patient with an abdominal aortic aneurysm, the systolic blood pressure in his thigh may be substantially lower than the systolic pressure in his arm.

If an aneurysm results in retroperitoneal rupture, the patient may develop intense back pain and ecchymosis in the back or flank. If an aneurysm ruptures into the abdominal cavity, the patient will have massive bleeding and go into shock.

Diagnostic tests

Most aortic aneurysms are found during a routine physical examination or chest X-ray. A physician may also use ultrasound, CT, MRI, and aortoiliac angiography to diagnose the condition.

If the patient has an aortic aneurysm, a chest X-ray may show a widening of the mecamylamine silhouette and aortic arch. If the aneurysm is in the abdominal aorta, an abdominal X-ray may show calcification in the aorta's wall. If the patient reports thoracic pain, the physician also may use an ECG to rule out an MI.

If the physician suspects an aortic aneurysm, he may order ultrasonography to confirm the aneurysm and detect thrombus formation. He may order a CT scan to determine the anterior-to-posterior and cross-sectional diameters of the aneurysm. A CT scan also helps to detect a thrombus in the pouch of the aneurysm. The physician may use an MRI to help diagnose these aortic conditions. And he may use aortoiliac angiography, an invasive procedure for locating the aneurysm's exact position, to help determine whether other arteries that receive blood from the aorta are affected by the condition.

Treatment

Treatment of an aortic aneurysm may include drug therapy and surgery to prevent the aneurysm from rupturing and becoming a life-threatening complication. Commonly, a physician prescribes an antihypertensive drug to lower a hypertensive patient's blood pressure. He may prescribe a beta-blocker to reduce the pulsatile aortic flow by reducing myocardial contractility.

If the patient needs surgery to repair an aortic aneurysm, the surgical technique will depend on the type of aneurysm. For example, if the patient has a fusiform aneurysm, a surgeon may perform an aneurysmectomy by incising the diseased segment of the aorta and inserting a synthetic arterial graft. He then wraps the aortic wall around the graft and sutures it (see *Surgical repair of a fusiform aneurysm*).

If the patient has a saccular aneurysm, the surgeon may remove only the bulbous portion and suture the artery together. Or, after removing the bulbous portion, he may apply a synthetic patch over the defect.

Nursing considerations

If the physician has prescribed an antihypertensive drug to control hypertension, administer the drug, as ordered, and monitor your patient's blood pressure. During the acute phase of an aortic aneurysm, monitor the patient for rupture, which would cause him to progress into shock quickly. Assess him for rapidly declining blood pressure, changes in level of consciousness, cool and clammy skin, and decreasing urine output. Monitor his respiratory rate; it may increase to compensate for decreased circulating oxygenated blood, weakened pulses, and tachycardia.

If your patient undergoes surgery for an aortic aneurysm, focus on maintaining cardiopulmonary and renal function and graft patency postoperatively. Also, monitor him for complications of surgery, such as CVA, renal failure, MI, respiratory insufficiency, and neurologic dysfunction.

To assess cardiopulmonary status, monitor his vital signs, ECG, serum electrolyte levels, and ABG measurements. Assess all peripheral pulses and compare the pulse, warmth, and color in his arms. Monitor his central venous pressure (CVP) readings and treat him for low blood volume as needed. Perform neurologic checks every 30 to 60 minutes, assessing his level of consciousness, pupillary reaction to light, arm and leg movement, and hand grasps.

A thrombus or plaque that breaks loose from the aorta may impair renal perfusion. Hypotension also can reduce renal perfusion. So monitor your patient's blood pressure and CVP and administer fluids and volume expanders to ensure adequate renal perfusion. Monitor his urine output. Report an output of less than 30 ml/hour for 2 consecutive hours. Also, assess his serum BUN and creatinine levels for adequate renal function.

To assess graft patency, palpate the peripheral pulses distal to the graft. Immediately report to the surgeon a decreased or absent pulse accompanied by cool, mottled skin.

Protect graft patency by preventing hypotension and hypertension. Treat hypotension, which promotes thrombosis, with I.V. fluids, volume expanders, or blood products, as prescribed. Treat hypertension, which puts stress on the graft suture lines, with the prescribed diuretic or other antihypertensive drug.

To monitor your patient for graft infection, check his temperature and WBC count every 4 hours. Observe the operative site for signs of local infection, such as redness, warmth, edema, and purulent drainage. Administer a broad-spectrum antibiotic, as ordered, and encourage coughing and deep breathing.

After surgery, your patient is at risk for paralytic ileus resulting from bowel manipulation, anesthesia, pain medication, and immobility. Auscultate his abdomen for the return of bowel sounds. Monitor him for flatus and record his gastric output. Reposition him every 2 hours and encourage early ambulation.

TREATMENT OF CHOICE

Surgical repair of a fusiform aneurysm

To repair a fusiform aneurysm, a surgeon first resects the aorta at the site of the aneurysm. Next, the surgeon sews biologically neutral graft material in place to connect the two ends of the aorta. After cleaning any plaque and clotted blood off the resected section of the aorta, the surgeon wraps it around the graft material and sews it back in place.

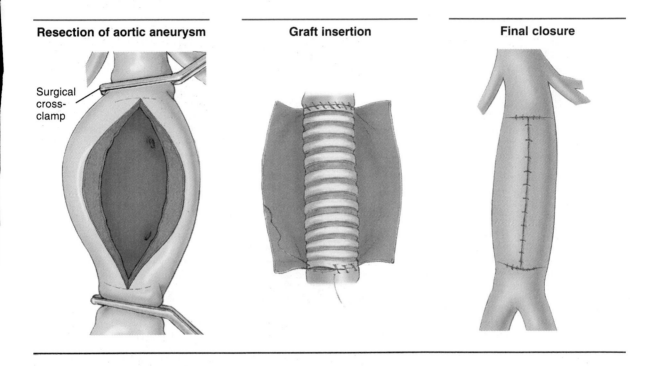

Resection of aortic aneurysm | **Graft insertion** | **Final closure**

Surgical cross-clamp

Patient teaching

Before your patient undergoes surgery, explain the procedure and outline what he can expect in the ICU, including cardiac, CVP, and pulmonary pressure monitoring and I.V. fluid administration. Also, tell him that he may need an arterial line, indwelling urinary catheter, and endotracheal tube.

After his surgery, explain that frequent assessment of vital signs and peripheral pulses is necessary to determine graft patency. Explain the need for early ambulation to prevent complications. Instruct him on coughing, deep breathing, and splinting the incision. Have him perform return demonstrations.

Whether your hypertensive patient had surgery or was successfully treated with drug therapy, he may be prescribed one or more antihypertensive drugs. Before he goes home, teach him the name of any prescribed drug and its dosage and therapeutic and adverse effects. Instruct him to take his blood pressure at home, and demonstrate how to take a pulse.

Discuss the signs and symptoms of a recurring aneurysm. Stress the need for him to promptly call his physician if signs or symptoms recur.

HYPERTENSION

Suggested Readings

Bates BA, Vickley LS, Hockelman RA. *A Guide to Physical Exam and History Taking.* 6th ed. Philadelphia: Lippincott-Raven Pubs; 1995.

Beilin LJ, Puddey IB, Burke V. Alcohol and hypertension: kill or cure? *J Hum Hypertens.* 1996;10 (Suppl 2):S1-S5.

Bronner LL, Kanter DS, Manson JE. Primary prevention of stroke. *N Engl J Med.* 1995;333(21):1392-1400.

Burt VL, Whelton P, Roccella EJ, et al. Prevalence of hypertension in the US adult population. Results from the third national health and nutrition examination survey, 1988-1991. *Hypertension.* 1995;25 (3):305-313.

Cuddy RP. Hypertension: keeping dangerous blood pressure down. *Nursing.* 1995;25(8):34-41.

Fauci A, Braunwald E, Wilson JD, Isselbacher KJ. *Harrison's Principles of Internal Medicine.* 14th ed. New York: McGraw-Hill, Inc; 1997.

Gurwitz JH, Avorn J, Bohn RL, Glynn RJ, Monane M, Mogun H. Initiation of antihypertensive treatment during nonsteroidal anti-inflammatory drug therapy. *JAMA.* 1994;272(10):781-786.

Heart and Stroke Facts. Dallas, Tex: American Health Association statistical supplement; 1996.

High Blood Pressure. American Heart Association; 1997.

Insel P. Hypertension: the silent killer. *Healthline Magazine.* 1995; 14(6):http://www.healthline.com.

Kannel WB, Wilson PW. An update of coronary risk factors. *Med Clin North Am.* 1995;79(5):951-971.

Kaplan N. Systemic hypertension: mechanisms and diagnosis. In: Braunwald E, ed. *Heart Disease: A Textbook of Cardiovascular Medicine.* 5th ed. Philadelphia: W.B. Saunders Co; 1996.

Kaplan N. Arterial hypertension. In: Klippel JH, Stein JH, eds. *Internal Medicine.* 5th ed. St Louis: Mosby, Inc; 1998.

Kaplan NM, Lieberman E. *Clinical Hypertension.* 6th ed. Baltimore: Williams & Wilkins; 1994.

Karppanen H, Mervaala E. Adherence to and population impact of non-pharmacological and pharmacological antihypertensive therapy. *J Hum Hypertens.* 1996;10(Suppl 1):S57-S61.

Kellick KA. Diuretics. In: Kuhn, M. *Pharmacotherapeutics: A Nursing Process Approach.* 4th ed. Philadelphia: F.A. Davis Co; 1997:774-808.

Laragh JH, Brenner BM, eds. *Hypertension: Pathophysiology, Diagnosis, and Management.* 2nd ed. Philadelphia: Lippincott-Raven Pubs; 1994.

Laslett L. Hypertension: Preoperative assessment and perioperative management. *West J Med.* 1995; 162(3):215-219.

Lewis CE. Characteristics and treatment of hypertension in women: a review of the literature. *Am J Med Sci.* 1996;311(4):193-199.

National High Blood Pressure Education Program: Group Report on Hypertension in the Elderly. National Heart Blood and Lung Institute, US Department of Health and Human Services, NIH Publication 94-3527; 1994.

Pagana KD, Pagana T. *Mosby's Diagnostic Laboratory and Test Reference.* 3rd ed. St Louis: Mosby, Inc; 1996.

Physical activity and hypertension. *Can Med Assoc J.* 1995;153(10):1477.

Sadowski AV, Redeker NS. The hypertensive elder: a review for the primary care provider. *Nurse Pract.* 1996;21(5):99-102.

Skidmore-Roth L. *Mosby's Nursing Drug Reference.* St Louis: Mosby, Inc; 1998.

Superko HL, Myll J, DiRicco C, Williams PT, Bortz WM, Wood PD. Effects of cessation of caffeinated-coffee consumption on ambulatory and resting blood pressure in men. *Am J Cardiol.* 1994;73(11):780-784.

Treadway KK. Evaluation of hypertension. In: Goroll AH, May LA, Mulley AG. *Primary Care Medicine: Office Evaluation and Management of the Adult Patient.* 3rd. Philadephia: Lippincott-Raven Pubs; 1995:89-94.

Whelton PK. Primary prevention of hypertension: rationale, approaches, realities and perspectives. *J Hum Hypertens.* 1996;10(Suppl 1):S47-S50.

Index

i indicates an illustration; t indicates a table.

G H I

M N

O P

U V W

i indicates an illustration; t indicates a table.